TEXTBOOK OF HISTOLOGY

TEXTBOOK OF
HISTOLOGY

William F. Windle

Denison University and
Department of Anatomy
Center for the Health Sciences
University of California at Los Angeles

Fifth Edition

McGraw-Hill Book Company

New York St. Louis San Francisco Auckland Düsseldorf
Johannesburg Kuala Lumpur London Mexico Montreal New Delhi Panama
Paris São Paulo Singapore Sydney Tokyo Toronto

TEXTBOOK OF HISTOLOGY

1 2 3 4 5 6 7 8 9 0 KPKP 7 9 8 7 6

This book was set in Times Roman by Textbook Services, Inc.
The editors were William J. Willey and Richard S. Laufer;
the cover was designed by Anne Canevari Green;
the production supervisor was Thomas J. LoPinto.
Kingsport Press, Inc., was printer and binder.

Library of Congress Cataloging in Publication Data

Windle, William Frederick, date
    Textbook of histology.

    First-2d ed. by J. F. Nonidez and W. F. Windle.
    Includes index.
    1. Histology.   I.   Nonidez, José Fernandez, date.
Textbook of histology.   II.   Title.
[DNLM: 1. Histology. QS504 W765t]
QM551.N76 1976   611'.018   75-24913
ISBN 0-07-070977-7

Contents

Preface

Textbook of Histology, fifth edition, has been largely rewritten and is a new book, although it does contain some passages and a good many of the best illustrations of the fourth edition. It is neither an outline nor a synopsis of histology, but rather intermediate between a brief coverage and a "big book." It provides complete coverage of functional microscopic anatomy, aiming at the same time to be concise.

The first edition of *Textbook of Histology,* written in collaboration with the late José Nonidez, was designed for abbreviated courses. It was first used in the medical and dental schools at the University of Pennsylvania where the number of hours assigned to the teaching of histology was limited. Today there is more ground to be covered and generally no more time to do so. The desirability of a concise text would seem to be even greater today than it was twenty-five years ago.

The character of histology has undergone far-reaching changes since the first edition came off the press. A revolution in medical science has occurred that has modified the approach to study of the structure of human tissues and organs. Morphology has taken on new meanings in relation to function. The teaching of histology in departments of physiology in English universities was prophetic. Not only are the two subjects interrelated, but they compose, along with biochemistry, the indispensable foundation of clinical medicine. The present edition of *Textbook of Histology* embodies this view.

The revolution in medical science has brought new technical procedures, the application of which has broken down lines between traditional microscopic anatomy and cellular and molecular biology. One can no longer deal with such organs as the endocrine glands simply by describing their structure. Neuroendocrinology has acquired greater emphasis. Knowledge of the heart surely has become as important as that of the liver. The thymus and other lymphatic organs have taken on new significance in terms of recent advances in immunology. If histology is defined as the study of microscopically visible structures, one must now include such things as antibodies.

Advances in knowledge of functional histology have taken place so rapidly that it has been difficult to keep up with them and maintain an authoritative position on every aspect of the subject. Each chapter was, for that reason, submitted for critical review to colleagues who have specialized in the particular subject.

A temptation to enlarge this book by profusely illustrating it with electron micrographs was resisted. The teaching of histology and microscopic anatomy still relies basically on light microscopy, to which electron micrographs add a dimension. There are several excellent atlases of fine structure of cells and tissues that can be employed as adjuncts to study with the conventional compound microscope. They are listed at the end of Chapter 2.

References to the literature have been limited mainly to recent articles reflecting current advances in biomedical science. Where possible, citations of readily accessible reviews have been given preference. Readers wishing to pursue the literature on a particular topic will find keys to other articles in the suggested readings.

The nomenclature of the Paris revision of *Basle Nomina Anatomica,* and particularly the preliminary recommendations of the committee on *Nomina Histologica,* have been followed, using anglicized words for the most part. A few common English terms have become so thoroughly established by use that they must be retained, and in these instances, the Latin terms appear in parentheses after the common names. One of the notable changes brought about by the Paris revision was elimination of the last vestiges of names of discoverers of anatomical components. This policy in respect to the use of eponyms has been followed. Where association of a person's name has persisted in common usage, rather than risk confusion by eliminating it immediately, a footnote has been added. In the few instances when no acceptable descriptive terms have become established, such as in the case of haversian canal, paneth cell, and golgi complex, eponyms have been retained without capitalization.

The student should be encouraged to use the descriptive terms that were officially adopted by international commissions supported by the American Association of Anatomists. There would seem to be no valid reason to continue to employ terms discarded by such commissions. The historical reason for retaining eponyms is appreciated, but history can be served better by separate consideration. Who takes the trouble, when using terms such as glands of Littré, capsule of Glisson, or even Eustachian tube, to find out what contributions to histology, if any, were made by learned doctors whose names have been carried down the years?

Acknowledgments

This *Textbook of Histology* was made possible by the generous provision of facilities at Denison University and at the Center for Health Sciences of the University of California at Los Angeles. Indirect aid through research grants HD-05929 and NS-11507 to the former institution from the National Institutes of Health is acknowledged.

I am grateful to colleagues who reviewed and criticized chapters in manuscript, and in many other ways helped in revision. Without identifying their specific contributions—for I do not want them to be blamed for any of my own errors and misunderstandings—I extend thanks to G. W. Bernard; M. A. B. Brazier; C. D. Clemente; E. L. Cooper; V. B. Eichler; M. E. Gertler; R. A. Gorski; L. Guth; P. H. Guth; H. Latta; H. A. Meineke; F. R. Miller; W. Montagna; J. S. Munroe; G. R. Norris; D. C. Pease; C. W. Sawyer; R. L. St. Pierre; B. Towers; and E. Zimmerman.

It is a pleasure to acknowledge the helpful cooperation of Louise Darling and her staff of the Biomedical Library at the University of California at Los Angeles. The preparation of manuscripts was skillfully done by Sara Kirby at Denison. New drawings and diagrams were made by C. H. Poole at New York University Medical Center, and are identified by his initials in parentheses after the figure legends. Previous artists' drawings are identified as follows: W. E. Loechel (WEL); J. F. Nonidez (JFN); and Mary W. Skyer (MWS).

A number of new photomicrographs and electron micrographs were provided for this fifth edition. The sources are acknowledged in the figure legends. I am pleased to name with thanks the following contributors: H. C. Anderson; M. W. Brightman; R. R. Cardell, Jr.; R. R. Cooper; L-T. Chen; W. H. Crosby; E. W. Dempsey; B. Droz; P. A. Farber; D. W. Fawcett; R. A. Good; J. L. Gowans; L. Guth; D. Hull; J. Ariens Kappers; J. Kempa; T. H. Lentz; A. A. Like; V. T. Marchesi; D. S. Maxwell; L. Orci; S. L. Palay; E. Puchala; J. J. Pysh; C. S. Raine; T. S. Reese; H. J. Romijn; J. Rosenbluth; S. J. Singer; S. E. Svehag; M. Tavassoli; G. Van Wagenen; S. M. Walker; E. R. Weibel; L. Weiss; C. Wolff; and A. A. Zalewski.

Finally, I appreciate the many helpful suggestions and criticisms of my wife, Ella H. Windle, without whose interest in the project the task would have been much more difficult.

William F. Windle

TEXTBOOK OF
HISTOLOGY

Chapter 1

Tissues

Histology (Gr. *histos,* tissue; *logia,* knowledge) in a broad sense is the study of tissues of living things, consideration being limited in this book to those of animals, especially man. Construction of simple lenses in the seventeenth century enabled scientists to examine tissue elements that are invisible to the naked eye, and, for the last hundred years or more, histology has implied the study of tissues with a microscope. Although histologists are concerned primarily with structure, they try to interpret the images in functional terms. Histology is as much a part of physiology as it is of morphology. Knowledge of it is basic to the study of medicine.

Ideally, one should study living tissues, and this can be done to a limited extent. Scrapings from the mouth, drops of blood from a finger, and even bits of tissues from a freshly killed animal, when spread upon microscope slides, will serve the purpose. A more sophisticated procedure is that of tissue culture. Time-lapse motion pictures of cellular activities in tissue cultures can be used. This technique, being the opposite of slow-motion photography, speeds up the activities of cells and enables one to get a direct impression of such activities of single cells as locomotion, food ingestion, and the cytoplasmic movement of intracellular constituents. One soon exhausts the possibilities of fresh-tissue histology and comes to rely on sections cut from preserved specimens.

HISTOLOGIC TECHNIQUE

The preparation of sections of tissues and organs for study under the micro-scope, known as histologic technique, requires some skill and much time. Methods are fully described in treatises devoted to that subject. It is doubtful if any word picture, even of the more common procedures employed to make stained microscope slides out of pieces of fresh organs, can substitute for first-hand observation of the process.

In order to observe structures with the microscope, the tissue must be cut into slices that are thin enough to allow light to pass through them. To do this, one uses a "microtome" which is similar to the machine used by the butcher for slicing meat, except that it permits one to obtain thin slices. To prepare such sections, the tissue must be hardened so that it will not be compressed by the microtome knife blade. This hardening can be accomplished by either freezing the tissue and cutting the sections at a temperature below 0°C or embedding the tissue in a substance that will harden at room temperature.

Reduced to barest essentials, histologic technique is as follows: (1) Tissues are killed, or "fixed," by subjecting them to the action of protoplasm-coagulat-ing chemical solutions, such as formaldehyde. Rapidity of action is essential; perfusion through vascular channels is preferable to immersion of pieces. (2) Water is removed from them with alcohol, and through an intermediate solvent, they are infiltrated with paraffin or celloidin, which solidifies to form blocks containing the tissues. (3) Slices as thin as 2 to 5 μm, but usually 10 μm or more, are shaved from these blocks with a microtome. (4) These slices or sec-tions of tissues are stained either before or after being affixed to glass slides. Staining is done with one of a great variety of dyes or with certain metallic salts. Some components of cells, notably nuclear chromatin, are said to be "basophilic" because they have affinity for basic dyes, such as hematoxylin. Other components of cells and intercellular substances are said to be "acidophilic" because they stain with the acid dyes, such as eosin. (5) The stained slices are rendered transparent with oils or solvents, such as xylol. They are finally covered with a drop of transparent mounting medium having nearly the same refractive index as the glass slide and cover slip between which they are preserved.

After all this, it is surprising that the final preparation bears as close a re-semblance to living tissue as it does. Standardized procedures, properly con-trolled, will constantly give uniform results which can be interpreted in terms of living tissues. The histologic technique outlined above is that used for most preparations studied in the classroom. There are numerous other techniques, employed essentially in histologic research and coming infrequently to the at-tention of the student. Biochemical and physiologic properties of living cells can be inferred from reactions between staining agents and fixed protoplasm. Histochemistry is an aspect of histology to which reference will be made throughout this book.

Many dyes besides hematoxylin and eosin are used to stain components of tissues. A number of histochemical methods are employed to color specific

chemical substances selectively. Among the methods in common use
to localize deoxyribonucleic acid (Feulgen reaction), certain polysacc
(periodic acid Schiff reaction), lipids (the Sudan dyes), enzymes (techniqu
acid and alkaline phosphatases), glycogen (Best's carmine), and elastic t.
(orcine).

Fluorescent microscopy adds another dimension to histologic study. It
depends on employment of fluorescent dyes (i.e., substances that change ultraviolet wavelengths to those of the visible spectrum) and on the binding of these
dyes to specific cell components. The technique has been used to study antigens and antibodies, binding sites of which become visible microscopically
under ultraviolet light.

Another approach to studying function of cellular components is through
the method of differential centrifugation. In a suspension of homogenized cells,
the heaviest components go down first; the lightest, last. Thus are separated in
relatively pure form such constituents as nuclei, mitochondria, microsomes
(which are fragments of the endoplasmic reticulum), ribosomes, and protein
macromolecules. Each can be analyzed by methods of biochemistry.

It is not necessary, in every case, to go through the routine of fixation,
dehydration, and embedding tissues to prepare sections for histologic examination. A more rapid method is that of freezing the specimen and sectioning it
before proceeding to staining. A variant involves quickly freezing at very low
temperature, then evaporating the water of the piece of tissue in a high vacuum.
This process is known as "freeze-drying."

Radioautography is another research method. Some radioactive substance, such as tritiated thymidine, is administered to living tissues, after which
its selective incorporation into cells or intercellular material can be detected in
histologic sections. The sections are coated with photographic emulsion, and
the radioactive substance causes reduction of fine silver halide grains to metallic silver which is visible under the microscope (also in electron micrographs).

MICROSCOPES

The standard instrument for studying histology is the compound microscope
which employs a source of visible light to transilluminate the histologic specimen. Three essential optical parts of the microscope are a substage condenser
to concentrate light upon the specimen, an objective lens that can be focused on
parts of the specimen and magnifies them, and an ocular lens to further enlarge
the image produced by the objective lens. The ocular lens is the "eyepiece"
through which one sees the magnified portion of the specimen. The image also
can be projected through it onto photographic film to produce a photomicrograph.[1]

The effectiveness of the optical system depends on its light-gathering abili-

---

[1]A photomicrograph is a photograph of a magnified image of a minute object, whereas a
microphotograph is a minute photograph of any object.

ty. It must be able to differentiate between closely adjacent points in the specimen being examined. Numerical aperture is a measure of the light-gathering ability of optical components. The high-quality lenses of modern compound microscopes have resolving powers of 0.25 to 1.8 μm.

Magnifications achieved by the microscope depend on the combination of the objective and ocular lenses employed. The initial magnification of the best oil-immersion objective lens is 100 times; when the image it forms is further magnified by an ocular lens, it may become 1,500 times; this is about the most one can expect without loss of detail. A photomicrograph taken with that combination of lenses can be enlarged, but without increasing resolution.

The possibility of obtaining greater resolution photographically is enhanced by using light of short wavelength. Ultraviolet light, requiring lenses made of quartz instead of glass, can lead to resolution of details in the range of 0.1 μm.

A number of other modifications of the standard compound microscope are in use for histologic studies. These involve altering the light paths through the specimen. The phase-contrast microscope is usually employed with living, or at least unstained, tissue, and provides contrast between components that have different refractive indices. A more effective instrument, the interference microscope, uses two light beams that are combined in the image plane to enhance contrasts. The dark-field microscope depends on use of oblique illumination and a special condenser; no light reaches the eyepiece except that reflected from small components (e.g., chylomicrons in blood) in the field of the specimen, which appear as bright objects against a black background. Another type of microscope uses polarized light obtained with Nicol prisms interposed in the path of light. By rotating the upper prism, one can analyze differences in refraction of light passing through the specimen. Observation of the birefringence of cross striations of muscle fibers is one example of application of the polarizing microscope. These optical systems are useful for special purposes, but none contributes toward increasing the resolving power of the microscope that uses visible light.

The wavelength of light limits the resolving power of the compound microscope. To increase the resolving power, one must use a system employing emissions of short wavelength. This is accomplished with high-speed beams of electrons, the path of which can be controlled with electrostatic or electromagnetic fields in a transmission electron microscope. Figure 1.1 compares diagramatically the path of electrons with that of light rays in the two types of microscope. The final electronic image can be viewed only with a fluorescent screen or photographically. Electron beams of high velocity have much shorter wavelengths than do beams of light. It is possible to attain resolutions in the order of 0.002 μm (20Å) or less.[2] Magnifications up to 20,000 times or more can be obtained on the photographic film and further enlarged.

[2]Note that 1 mm $= 10^3$ μm $= 10^6$ nm $= 10^7$ Å.

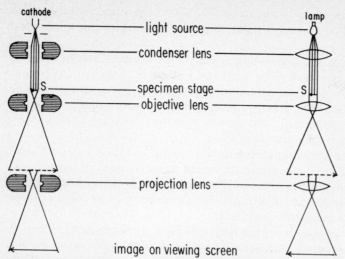

Figure 1-1 Diagram comparing light microscope with transmission electron microscope. *(CHP)*

It is easy to remember the following approximate resolving powers: 200 μm by the human eye; 0.2 μm by the light microscope; and 0.002 μm by the transmission electron microscope. Some size relationships are illustrated in Fig. 1.2.

Histologic techniques for electron microscopy differ from those for light microscopy. Very small pieces of tissue must be selected. Fixation is often done with glutaraldehyde and osmium, and embedding employs epoxy resin. The hardened blocks are sectioned with a glass or a diamond knife at 0.1 μm or less. Electrons do not satisfactorily penetrate thicker tissue slices. Osmic acid and certain heavy metallic compounds are used to "stain" the specimens, i.e., to introduce electron density selectively to cellular components. The sections are placed on a grid which is then inserted into the instrument and a high vacu-

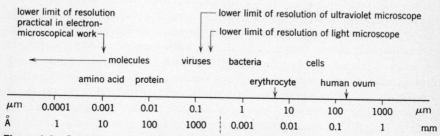

Figure 1-2 Comparison between the diameter of molecules, viruses, bacteria, and cells; the lower limits of resolution are indicated for microscopes employing visible light, ultraviolet light, and electron beams.

um is created before the flow of electrons is started. The usual voltage is less than 100,000 volts, but some specially designed instruments now utilize 1 million volts.

A different image-producing system is used in the scanning electron microscope. Specimens do not have to be sectioned. Metallic coatings of their surfaces are formed by a process of sublimation, producing replicas which can be placed in the microscope. The electron beams are reflected from the surface of the replica to a photographic film. The resulting photomicrograph exhibits a remarkable three-dimensional effect (Fig. 7.2).

Specimens for the scanning electron microscope need not be completely anhydrous. It is possible, furthermore, to freeze minute pieces of tissue, fracture them, and form metallic replicas of fracture planes. By this freeze-etching method, one can obtain images of intracellular components. The fracture often occurs through unit membranes (Fig. 2.8).

The techniques of electron microscopy have opened new vistas in cytology and clarified others that were at best only dimly perceived before. Nevertheless, they do not supplant study of prepared slides of stained tissues—the conventional material of light microscopy. The fine detail revealed in electron micrographs will only be confusing unless one has a sound background of light-microscope histology.

CLASSIFICATION AND COMPOSITION OF TISSUES

Tissues of higher animals are made of six types of material, but not all are found in every tissue. First of these are the "living cells," occupying a prominent place in all tissues. "Dead cells" are another. They are limited mainly to the surface of the skin, the hair, and nails. Three other types are nonliving materials produced by cells. These are "fibers," the main constituents of connective tissues; "ground substances," likewise in connective tissues; and "cuticles," the most important example being enamel of the teeth. Finally, there is "tissue fluid," largely water.

Four fundamental tissues make up the body. The sheets of cells covering surfaces, lining cavities, and arranged as secreting clusters constitute **epithelial tissue**. The highly fibrous and only slightly cellular supporting, connecting, and padding materials, including bones, cartilages, tendons, and fat, are collectively designated **connective tissue**. The elongated elements concerned with contraction form **muscular tissue**. Collections of cells with long processes specialized for reception of stimuli and conduction of impulses, together with other developmentally related elements, build **nervous tissue**. The circulating cell-containing fluid within vascular channels may be considered a fifth tissue, the **blood**, although it is actually a specialized part of connective tissue. These are rather arbitrary divisions, for no tissue exists in pure form. Epithelium contains nerves. Connective tissue has nerves and blood vessels. Muscular tissue could not function without both these, plus connective-tissue sheaths. The term "tissue" also is applied to subtypes of the four fundamental ones. Examples are reticular tissue, adipose tissue, and lymphatic tissue. Characteristics of each will be described in succeeding chapters (Table 1.1).

In histology it is essential to study each tissue separately, but one must bear in mind that all are interdependent. Consideration of such a component of the body as a muscle can be divided into the histology of its principal tissue, which is muscular tissue, and the microscopic anatomy of it as in an organ performing a certain function by the interaction of all its tissues. Two useful terms with which to become acquainted are **parenchyma** and **stroma.** In our example, the parenchyma is muscular tissue, i.e., the essential and proper tissue, and the stroma is the connective tissue holding functional elements apart and forming a framework over which nerves and vessels can reach them. All organs are composed of parenchymal and stromal tissues.

Table 1.1 Characteristics of Tissues

	Epithelial	Blood	Connective	Muscular	Nervous
Names of principal cells	Squamous, columnar	Erythrocytes, leucocytes	Fibrocytes, macrophages	Smooth, skeletal, cardiac	Neurons, neuroglia, neurolemma
Prevalent shapes of cells	Polyhedral	Discoid, ovoid	Stellate, fusiform, irregular	Elongated	Multipolar, unipolar, with long processes
Cell surface	Microvilli, cilia	Plasma membrane only	Plasma membrane only	Sarcolemma	Plasma membrane only
Cytoplasmic fibrils	Tonofibrils	None	Fibroglia in some	Myofibrils	Neurofibrils, gliofibrils
Other specific features	Secretion granules	Hemoglobin, specific granules	Few granules, pigment	Striations, intercalated discs	Chromophil substance
Interstitial fibers	None	None (fibrin)	Collagenous, reticular, elastic	None	None
Interstitial matrix	Basal lamina	None	Ground substance, cartilage and bone matrix	Basal lamina of sarcolemma	Practically none in brain
Interstitial fluid	Little	Blood plasma	Considerable	Little	Cerebrospinal fluid

It will simplify the study of histology to consider the components of tissues in three categories: cells, intercellular fibers and ground substances formed by cells, and water within and outside the cells.

Cells   These are the vital units of all tissues. They not only constitute building blocks but also produce and regulate the formation of noncellular components of tissues. We shall address ourselves to the study of cells, i.e., cytology, in Chap. 2.

The cell is still considered the unit of structure of living matter, although the question whether viruses are living elements is a valid one. Tissues are structures that contain more than one type of cell and are specialized to perform a specific function. Organs are structures composed of more than one type of tissue and are therefore specialized to perform still more complex functions.

Cells utilize energy coming from outside the body in the form of carbohydrates, fats, and proteins. The ultimate source of energy is sunlight, but only in cells of green plants is that employed directly. Structure of the intracellular machinery for using basic material, converting one form of energy to another, synthesizing complex protein molecules, such as enzymes, and discharging them from the cell has been brought into clearer focus with the development of electron microscopy. From cells of one tissue to those of another, remarkable similarities in fundamental fine structure exist; and yet, functions of diverse nature are performed.

Intercellular Components[3]   Cells produce materials with which the body is held together, as it were. Among these are the fibers in some amorphous ground substances.

Fibers are made up of protein macromolecules. There are three varieties, known as collagenous, reticular, and elastic. All are formed by cells of connective tissue. They are the major components of connective tissue and are considered in Chap. 4.

Ground substances, composed of protein-polysaccharide and protein-lipid complexes, are amorphous and difficult to see in routine preparations with the light microscope, although techniques of histochemistry can reveal them in many tissues. Those composing the matrix of cartilage and bone are readily demonstrable. In the skeleton, the ground substance has a solid consistency and provides shape and strength to bones. In young connective tissue it is like a thin jelly permeating the whole tissue. This substance tends to become more viscid in the adult and is confined to the vicinity of fiber bundles or along the bases of epithelial cells.

Finally, there are the **cuticles** formed by cells and separable from them. They occur only on the surface of certain epithelial cells and will be considered with the organs in which they are present.

---

[3]*Intercellular* means between cells while *intracellular* means within a cell. One must be careful not to confuse these terms.

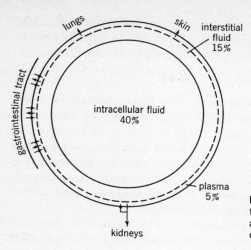

Figure 1-3 Schematic diagram of the three body-fluid compartments and the amounts of water in each in terms of percentages of body weight.

Fluids   Water plays a fundamental role in the structure of the body.[4] The amount of water is proportionally great in some tissues, such as blood and brain, whereas muscle has less, and adipose tissue the least. Water exists either in bound form in the protoplasm of cells, as colloidal gels, or as true solutions intercellularly. Vital processes take place in the aqueous media of the cells and intercellular substances.

The quantity of water in the body varies with age, sex, and adiposity. It forms 50 to 70 percent of the body of adult males, and 45 to 65 percent in adult females. Obese individuals may have water content as low as 40 percent of their body weight. The water content of the newborn, on the other hand, may be as high as 80 percent.

WATER AND ELECTROLYTE BALANCE

The fluids of the body occupy three hypothetical "compartments." One of these is within the cells; one is outside the cells in intercellular spaces; and the other is an extracellular compartment in vascular and lymphatic systems. The fluids of the three compartments are designated **intracellular fluid, interstitial fluid,** and **extracellular fluid.** The interstitial compartment may be subdivided into hardly perceptible tissue spaces containing tissue fluid proper and certain discrete spaces around the brain, in joints, and in the thorax and abdomen, all of which contain special tissue fluids of a second order. The three compartments are represented schematically in Fig. 1.3.

If mean water content is 60 percent of body weight, the body of a person

[4]A precise fluid balance must be maintained if the organism is to survive, and many specialized functions of tissues have evolved in response to that requirement. An important aspect of histology is the study of those structural specializations that subserve the function of maintaining fluid balance. For this reason, the subject is considered in some detail in this introductory chapter.

weighing 70 kg has 42 liters of water, of which 28 liters are intracellular, 10.5 liters are interstitial, and 3.5 liters are extracellular (plasma). A delicate balance exists between the constituents of the three compartments. Semipermeable membranes separate one from another, being more tenuous in some locations than in others.

The daily intake of water must be equal to the amount leaving the body; otherwise dehydration (loss of water) or edema (accumulation of water) of the tissues will occur. The healthy body, under mean conditions of exercise and ambient temperature, exchanges 2 to 3 liters of water each day. Water enters the body as imbibed fluids, as preformed water in food, and as water formed in the body by oxidative processes. Water leaves the body through the kidneys in urine, from the skin in perspiration and sweat, from the lungs as vapor, and in the feces. Figure 1.4 illustrates the typical relationships.

Another situation to consider in evaluating water balance is the relationship between alimentary secretion and absorption (Fig. 1.5). An adult secretes about 8.2 liters of fluid, including 1.5 liters of saliva, 2.5 liters of gastric juice, 1.2 liters of bile and pancreatic juice, and 3 liters of intestinal juice per day. All but the small amount eliminated in feces (0.15 liter) is absorbed by the intestinal mucosa. Absorption failure without compensatory fluid and electrolyte replacement can be disastrous.

The fluids of the body are essentially solutions of electrolytes, that is, of chemical compounds that dissociate in water into charged ionic particles. The principal ones having positive charges (cations) are sodium (Na^+), potassium (K^+), calcium (Ca^{2+}), and magnesium (Mg^{2+}). Those with negative charges (anions) are chloride (Cl^-), bicarbonate (HCO_3^-), phosphate (HPO_4^{2-}), sulfate (SO_4^{2-}), and protein. The fluids of the three compartments differ in their ionic profiles as shown in Table 1.2 and Fig. 1.6. There is a significant difference between plasma and interstitial fluid only in the concentration of protein. These two fluids, however, differ markedly from intracellular fluid in which, among other contrasts, potassium ionic concentration is notably high. The high

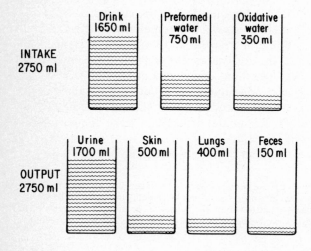

Figure 1-4 Water intake versus output per day under conditions of normal health and mean ambient temperature. *(CHP)*

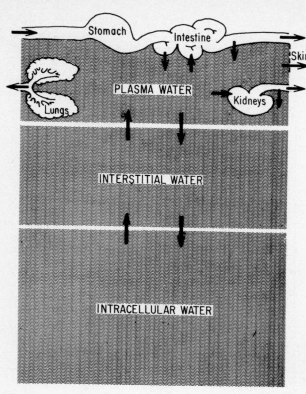

Figure 1-5 Routes of passage of water into and out of the body in achieving normal water balance. Redrawn from S. M. Brooks. *(CHP)*

Table 1.2   Ionic Profile of the Body Fluids in Milliequivalents per Liter*

Ion	Plasma	Interstitial	Intracellular
Na^+	142	145	10
K^+	4	4	160
Ca^{2+}	5	5	2
Mg^{2+}	2	2	26
Cl^-	101	114	3
HCO_3^-	27	31	10
HPO_4^{2-}	2	2	100
SO_4^-	1	1	20
$Protein^-$	16	1	65

*Ionic concentration is expressed in terms of milliequivalents per liter (meq/l). One milliequivalent is the amount of an ion that exactly reacts with or replaces one milliequivalent of another ion.

$$Milliequivalent = \frac{atomic\ weight}{ionic\ charge \times 1,000}$$

thus,

$$1\ meq\ of\ Na^+ = \frac{23}{1 \times 1,000} = 0.023\ g$$

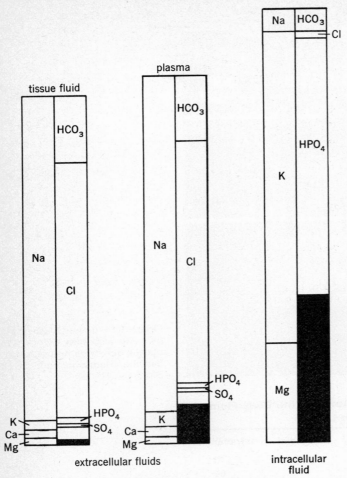

Figure 1-6 Principal solutes of body fluids. Columns on left indicate cation concentrations; those on the right anion concentrations. Black refers to protein; unlabeled white, to other ions. Note the marked difference between extracellular fluids and intracellular fluid.

cellular concentration of potassium is achieved by means of an active transport process at the cell membrane by which Na^+ ions are continuously pumped out of the cell and K^+ ions into it in order to maintain the necessary intracellular and extracellular concentrations of these cations.

The electrolyte balance between plasma and interstitial fluid on one hand and intracellular fluid on the other is critical and is maintained by adequate functioning of kidneys, lungs, intestinal mucosa, and sweat glands. It is noteworthy that excessive loss of sodium chloride can occur through the skin during exercise under high temperatures.

Equilibrium in passage of water across the semipermeable membranes separating the three fluid compartments does not depend solely upon the concentrations of electrolyte particles. It depends also on the osmolarity of the solutions on either side of the membranes, that is, on the force with which water flows from the side of lesser density to that of greater density of particles.

Healthy conditions in the three hypothetical compartments require maintenance of a state of acid-base balance. There is a ratio of 20 to 1 between bicarbonate and carbonic acid that keeps the pH value of blood at 7.35 to 7.45. Deviation toward acidity of as little as 0.35 point (acidosis) can result in death. Deviation toward alkalinity of 0.35 point or more (alkalosis) likewise results in death. Acid-base balance is maintained by the lungs which reduce the level of carbonic acid of the blood by emitting carbon dioxide, and by the kidneys which, upon demand, can conserve bicarbonate as well as hydrogen ions in response to changes in the 20-to-1 ratio (Fig. 1.7).

This brief account of the body fluids emphasizes the point that water, invisible in histologic sections, plays an important part in bodily activities. Indeed, it serves as the medium for all physiologic processes. Tissue fluid and the plasma constitute the internal environment of the body. They provide a liaison with the outer world. Not much of a problem presents itself to lower organisms living in sea water. Terrestrial life became possible only because the organism was able to find a means of maintaining a constant environment for the life processes of its cells irrespective of most external changes. **Homeostasis** is the term applied to this constancy of the internal environment.

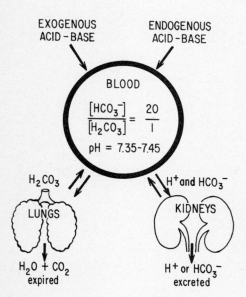

EXOGENOUS ACID-BASE

ENDOGENOUS ACID-BASE

BLOOD

$$\frac{[HCO_3^-]}{[H_2CO_3]} = \frac{20}{1}$$

pH = 7.35-7.45

H_2CO_3

LUNGS

$H_2O + CO_2$ expired

H^+ and HCO_3^-

KIDNEYS

H^+ or HCO_3^- excreted

Figure 1-7 Regulation of blood pH. Even though acidic and basic substances regularly enter the plasma compartment, the pH remains constant so long as the lungs and kidneys maintain a bicarbonate to carbonic acid ratio of 20 to 1. Redrawn from S. M. Brooks. *(CHP)*

SUGGESTED READING

Baker, J. R.: *Cytological Technique. The Principles Underlying Routine Methods,* 5th ed. John Wiley & Sons, Inc., New York, 1966.

Brooks, S. M.: *Basic Facts of Body Water and Ions,* 3d ed. Springer Publishing Co., Inc., New York, 1973.

Dupouy, G.: Three-megavolt Electron Microscopy. *Endeavour,* vol. 32, pp. 66–70, 1973.

Everhart, T. E., and G. T. L. Hayer: The Scanning Electron Microscope. *Scientific American,* vol. 226, no. 1, pp. 55–69, January, 1972.

Gray, P.: *The Use of the Microscope.* McGraw-Hill Book Company, New York, 1967.

Mercer, E. H., and M. S. C. Birbeck: *Electron Microscopy. A Handbook for Biologists,* 3d ed. Blackwell Scientific Publications, Ltd., Oxford, 1972.

Pearse, A. G. E.: *Histochemistry: Theoretical and Applied,* 3d ed. Little, Brown and Company, Boston, 1968.

Snively, W. D. J.: *Sea Within. The Story of Our Body Fluid.* J. B. Lippincott Company, Philadelphia, 1960.

Cells

All tissues of the body are composed of cells and the products of cells. The animal cell, in its simplified and ideal form, is a spherical mass of protoplasm, bounded by a delicate plasma membrane and containing various microscopic and submicroscopic structures. The largest of these, and the most conspicuous, is the nucleus.[1] The rest of the protoplasm is called cytoplasm. A number of minute organelles are encountered in the cytoplasm. Many of them, being less than 0.2 μm in diameter, are below the limit of resolution of the light microscope. The electron microscope must be employed to see the smaller substructures in the cell.

LIVING CELLS

Some idea of the appearance of protoplasm can be gained by studying living cells; two are illustrated in accompanying photomicrographs (Fig. 2.1 and 2.2). Protoplasm exists as a colloidal solution, the state of which can vary from a sol to a gel and vice versa.

[1]A nucleus is absent from some organisms. Cells lacking nuclei, the bacteria and blue-green algae, are called "prokaryotes." Those with nuclei in all other forms of plant and animal life are called "eukaryotes."

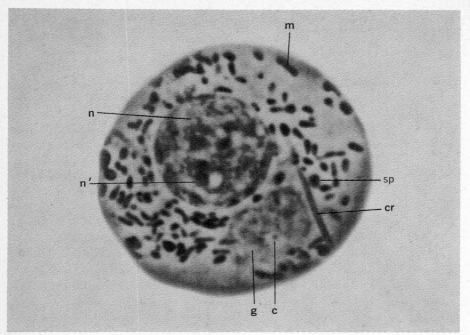

Figure 2-1 Living cell; a myelocyte of bone marrow. The large central body, *n*, is the nucleus containing a nucleolus, *n'*. Dark elongated bodies, *m*, are mitochondria; rounded ones, *sp*, are the specific granules, lysosomal in nature, that will become more numerous as the cell matures into a granular leucocyte. The light hazy region, *g*, is the golgi complex, in which the centrosome can be seen as a light spot containing a dark dot, a centriole, *c*. A crystalloid inclusion, *cr*, is present in the cytoplasm. Photographed with phase-contrast optics and reproduced at ×3,000. *(Contributed by P. H. Ralph.)*

Macromolecules are fundamental components of this colloidal substance. They are large combinations of smaller organic units, called monomers, that are attached to one another in repetitive fashion by chemical bonds. Besides macromolecules, there are smaller organic and inorganic units, notably potassium and magnesium ions, phosphate and bicarbonate anions, and many trace elements. Water forms three-fourths of the substance of protoplasm, largely in a bound form. The principal large organic molecules are polysaccharides, proteins, nucleic acids, and lipids.

Polysaccharides include glycogen, a number of protein-polysaccharides, and the hyaluronic and chondroitin sulfuric acids of connective tissue and cartilage. Glycogen, a polymer of D-glucose, is an all-important energy material for cellular activities.

Proteins are long-chain macromolecules composed of specified numbers of amino acids linked together in precisely determined polypeptide sequences. Structural protein precursors are synthesized in the cytoplasm of the cell in forms that can be transported to intercellular spaces. Among the proteins produced by cells are enzymes, which are catalytic substances controlling activities of cells, and also antibodies and certain hormones. In number and variety, the proteins far exceed other cellular macromolecules.

Nucleic acids constitute a third class of macromolecules. They are polymers of nucleotides, two types being recognized. **Deoxyribonucleic acid (DNA)** is found mainly in the nucleus, but in lesser amount in mitochondria. **Ribonucleic acid (RNA)** occurs in several forms in the cytoplasm and nucleus of the cell. Both DNA and RNA are constructed of pentose sugar groups alternating sequentially with phosphate groups. Attached to deoxyribose are four base groups, namely adenine, thymine, guanine, and cytosine, sequentially arranged in a precise manner; the arrangement is such that two polynucleotide chains coil around a central axis to form the double helix of DNA. The sugar of RNA, ribose, has uracil in place of thymine. The DNA molecule constitutes the genetic material of the cell. It and the several kinds of RNA are given further consideration later in this chapter.

Lipids are smaller molecules found in protoplasm. Some, especially

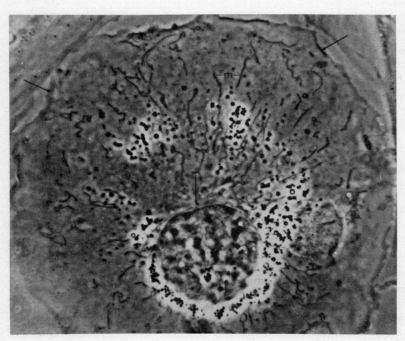

Figure 2-2 Living cell cultured from the spleen of a salamander. Note the undulating cell border, *black arrows,* filamentous mitochondria, *m,* and centrosome with centriole, *white arrow,* just above the nucleus. Photographed with phase-contrast optics, × 1,500. *(Contributed by R. Buchsbaum.)*

triglycerides, occur as visible particles or droplets in the cytoplasm. Others exist in combination with proteins and form some of the cytoplasmic organelles, particularly the membranous ones.

Characteristics of Protoplasm   Living protoplasm is not static. In tissue cultures, its inherent viscosity can be seen to fluctuate locally in the cell, resulting in streaming movements. Undulations of the cell surface and pseudopodia formation result in amoeboid movements in such cells as leucocytes. Less evident activity at the surface makes it possible for the cell to engulf droplets of fluid or even particles from surrounding media, the processes being known as pinocytosis (cell drinking) and phagocytosis (cell eating). Movement of substances into the cytoplasm is accomplished by endocytosis; movement out of the cytoplasm, by exocytosis.

Among the more pronounced protoplasmic movements are those involved in the extension of long cell processes. Cell locomotion and cell elongation are fundamentally different.

Other characteristics of protoplasm are its irritability, conductivity, contractility, and capacity to reproduce and give rise to other protoplasmic units. The fundamental properties are common to almost all cells, but in the course of evolution, some have become specialists in contraction, conduction, secretion, or some other function.

Since protoplasm is a colloidal system, its appearance is changed radically when its solutes are salted out by subjecting it to chemical fixing agents, when water is removed by drying it, or when its vital activities are arrested by subjecting it to high or low temperatures. Consider the difference in appearance of the colloidal albumen of a hen's egg before and after coagulation by boiling. There is as great a difference between protoplasm before and after chemical fixation.

CELL STRUCTURE, ORGANELLES

The cells of the human body have various shapes and sizes (Fig. 2.3). Under the light microscope, those in layers and compact masses are seen to be polyhedral, owing to mutual pressure. When spheres are arranged in a single layer, each borders upon six neighbors and, under pressure, becomes a polyhedron with eight sides. Superimposition of layer upon layer leads to formation of 14-sided polyhedrons (tetrakaidecahedrons), conforming to an ideal geometric design which encloses the greatest mass with the least surface. Few cells conform to this ideal. Elongation is a modification favoring contractility and conductivity, as in muscle and nerve cells. Stellate forms provide an increased surface, as in fixed macrophages and fibroblasts. Pressure of other cells or of intercellular structures produces irregular forms, as the cells of tendons. Flattened platelike cells distribute their masses over surfaces, as in the lining of closed body cavities and blood vessels. Cells that secrete tend to release the secretions through one region of the cytoplasm and acquire a fixed

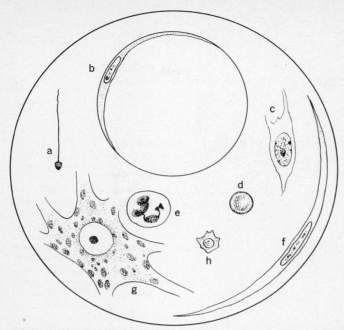

Figure 2-3 Diagram illustrating variations in relative size and shape of mammalian cells, all drawn to the same scale, approximateiy ×900. The enclosing circle represents the outline of a mature human ovum. Within the circle are a sperm cell, *a;* lipocyte, *b;* fibrocyte, *c;* erythrocyte, *d;* leucocyte, *e;* smooth-muscle cell, *f;* nerve cell, *g;* and neuroglia cell, *h. (WEL)*

polarity. Cells that store fat, and do not move about, most closely conform to the spherical or 8-sided or 14-sided shapes.

Cells vary in size from about 4 μm in diameter to those visible to the naked eye (100 μm). Some attain a length of more than a meter, as in the nervous system. However, there is no correlation between body size and cell size. The cells of the giant are as small as those of the dwarf.

Although cells display great diversity of shape and size, and tissues composed of them have widely different functions, they are individually remarkably similar in respect to their fundamental biochemical activities. Correlatively, the same submicroscopic structures are represented in nearly all animal cells. Indeed, the similarity between animal and plant, and even some bacterial cells, in respect to some of the organelles, is striking. Cell organelles have distinguishing morphologic characteristics. Observations of many kinds of cell have been combined in a diagrammatic representation of a typical cell in Fig. 2.4.[2]

Unit Membrane   The cell surface and many of the organelles in the cytoplasm are formed by unit membranes. These are liquid mosaics consisting of

[2]Atlases of electron micrographs can be used for studying fine structure just as collections of microscope slides serve for general histologic study. Several are listed at the end of this chapter.

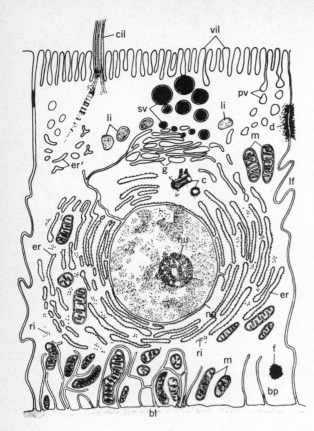

Figure 2-4 Schematic representation of a cell (epithelial) showing organelles. Plasmolemma bounds microvilli, *vil,* lateral folds, *lf,* and basal processes, *bp.* The nucleus, containing a nucleolus, *nu,* is enclosed by the nuclear envelope with pores, *np.* Other organelles and inclusions are granular endoplasmic reticulum, *er;* agranular endoplasmic reticulum, *er';* ribosomes, *ri;* golgi complex, *g;* mitochondria, *m;* lysomes, *li;* centrioles, *c;* pinocytotic vesicles, *pv;* secretory vesicles, *sv;* desmosome, *d;* lipid inclusions, *f.* One cilium, *cil,* with basal bodies is shown. Beneath the cell is a basal lamina, *bl. (Slightly modified from E. De Robertis and A. Pellegrino de Iraldi.)*

phospholipid bilayers in which the polar heads of the molecules, being hydrophilic, face, for example, the fluid of intercellular space on one side and that of the cytoplasm on the other, and in which hydrophobic fatty-acid chains extend inward from both sides. Figure 2.5 is a model of the presumed arrangement. Figure 2.6 is an electron micrograph showing two unit membranes in close apposition, each of which appears to consist of two dense layers (the hydrophilic portions) and a light layer (the hydrophobic fatty-acid portions of the molecules) sandwiched between. The thickness of unit membranes varies somewhat, 70 to 100 Å being the usual range. Globular protein molecules about 85 Å in diameter may be more or less embedded in the membrane, as illustrated in Fig. 2.7.

Plasmolemma   The unit membrane forming the surface boundary of a cell is called the plasmolemma.[3] In cross section, it cannot be seen with the light mi-

---

[3]Spelling after *Nomina Histologia*: the letter *o* always precedes the suffix *-lemma.*

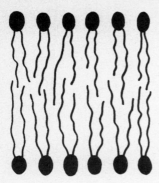

Figure 2-5 Schematic cross-sectional view of a phospholipid bilayer. Filled circles represent polar heads of the molecules that are in contact with water. Wavy lines represent the fatty-acid chains. *(Redrawn from S. J. Singer and S. L. Nicolson.) (CHP)*

croscope. Visible cell borders are composite structures made up of plasmolemma and associated ground substance or other surface coatings.

The structure of the plasmolemma varies from one type of cell to another in respect to the number and arrangement of 85Å protein particles protruding from its surface. Figure 2.8 shows a platinum-shadowed replica of the erythrocyte surface on which such particles are especially abundant. Metabolically inactive cells show few particles. It is believed that the particles in the mosaic represent sites related to specific functions of the plasmolemma.

The plasmolemma plays an active part in movement of substances between the cell interior and the intercellular spaces and extracellular environment, e.g., in processes of **endocytosis** and **exocytosis**. It has a selective action. It is able, for example, to bring potassium ions from the intercellular spaces,

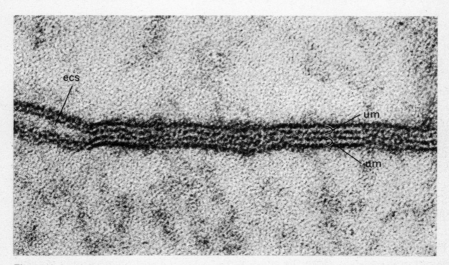

Figure 2-6 Unit membranes, *um,* in close approximation, though separated by a narrow extracellular space, *ecs,* at a gap junction between two neuroglia cells in the mouse brain. Electron micrograph, × 400,000. *(Contributed by T. S. Reese and M. W. Brightman.)*

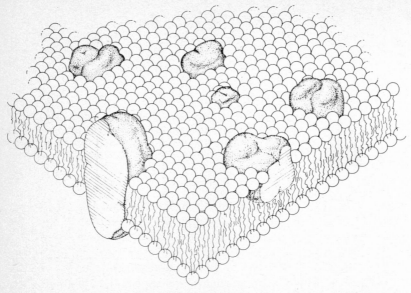

Figure 2-7 Lipid-globular-protein mosaic model of a unit membrane in three-dimensional cross-sectional view. The basic elements are shown as open circles and wavy lines. The solid bodies with stippled surfaces represent the globular integral proteins embedded in the membrane. *(Contributed by S. J. Singer and G. L. Nicolson, Science, 175:720–731, 1973.)*

where they are present in low concentration, into the cytoplasm, where their concentration is high. It can "pump" sodium ions against a gradient in the reverse direction.

Cells of certain tissues have little or no contact with each other, some being surrounded by fluid, ground substance, or fibers. Other types of cell, for example, those of epithelia, are arranged in compact groups. The borders of adjacent cells commonly have junctional specializations involving the plasmolemma. These bind neighboring cells to each other and provide for communication between them. Junctional complexes, or structures, are prominent features of epithelial cells and are described in Chap. 3.

Cells that present free surfaces to their environments commonly exhibit processes that vary in length and density of distribution in different types of cell and in different locations. Closely packed microvilli form striated borders. These are well developed on cells lining the intestines (Fig. 3.11). Cilia and flagellae are longer and more highly specialized projections from free surfaces of cells. They are described later in this chapter.

Invaginations of the Plasmolemma Two types of vesicle are related to the process of endocytosis. Both the pinocytotic vesicles and phagosomes involve budding from the plasmolemma. Others make their appearance at points where substances are being extruded through the plasmolemma by exocytosis.

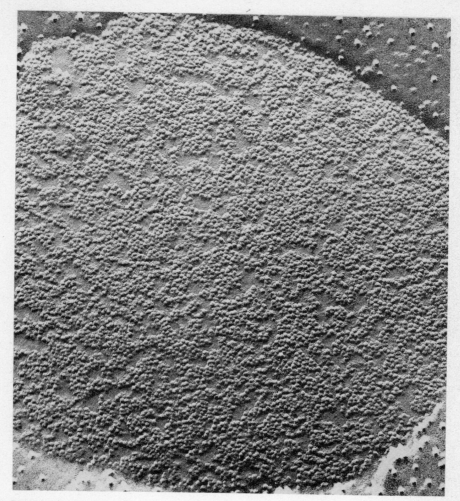

Figure 2-8 Platinum replica of freeze-etched erythrocyte membrane, showing distribution of binding sites to which protein molecules are attached. Electron micrograph, ×85,000. *(Contributed by V. T. Marchesi, Federation Proceedings, 32:1833–1837, 1973.)*

Pinocytotic vesicles are formed in cells by dimpling of the plasmolemma. The resulting "caveolae" then pinch off to become vesicles. Energy is expended in this process. Globular protein particles of 85 Å diameter form in rings around the openings of the caveolae (Fig. 2.9).

Pinocytosis was first observed in tissue cultures with the light microscope, the vesicles being considerably larger than most of those revealed with the electron microscope. Indeed, the latter are sometimes called "micropinocytotic" vesicles. Pinocytosis is one of the principal mechanisms of transporting large

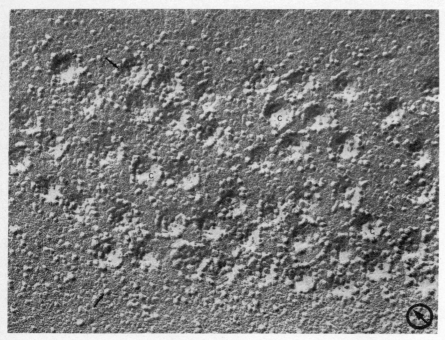

Figure 2-9 Membrane-associated particles, *arrows,* some of which surround pinocytotic "caveolae," *c,* on fracture face of a smooth-muscle cell. Electron micrograph of a platinum replica prepared by the freeze-fracture technique. (Arrow through circle indicates direction of the shadowing.) Micrograph, ×115,000. *(Contributed by L. Orci.)*

molecules into cells. Figure 11.4*B* shows pinocytotic vesicles in the wall of a small blood vessel. As vesicles pass through the outer zone of thicker cells, they may merge with other membranous organelles.

Phagosomes are formed similarly, but involve ingestion of extracellular particulate matter. The disposition of material engulfed by the cell is different from that coming in via pinocytotic vesicles. Phagosomes become associated with membranous organelles in the cytoplasm that contain enzymes necessary for digestion of the foreign material.

Lysosomes These are vesicles less than 0.5 μm in diameter, as a rule. Their appearance in electron micrographs varies considerably (Fig. 2.10). Somewhat similar "multivesicular bodies" are thought to be related to them. Lysosomes appear to be formed by a process similar to that resulting in production of secretory granules. They remain in the cell instead of being extruded. Lysosomes contain hydrolytic enzymes in a medium that is more acid than the surrounding cytoplasm. When they come in contact with phagosomes, the membranes of the two organelles coalesce, and this permits the enzymes to enter the phagosomes and lyse the contents of the latter. Should lysosomal

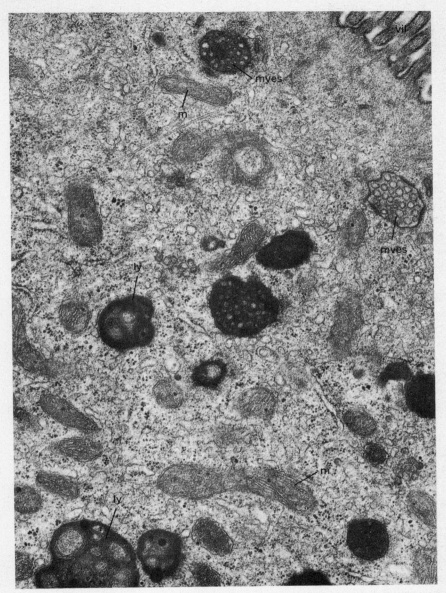

Figure 2-10 Lysosomes, *ly*, and multivesicular bodies, *mves*, near the surface of a cell in the intestinal epithelium (toad). Microvilli, *vil*, and mitochondria, *m*, are present. Electron micrograph, ×30,000. (*Contributed by J. Rosenbluth.*)

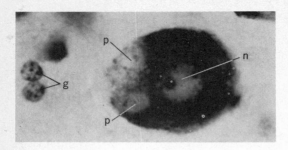

Figure 2-11 Nerve cell in the brain of a 7-year-old guinea pig. Masses of lipofuscin bodies, *p*, have accumulated in the cytoplasm at one side of the nucleus, *n*. The masses are known as "pigment of aging." Small nuclei belong to neuroglia cells, *g*. Photomicrograph of thionine-stained preparation, × 600. *(Contributed by H. H. Wilcox.)*

membranes rupture into the cytoplasm, their digestive enzymes would cause autolysis of the cell, an activity that apparently does take place in dying cells.[4]

Material that is resistant to digestion by lysosomal enzymes may remain in the cell indefinitely in membrane-bounded **lipofuscin bodies**. These accumulate and, with aging, become clumped in masses (Fig. 2.11). Pigments of different type, notably melanin, occur in certain cells in the skin, iris, and retina.

Endoplasmic Reticulum   A system of membranous organelles, mainly in the form of tubules and parallel arrays of flat cisternae, composes the endoplasmic reticulum. It is present, at least in small amounts, in nearly all cells and is closely associated with other membranous organelles, particularly the golgi complex. Its elements interconnect or anastomose. Two varieties of the endoplasmic reticulum are designated as granular and agranular, according to whether they have ribosomes attached along the outer surfaces of their membranes. Both types may be found in the same cell.

Cell fractionation experiments employing differential ultracentrifugation produce fragments of the endoplasmic reticulum called "microsomes." These ribosome-studded vesicles are partially artifactitious.

Agranular endoplasmic reticulum is the variety lacking ribosomes. Figure 2.12 shows it in a liver cell where it is composed of tortuous anastomosing tubules. It occurs abundantly in another form in muscle cells where it is called "sarcoplasmic reticulum" (Fig. 9.12). A long, tubular variety has been revealed in nerve axons by high-voltage, thick-section electron microscopy (Fig. 14.8).

Functions other than that of protein synthesis are ascribed to the agranular endoplasmic reticulum. The close association of this organelle to clusters of glycogen particles in the cytoplasmic matrix of various types of cell, especially in the liver (Fig. 2.12), suggests a role in carbohydrate metabolism. It appears also to be associated with lipid and cholesterol metabolism and transport, and, in certain endocrine organs, with steroid-hormone synthesis. In muscle, it has to do with calcium-ion transfer during contraction and relaxation. The

[4]Advantage is being taken of these phenomena in attempting to introduce cytotoxic chemicals into cancer cells. Such chemicals first are bonded to substances that are readily phagocytized by the cancer cells. Subsequently, it is hoped, action of lysosomes will release the chemicals, and death of the cancer cell will occur.

agranular endoplasmic reticulum, consisting of long tubules, is believed to provide a means of transporting substances formed by the cell for its own use to distant parts of the cell, a function that is especially well defined in nerve-cell processes.

Granular endoplasmic reticulum, so named because its membrane is studded with minute ribonucleoprotein granules, i.e. ribosomes, has a structural organization quite different from that of the agranular variety. It consists of intercommunicating vesicles and flat lamellae commonly arranged in parallel arrays.

This organelle is seldom seen in rapidly dividing embryonic cells, but is one of the most prominent features of many types of cell in adults. Its organization is diffuse in some cells, but is concentrated in discrete clumps at the basal pole of actively secreting gland cells. Because of the basophilia of its attendant ribosomes, masses of it are visible with the light microscope as "chromophil substance" (Fig. 14.4A). The striking appearance of the granular endoplasmic reticulum is shown in an electron micrograph at moderately low magnification (Fig. 2.13). More details of its structure are visible in Fig. 2.14 at the same magnification used to show agranular endoplasmic reticulum in Fig. 2.12.

Proteins are synthesized by ribosomes adherent to outer surface of the membrane of the granular endoplasmic reticulum. They are selectively passed

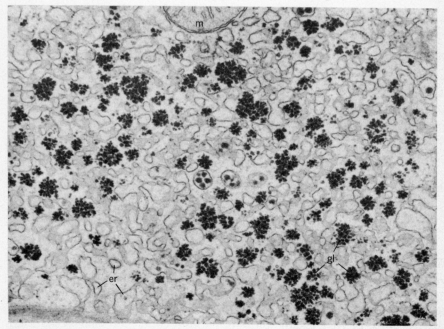

Figure 2-12 Agranular endoplasmic reticulum, *er,* in a hepatocyte (rat). Clumps of glycogen granules, *gl,* are darkly stained. Part of one mitochondrion, *m,* is visible at the top of the figure. Electron micrograph, about ×33,000. *(Contributed by G. E. Palade.)*

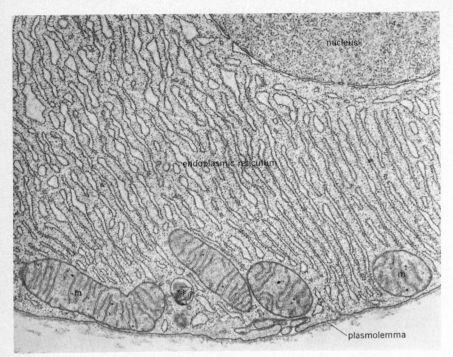

Figure 2-13 Basal portion of a pancreatic exocrine cell (rat) showing compact parallel arrays of granular endoplasmic reticulum. Mitochondria, *m*. The nucleus is visible at the top, and the superficial region of the cell is seen at the bottom. The asterisk marks a multivesicular body. Electron micrograph, ×12,500. *(Contributed by G. E. Palade.)*

into the interior of the vesicular lamellae. These channels isolate them from the cytoplasmic matrix and transport them to a center, the golgi complex, for their further chemical elaboration to become secretory products or other exportable proteins. The transfer is effected in membranous agranular **transfer vesicles** (Fig. 2.19).

Ribosomes and Polysomes   These minute bodies are associated structurally and functionally with the endoplasmic reticulum. Actually, they are particulate organelles of uneven contour without membranous boundaries (Fig. 2.15). Each ribosome has a diameter in the range of 200 Å and is composed of two subunits that have been shown to have different sedimentation rates by ultracentrifugation (60 S and 40 S). Chemically, ribosomes are made up of **ribosomal ribonucleic acid** (rRNA) and protein. They impart basophilia to the cell cytoplasm, the intensity of which depends on their concentration.

Ribosomes are present in all cells except erythrocytes. They occur individually and as clusters, rosettes, or spiral formations, called **polysomes,** dispersed throughout the cytoplasmic matrix or attached along the membranes of the en-

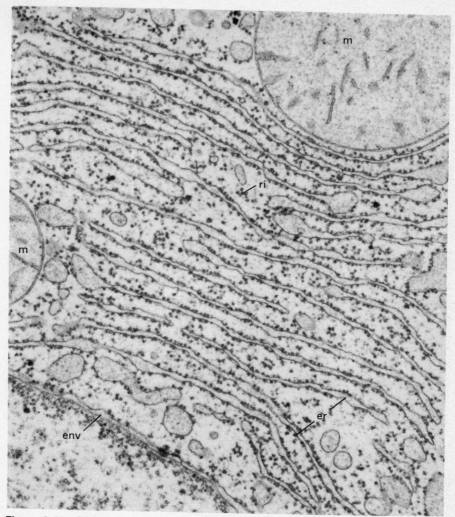

Figure 2-14 Granular endoplasmic reticulum, *er*, in the cytoplasm of a hepatic cell (rat). Compare with Fig. 2-12. Note the parallel arrays of flattened vesicles studded with ribosomes, *ri;* some ribosomes lie free in the matrix. Parts of the nuclear envelope, *env*, are shown. The mitochondria, *m*, have few cristae. Electron micrograph, ×33,000. *(Contributed by G. E. Palade.)*

doplasmic reticulum (giving the latter a granular appearance) by their larger subunits.

Polysomal ribosomes, varying in number, are attached to thin (15 Å diameter) filaments by another variety of nucleic acid, called **messenger ribonucleic acid** (mRNA), as illustrated in Fig. 2.15. Free polysomes are responsible for synthesis of proteins for growth and intrinsic activities of the cell. Those at-

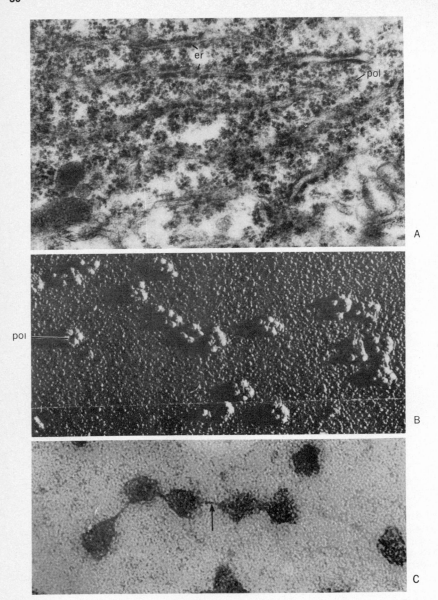

Figure 2-15   Ribosomes in groups forming rosettes called polysomes, *pol*. *A*. Polysomes between lamellae of endoplasmic reticulum, *er,* in a nerve cell of the spinal cord (neonatal rat).
Electron micrograph, about × 100,000. (Contributed by E. Puchala.) *B*. Polysomes (rabbit)
spread on a grid and prepared by shadowing technique; *C* ribosomes uncoiled along a filament of mRNA *(arrow)*. *B* and *C*. Electron micrographs, about × 400,000. *(Contributed by A.
Rich.)*

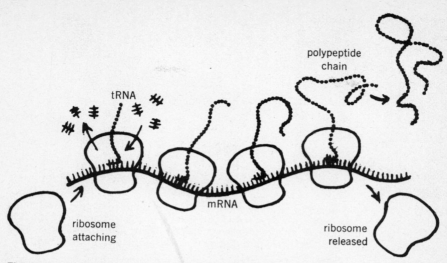

Figure 2-16 Diagram illustrating protein synthesis. Ribosomes become attached to a filamentous molecule of mRNA. Molecules of tRNA, linked with specific amino acid, bring the required information to mRNA for the type of protein to be synthesized. The ribosomes move along the strand of mRNA putting together amino-acid sequences; the longer the molecule of mRNA, the more ribosomes are in a polysome, and the greater the number of amino acids assembled in the final polypeptide chain. (*Modified from* Bailey's Textbook of Histology, *16th ed. W. M. Copenhaver, R. P. Bunge, and M. B. Bunge (eds.), The Williams & Wilkins Company, Baltimore, 1971.*)

tached to membranes of the endoplasmic reticulum engage in synthesis of proteins exported by the cell, such as enzymes, antibodies, and structural proteins. The ribosomes are sites where amino acids are incorporated into peptides.

The nucleic acid of ribosomes (rRNA) is produced in the nucleolus, exiting from the nucleus through the nuclear envelope into the cytoplasm. The fine filamentous messenger form (mRNA), along which ribosomes are aligned as polysomes, arises in the nucleus and moves into the cytoplasm. A soluble form of ribonucleic acid of low molecular weight, called **transfer ribonucleic acid** (tRNA), likewise comes from the nucleus.

Specific amino acid molecules are carried by transfer ribonucleic acid to the strand of messenger ribonucleic acid of the polysome, where they are placed in proper sequence to form the specific protein being synthesized by that particular polysome. The ribosomes appear to move along the filament, as illustrated schematically in Fig. 2.16, assembling amino acids into polypeptide chains. In doing so, they impart the information encoded by the messenger ribonucleic acid to the protein which is being produced. The length of the protein molecule is related to the number of ribosomes in a polysome.

Intracellular Reticular Apparatus This organelle, generally called the golgi apparatus or **golgi complex**, is found in a wide variety of cells. It is located next to the nucleus in close association with the centrosome of actively secret-

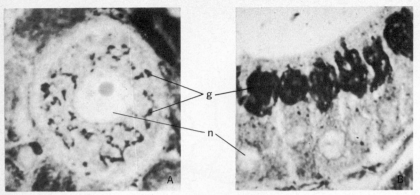

Figure 2-17 The golgi complex, *g*, as observed through the light microscope: *A*, arranged diffusely in a spinal ganglion cell; *B*, concentrated between the nucleus, *n*, and free surface in simple columnar epithelial cell. The organelle is stained black with osmic acid. Photomicrographs: *A*, ×900; *B*, ×1,500. *(Contributed by G. L. Rasmussen and H. Elftman.)*

ing cells, such as those of glands and plasmocytes. Its arrangement is diffuse in large nerve cells. The golgi complex can be visualized under the light microscope, after special staining with silver salts or osmic acid, either as a light region in the cytoplasm or as a blackened reticulum (Fig. 2.17).

The golgi complex consists of an array of smooth-surfaced, flattened cisternae with bulbous ends (Fig. 2.18). Occasional points of communication with the lamellae of granular endoplasmic reticulum are encountered (Fig. 2.19). More commonly, transfer vesicles bud off the latter and move with their contents to the cisternae of the golgi complex where the two elements become confluent. It receives proteins in solution from the granular endoplasmic reticulum and concentrates and modifies them in its bulbous **condensing vesicles.** It delivers the concentrated substances in membrane-bounded packages to the periphery of the cell, for example, zymogen granules of gland cells or specific granules of certain leucocytes. The process of concentration of protein-containing material is associated in some types of cell with incorporation of carbohydrate molecules to form glycoproteins. Mucous secretions are examples of this.

Annulate Lamellae   This organelle, composed of several parallel agranular membranes with irregularly spaced pores, is sometimes encountered near the nucleus of developing cells.

Microtubules   The microtubules are organelles of indefinite length, averaging 240 Å in diameter. In cross sections each appears to consist of 13 helically arranged subunits measuring individually about 40 or 50 Å in diameter. Microtubules are present in all nucleated cells. They increase numerically and attain considerable prominence in the spindle formations of dividing cells

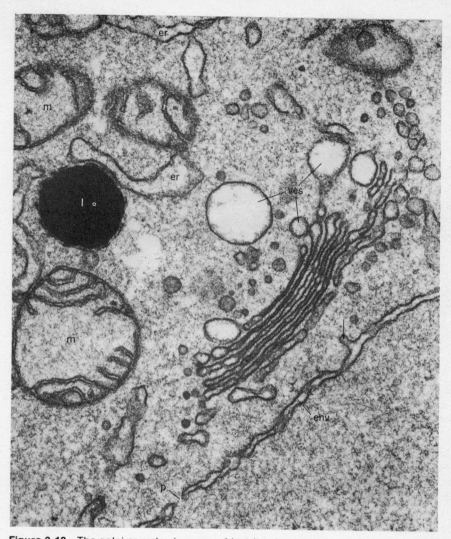

Figure 2-18 The golgi complex in a neuroblast (toad) consists of parallel arrays of smooth-surfaced cisternae, some with swollen ends, and vesicles, *ves,* of several sizes, containing secretion products. It lies next to the nucleus which is bounded by the nuclear envelope, *env,* in this case showing nuclear pores, *p,* and a communication (*arrow*) with other components of the internal membrane system. Other structures shown are mitochondrion, *m,* endoplasmic reticulum, *er,* and a lipid inclusion, *l.* Electron micrograph, × 40,000. *(Contributed by J. Rosenbluth.)*

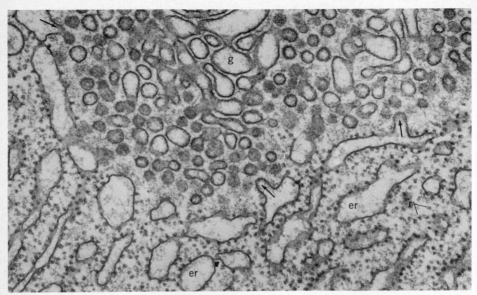

Figure 2-19 Agranular transfer vesicles of the golgi complex, *g*, confluent (*arrows*) with those of the granular endoplasmic reticulum, *er*, in a pancreatic cell (rat). Electron micrograph, ×45,000. *(Contributed by G. E. Palade.)*

(Fig. 2.33). They radiate from centrioles, form the cores of cilia and flagellae, and occur in scattered clusters or singly elsewhere in the cytoplasm. Their presence in the long processes of nerve cells is noteworthy (Fig. 14.21).

Microtubules provide a sort of framework for the cell, making possible the maintenance of a given shape. Furthermore, they may direct intracytoplasmic transport of macromolecules. The protein of which they are composed resembles the muscle protein, actin, in respect to amino-acid sequences, and it is possible that intracellular movement may be a function of some microtubules.

Chemically, microtubules are polymers of the protein "tubulin." When cells are experimentally homogenized, their microtubules cannot be recovered intact by ultracentrifugation, but tubulin subunits can be isolated and polymerized in the test tube by removal of calcium from the medium.

Centrioles are made up of short microtubules. They have long been recognized for their association with the mitotic apparatus of the cell during division, but are found also in the ciliary basal bodies of some epithelial cells, and have been recognized in many other cells. Centrioles occur in pairs just visible in living cells examined with phase-contrast optics (Fig. 2.1) and in fixed cells stained with iron hematoxylin, but their fine structure can be visualized only in electron micrographs (Fig. 2.20). They are located near the nucleus and are frequently surrounded by cisternae of the golgi complex.

Centrioles are short cylinders, about 150 μm in diameter, closed at one end. One member of each pair lies at right angles to the other. Each consists of

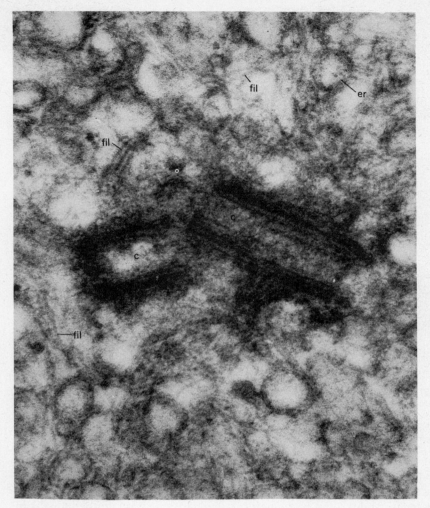

Figure 2-20 Two centrioles, *c,* in the centrosome of a mouse fibroblast in the resting stage. The centriole at the right was sectioned longitudinally, that at the left obliquely, displaying some of the coarse microtubules. Many fine microfilaments, *fil,* traverse the matrix among microvesicles of the endoplasmic reticulum, *er.* Electron micrograph, × 143,000. *(Contributed by W. Bernhard.)*

a pinwheel-shaped arrangement of nine groups of three short microtubules (Fig. 2.21*A*). In ciliary basal bodies, the components of one centriole are continued into the cilium.

The cytoplasm immediately around the pairs of centrioles has a rather clear appearance. It is designated the central body, or **centrosome**. Close to each centriole, some electron-dense material in clumps is associated with each group of three tubules. These clumps are called "pericentriolar satellites." The material may be concerned with replication of the centriole.

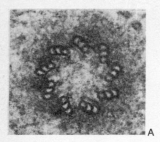
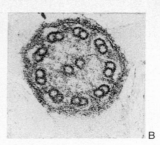
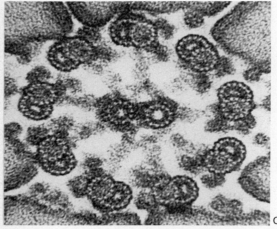

Figure 2-21 Cross sections of a centriole from a cell in the lens of a newborn rat, *A;* of a cilium from an epithelial cell of a mammalian uterine tube, *B;* and of a flagellum from principal piece of sperm of a guinea pig, *C.* Note the protofilaments in the walls of the microtubules of *C.* Electron micrographs, *A,* × 140,000; *B,* about × 140,000; *C,* about × 380,000. [*A* contributed by K. R. Porter. *B* and *C* contributed by D. W. Fawcett, from preparations of E. Anderson (*B*) and D. Phillips (*C*).]

Cilia and **flagellae** are motile processes of cells, the former measuring 5 to 10 μm in length and 0.5 μm in diameter. Cilia are present on epithelial cells in parts of respiratory and genital passages. Modified cilia on olfactory cells serve as sensory receptors. Flagellae are longer and are represented by sperm tails (Fig. 2.21*C*). Both types of processes are covered by extension of the plasmolemma.

The core of each cilium contains nine pairs of microtubules arranged cylindrically, with two separate microtubules in the center (Fig. 2.21*B*). The cylindrical group extends from the cilium down into the outer zone of the cell as a basal body, but the separate central microtubules end at the level of the cell surface. Rootlets of the basal body may exhibit cross striations (Fig. 2.22).

Microfilaments   Like microtubules, microfilaments are distributed widely among many types of cell, occurring in networks, bundles, and parallel arrays. They are of indefinite length and vary in diameter from 30 to 50 Å. The periph-

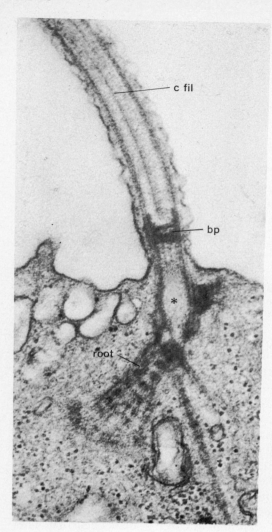

Figure 2-22 A cilium sectioned longitudinally. Central filaments, *c fil*, terminate just above the basal plate, *bp*, below which is the basal body (asterisk in basal body), with its striated rootlets, *root*. Electron micrograph, ×100,000. *(Contributed by R. M. Steinman and D. W. Fawcett.)*

eral cytoplasm of cells often shows great numbers of thin microfilaments forming meshworks. Processes of nerve cells and neuroglia cells characteristically have parallel arrangement of bundles (Fig. 14.13).

The term **filament** is reserved for structures of submicroscopic dimensions. These may be assembled into **fibrils**, which are structures of much greater magnitude. Fibrils are visible under the light microscope, and some bear specific names, for example, "myofibril" of muscle cells. Other fibrils, particularly in neurons and neuroglia cells, represent artifactitious condensations of groups of filaments, formed during fixation, and cannot be identified as entities in electron micrographs. The term **fiber** is reserved for even larger components of tissue, whether cellular or extracellular.

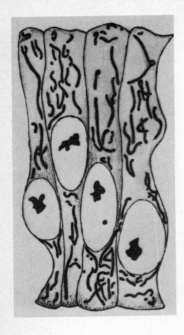

Figure 2-23 Filamentous mitochondria in the cytoplasm of a cell in the intestinal epithelium of a chick. About ×1,200. *(JFN)*

Mitochondria   Minute bodies observed in the cell more than a century ago became known later as mitochondria. These organelles can be observed in living cells by phase microscopy, and also after supravital staining. Figures 2.1 and 2.2 show different forms of mitochondria in two types of cell. Figure 2.23 illustrates their appearance and distribution in another.

Most mitochondria are 0.5 μm or less in diameter and vary in length from 2 μm up to 80 or 100 μm, depending on functional state as well as location. Some are ovoid bodies or short rods, others are elongated and tortuous. In living cells they appear to be engaged in active motion, twisting, swelling and contracting, and shifting their position in a saltatory manner (particularly in processes of nerve cells). Mitochondria tend to congregate at sites of high cellular activity, e.g., where active transport, secretion, or contraction is occurring. They form close relationships with folds of the plasmolemma, lamellae of the endoplasmic reticulum, and cisternae of the sarcoplasmic reticulum.

Figure 2.24 and other illustrations (Figs. 2.14 and 2.18) show the fine structure of mitochondria. They are membranous organelles, but it is doubtful that they have points of confluence with other membranous organelles or with the plasmolemma, even though some are found in close proximity to them. Each is bounded by an outer membrane, 70 Å thick, which has no ribosomes adherent to its surface. An inner membrane, separated from the outer one by a space of 80 Å, is thrown into folds, called **cristae**, and sometimes into tubular processes. These folds and processes vary greatly in form and number, depending on how actively the mitochondrion is functioning. The internal surface of the inner membrane and its projections appear to be studded with particles

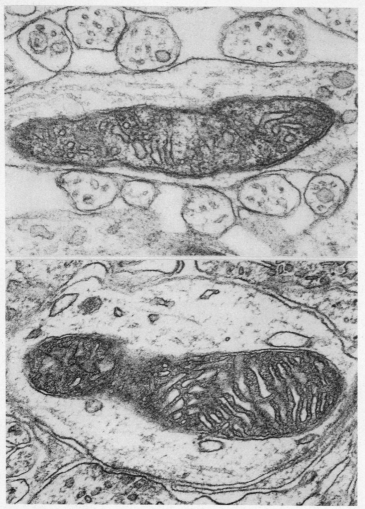

Figure 2-24 Mitochondria in the central nervous system of a four-day-old, *A*, and a 35-day-old rat, *B*. Cristae are more numerous in the older specimen. Electron micrographs, ×35,000. *(Contributed by J.J. Pysh.)*

measuring about 85 Å in diameter.[5] These are presumed to be globular protein macromolecules, the enzymes that are fundamental elements in mitochondrial activities.

The **matrix** substance in mitochondria often presents a finely granular appearance in electron micrographs. A variable number of dense granules 300 to 500 Å in diameter is found in it. The matrix also contains strands of DNA and

[5]There is some doubt that these exist as "lollipop" structures in life.

granules of RNA, the latter being smaller than the ribosomes in the cytoplasm. Thus, the mitochondrion has built into it the means of synthesizing protein (enzymes) and of genetic replication. It is, to a high degree, an autonomous unit.

These organelles provide the main source of energy for cellular activities. They are the cell's power supply. The enzymes required in the citric-acid cycle (Krebs cycle) are located in the mitochondrial matrix. They involve breakdown mainly of carbohydrates and fatty acids. Oxidative enzymes for the processes of oxidative phosphorylation are thought to be located in the particles on the mitochondrial cristae. These enzymes result in conversion of adenosine diphosphate (ADP) to adenosine triphosphate (ATP), a source of high energy that can be stored for such cellular activities as protein synthesis and muscle contraction. The degree of complexity of the arrays of cristae varies with the rate of production of this material.

The relationship of this complex organelle to the cell in which it occurs has been an enigma for many years. Mitochondria have few of the fundamental characteristics of the other organelles. Indeed, they have many features of prokaryotic cells,[6] e.g., nonnucleated bacterial cells. Principal among these in both mitochondria and bacteria (*E. coli*) are an oxygen-metabolizing enzyme (superoxide dismutase), quite different from that occurring in other components of eukaryotic cells, and an amino-acid sequence remarkably similar to that in the prokaryocyte. Furthermore, mitochondria have DNA filaments dispersed throughout their matrix, as do bacteria. They are thereby able to replicate when the cell containing them divides.

In view of these observations it has been proposed that some ancestral form of life may have succeeded in engulfing a bacterial cell and putting its enzyme systems to work in respiring. In other words, a prokaryocyte may have been incorporated by a "lucky gulp" into the cytoplasm of a eukaryocytic cell, and found that the two could live symbiotically ever after!

Peroxisomes   These are **microbodies** bounded by a unit membrane, filled with finely granular electron-dense substances. They contain catalase and hydrogen peroxide–producing oxidases. Peroxisomes occur abundantly, closely associated with mitochondria, in cells engaged in conversion of lipids to sugars, as in liver, muscle, and adipose tissue.

Nucleus   The nucleus is the largest organelle. It is vital to the cell, which is incapable of dividing without it. Nonetheless, some cells perform their functions for a long time without a nucleus.

The nucleus of the fixed cell is prominent except during cell division. It varies in appearance in cells of different types and to some extent with different fixing reagents. Although spherical and ovoid nuclei predominate, some cells have elongated nuclei and others polymorphic ones (Fig. 2.25). There tends to be a constant relation between nuclear size and cell size; large cells have large

[6]See footnote 1.

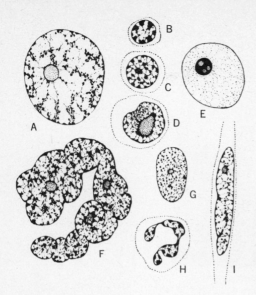

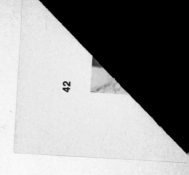

Figure 2-25 Variation in size, shape, and structure of nuclei: *A*, oocyte; *B*, lymphoctye; *C*, erythroblast from bone marrow; *D*, hemocytoblast from bone marrow; *E*, nerve cell of spinal cord; *F*, megakaryocyte of bone marrow; *G*, endothelium; *H*, neutrophil of blood; *I*, smooth muscle. × 1,200. *(JFN)*

nuclei, and small cells have small ones. Typically only one nucleus is present; however, binucleate cells are encountered in liver and sympathetic ganglia, and a multinucleate condition is found in certain phagocytes, osteoclasts, and especially in skeletal muscle where each fiber (cell) may have several hundred nuclei. A multinucleated nerve cell is shown in Fig. 2.26.

The nucleus appears under the light microscope to be bounded by a "nuclear membrane." Actually this consists of the submicroscopic **nuclear envelope** plus adherent ribosomes on the cytoplasmic side and chromatin on the inner face. The nuclear envelope is a component in the system of membranous organelles. It is composed of two unit membranes enclosing a narrow cavity. The inner and outer membranes fuse at regular intervals where there are circular **nuclear pores** 500 to 700 Å in diameter, bridged by thin diaphragms, seen in Fig. 2.27 (also Fig. 2.18). The outer membrane of the envelope exhibits occasional points of continuity with cisternae of the endoplasmic reticulum and, in those cells richly supplied with granular endoplasmic reticulum, is studded with ribosomes. The nuclear envelope disappears during cell division and is re-formed afterward by the endoplasmic reticulum. It is too thin to be resolved by the light microscope, but a nuclear boundry made up of its membranes and adherent particles is commonly seen.

The substance of the nucleus consists of nuclear matrix, chromatin, and nucleoli. The **matrix** is unstained and resembles a clear fluid when viewed by light microscopy, but consists of submicroscopic granules of interchromosomal substance. The nuclei of cells engaged actively in protein synthesis have nuclei with a great deal of matrix, which gives them a light appearance (Fig. 2.25*E*). Darkly staining nuclei, for example, those in lymphocytes, are indicative of a low activity level.

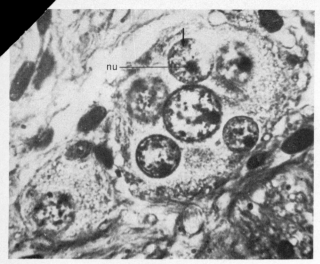

Figure 2-26 Multinucleated nerve cell in a human female autonomic ganglion; parts of six nuclei are visible. A nerve cell with a single nucleus appears at the lower left. The nucleolus, *nu*, of several nuclei is in the plane of section; a nucleolar satellite is marked by an *arrow*. Photomicrograph, × 900.

Chromatin is identified as deoxyribonucleoprotein. It stains intensely with basic dyes. Electron microscopy reveals dense regions in the nucleus that are believed to be the same as the chromatin clumps seen with light microscopy.

Chromatin consists of condensed portions of nuclear **chromosomes** of the interphase nucleus. The matrix contains the more dispersed parts of chromosomes. One of the female sex chromosomes never enters the dispersed phase, but remains as a compact body either adjacent to a nucleolus or against the nuclear membrane. This "sex chromatin" is visible in a nucleus in Fig. 2.26.

Nuclei of most cells contain a distinct homogeneous body, the **nucleolus** (Fig. 2.28), composed largely of RNA, and no DNA. It is easily seen in nuclei that have sparse chromatin, but in other nuclei is often confused with the larger clumps of chromatin known as "karyosomes." Electron micrographs reveal no membranous boundary. The nucleolus consists of groups of particles which are coarser and darker than those of other parts of the nucleus and are arranged in skeins. Cells actively synthesizing protein and requiring much ribosomal RNA have larger nucleoli than those engaged in little activity of this kind. The nucleolus loses its identity during cell division.

Much of the material of the interphase nucleus, with a granular appearance in electron micrographs, actually belongs to dispersed chromosomes. Some represents ribonucleoprotein precursors of ribosomes that are formed in the nucleus and pass into the cytoplasm through nuclear pores.

Deoxyribonucleic acid of dispersed chromosomes is duplicated during the nuclear interphase. As a cell prepares to divide, the chromosomes begin to condense, and ultimately are recognizable as more discrete elongated basophilic

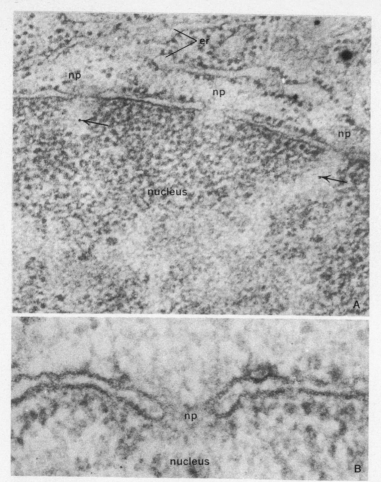

Figure 2-27 Nuclear pores. Section perpendicular to the nuclear surface of pancreatic acinous cell, *A*, and hepatic cell, *B*, from a rat. The nuclear envelope is interrupted by the nuclear pores, *np*. Regions of low density in the nucleus, marked by arrows, are designated "nuclear channels." Components of endoplasmic reticulum, *er*, are seen in the cytoplasmic matrix. Electron micrographs: *A*, × 80,000; *B*, × 190,000. *(Contributed by M. L. Watson.)*

structures. Figure 2.29 shows an electron micrograph of whole chromosomes, quite different in appearance from those seen in ultrathin sections.

Under the light microscope, chromosomes present two arms, often unequal in length, joined at a minute clear region, the **centromere**. Somatic chromosomes are paired, the members of the pair being joined at the centromere. "Acrocentric" chromosomes have one arm very short; "metacentric" chromosomes have arms approximately equal in length (Fig. 2.30). Constrictions in the arms occur in some.

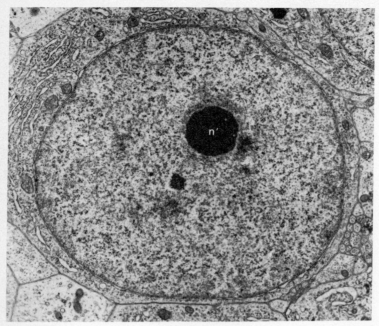

Figure 2-28 Nucleus of a nerve cell in the brain (toad) showing dispersed chromatin and a compact nucleolus, n'. Electron micrograph, ×20,000 *(Contributed by J. Rosenbluth.)*

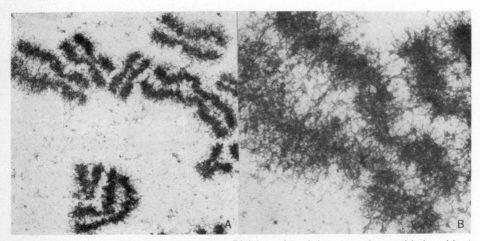

Figure 2-29 Whole human chromosomes. Division of each into two chromatids is evident. Coiling of the components is visible in *B*. Electron micrographs *A*, × 4,300, and *B*, × 13,000. *(Contributed by C. Wolff, G. Gilly, and C. Mouriquand*, Stain Technology, *vol. 49, pp. 133–136, 1974. With permission of The Williams & Wilkins Company, Baltimore.)*

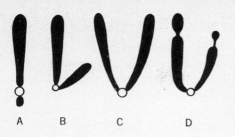

Figure 2-30 Diagrammatic representation of four chromosomes: *A,* acrocentric; *B,* submetacentric; *C,* metacentric; and *D,* metacentric with constrictions of arms. Clear circles are the centromeres. *(CHP)*

The number of chromosomes is constant for all body cells of each species. There are 46 in the human being, arranged in 22 homologous pairs plus the sex chromosomes, a pair of X chromosomes in females, and an X and a Y in males. Figure 2.31 shows a spread preparation of human male chromosomes.

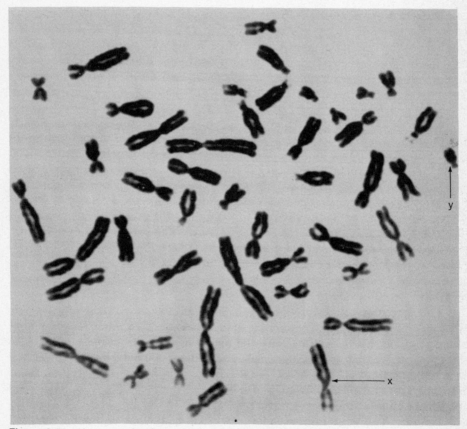

Figure 2-31 Human male chromosomes in metaphase. The X and Y chromosomes are indicated. Photomicrograph, ×900. *(Contributed by P. A. Farber.)*

CELL DIVISION

The process of division of the body cells, known as **mitosis**, involves not only the chromatic material of the nucleus, but also achromatic components of the **mitotic apparatus**. The latter term applies to the centrioles and associated microtubules. Each centrosome contains two centrioles with microtubules radiating from them to form **asters**. The fully developed mitotic apparatus has microtubules connecting the two asters and attaching to the chromosomes, forming a temporary organelle known as the **spindle**. The bundles of microtubules are called "spindle fibers."

The four phases of the process of mitosis are arbitrarily described; they are illustrated in Fig. 2.32. Mitosis occupies only a brief interval in the life cycle of most cells. The interphase is long. During it the nucleus is engaged in providing precisely defined ribonucleoprotein complexes to the cyptoplasm.

The **prophase** is that period during which the chromosomes become recognizable. Each consists of two identical rod-shaped bodies held together at the centromere. As these chromosomes shorten and become compact, the asters with their centrosomes move apart, and a spindle becomes evident (Fig. 2.33). The nuclear envelope and nucleolus disappear at the end of the prophase.

The **metaphase** is the stage during which the chromosomes are arranged at the equator of the cell. They appear as if suspended by threads, the microtubules, in a single plane midway between the two asters. This is illustrated diagrammatically in Fig. 2.32D. When viewed from one pole of the cell, chromosomes appear as in Fig. 2.32E.

The **anaphase** sees the complete separation of halves of each chromosome and their migration to opposite poles of the central spindle. In the diagram of Fig. 2.32, this is shown in F and G. Separation of the chromosomes begins at points of attachment of the mantle tubules. As the separating chromosomes move apart, tubular filaments are left behind them connecting one with another. The number of chromosomes at either pole of the cell at the end of the anaphase is the same as the number in the cell at the prophase.

The **telophase** is the reverse of the prophase. The chromosomes fade from view and are soon no longer identified as separate structures under the light microscope. The nuclear envelope and nucleolus re-form. Aster tubules disappear, and the cytoplasm constricts between the daughter nuclei. Thus, two new cells have been formed in place of one.

The time required for completion of one cell division varies with the type of tissue and the species. It is an hour or less in some; 2 or 3 hours is common. In tissue cultures of fibroblast cells, the prophase takes 30 to 60 minutes. The chromosomes remain in the equatorial plate at the metaphase for a time varying from only a minute or two to 15 minutes or more. The actual migration takes only 2 or 3 minutes. Thus the anaphase is brief. The telophase, from the arrival of chromosomes at the poles until the separation of the daughter cells, takes 3 to 6 minutes. The period of rest and growth varies between 30 minutes and 2 hours in these tissue-culture cells, but is ordinarily longer in vivo. From a con-

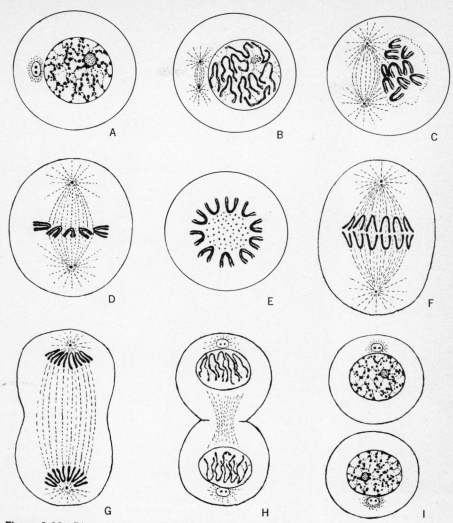

Figure 2-32 Diagram of mitotic cell division in animal cell: *A, B,* and *C,* prophase; *D* and *E,* lateral and polar views of metaphase; *F* and *G,* anaphase; *H* and *I,* telophase. *(JFN)*

sideration of these facts, it appears that the greatest number of mitotic figures encountered will be prophases. The actual pulling apart of the chromosomes is rarely seen.

Mitotic cell divisions take place in most tissues of the adult body. An unusual type occurs during maturation of the germ cells in the ovary and testis. It involves no splitting of the chromosomes, but a division of the homologous chromosomes. This process, in which there is a reduction to half the species number of chromosomes, is called **meiosis**.

Cell division may occur as a simple and direct splitting of the nucleus and

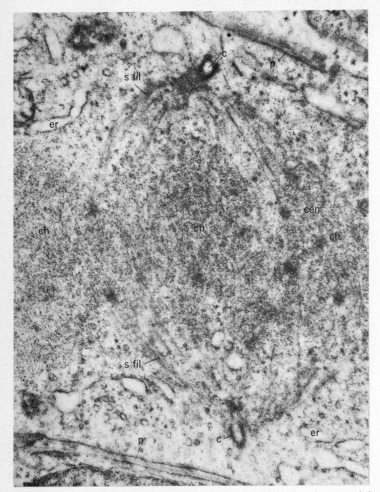

Figure 2-33   A dividing cell from the spleen of a chick, showing centrioles, *c,* at the poles of a mitotic figure. Tubular spindle "fibers," *sfil,* attached to centromeres, *cen,* of chromosomes. The chromosomes, *ch,* are represented by masses of granules in the central region. Vesicles of the endoplasmic reticulum, *er,* are present near the poles. Plasma membranes, *p,* are visible above and below the mitotic figure. Electron micrograph, × 18,000. *(Contributed by W. Bernhard.)*

cytoplasm by the process known as **amitosis**. It is probable that this takes place only in cells whose metabolism has been impaired and are on the verge of death.

GROWTH, AGING, AND DEGENERATION

Noncellular interstitial substances may increase in size by the addition of cellular secretions and water, but they do not grow in the true sense. Cells lacking nuclei may live a long time, but they do not grow. The nucleus is essential.

Growth is a vital phenomenon involving the synthesis of proteins and imbibition of water by them.

Growth may be uniform in all directions, as in the human egg, or it may be confined to one or two poles and involve flowing out of the protoplasm, as in nerve-cell processes. Increase in cell size can result from the combining of two or more small cells to make one big one, such as the giant, multinucleated, phagocytic, "foreign-body" cell. There is a limit beyond which a cell can no longer increase in size.

Cell division is essential for growth of the whole organism, but it cannot go on indefinitely without cell growth. The fertilized egg, a big cell to begin with, divides and redivides until a multicellular blastocyst has been formed which is scarcely larger than the original egg, but whose individual cells are much smaller. Some other cells grow and then divide into two daughter cells of ordinary mean size. In most instances, however, cells of mean size divide into smaller daughter cells, which then increase in size.

Cell division offers the means by which the body grows. Mitotic stages are encountered more frequently in tissues of young individuals or fetuses than in adults. The process of cell reproduction slows in normal tissues with advancing age.

Frequency of cell division in an organ depends largely upon the life span of its component cells, and varies widely. Nerve cells, for instance, live as long as the individual and are not replaced when destroyed. Cell divisions are not encountered in the nerve cells. On the other hand, there are cells with short lives that have to be replaced continuously. Cell division never ceases in the organs producing them.

Many cells of the adult have lost the power to divide. They are the definitive cells, such as those of the brain and muscles. A different category of cells is that whose members live a while and then divide to produce a definitive cell and another reproducer, continuing in this manner throughout life.

Some normal healthy tissues of the body are composed, in significant part, of cells that are in the process of dying or are actually dead. The gradual degenerative changes that ultimately benefit the organ as a whole are a part of normal histology. Such changes constitute physiologic degeneration.

The normal process of aging is a phenomenon differing from senility of pathologic basis; the term "senescence" is often used in connection with it. We are no sooner born than we begin to grow old. Some organs start to degenerate before birth. One notable example of this is the change that takes place in the umbilical arteries and the ductus arteriosus, which structures were of great functional value before birth but which are undesirable after birth.

Physiologic degeneration of cells begins before birth and extends throughout life. A few examples will be considered. The barrier between the external environment and the body protoplasm is the surface of the skin. This is a nonliving barrier formed by dry, dead, epithelial cells in the epidermis that have undergone cytoplasmic and nuclear transformations. Nuclei of living cells diminish in size, and their chromatin becomes denser and more deeply stained with hematoxylin. This process is known as "pyknosis." Dark granules of a substance which is the precursor of keratin manifest themselves in the cytoplasm and promptly coalesce as the cell dies and takes on a hyaloid or homogeneous appearance. Nuclei disappear. Growth and cell division in deeper layers maintain a constant supply of dying cells to provide a protective cornified layer, which is constantly sloughed away by abrasion, on the surface of the skin.

Another example of physiologic degeneration is seen in the cells of sebaceous glands, where a transition from large cells filled with lipid droplets and containing intact nuclei to dying cells with pyknotic nuclei occurs. When lipids replace the protoplasm, these cells disintegrate to release their oily substance through the neck of the gland along the shaft of a hair. Replacement from dividing cells at the periphery of the gland goes on constantly.

Physiologic degeneration will not be encountered in all tissues of the body but only in places where replacements are available—where young dividing cells can keep pace with the demand for their products. The process is characteristic of epithelial and connective tissues but is uncommon in muscle and absent in nervous tissues of the adult. The parenchymal cells of these tissues last a lifetime. Only with advancing years do they normally exhibit changes comparable with those seen in physiologic degeneration, namely, the accumulation of lipofuscin pigment or other cytoplasmic inclusions and pyknosis of the nucleus. When they degenerate, they are not replaced.

SUGGESTED READING

Abell, C. W., and T. M. Monahan: The Role of Adenosine 3',5'-Cyclic Monophosphate in the Regulation of Mammalian Cell Division. *Journal of Cell Biology*, vol. 59, pp. 549–558, 1973.

Bretcher, M. S.: Membrane Structure: Some General Principles. *Science*, vol. 181, pp. 622–629, 1973.

Brown, D. D.: The Isolation of Genes. *Scientific American*, vol. 229, no. 2, pp. 20–29, August, 1973.

deBruijn, W. C.: Glycogen, Its Chemistry and Morphologic Appearance in the Electron Microscope. *Journal of Ultrastructure Research*, vol. 42, pp. 29–50, 1973.

Carr, I.: The Fine Structure of Microfibrils and Microtubules in Macrophage and Other Lymphoreticular Cells in Relation to Cytoplasmic Movement. *Journal of Anatomy*, vol. 112, pp. 383–389, 1972.

Crick, F. H. C.: The Genetic Code. III. *Scientific American*, vol. 215, no. 4, pp. 55–62, October, 1966.

DeRobertis, E. D. P., W. W. Nowinski, and F. A. Saez: *Cell Biology*, 5th ed. W. B. Saunders Company, Philadelphia, 1970.

de Duve, C.: Biochemical Studies on the Occurrence, Biogenesis and Life History of Mammalian Peroxisomes, *Journal of Histochemistry and Cytochemistry*, vol. 21, pp. 941–948, 1973.

DuPraw, E. J.: *DNA and Chromosomes*. Holt, Rinehart and Winston, Inc., New York, 1970.

Fawcett, D. W.: *An Atlas of Fine Structure. The Cell: Its Organelles and Inclusions.* W. B. Saunders Company, Philadelphia, 1966.

Fox, C. F.: The Structure of Cell Membranes. *Scientific American,* vol. 226, no. 2, pp. 30–38, February, 1972.

Garrett, R. A., and H. G. Wittmann: Structure and Function of the Ribosome. *Endeavour,* vol. 12, pp. 8–14, 1973.

Kessel, R. G.: Annulate Lamellae. *Journal of Ultrastructure Research, Suppl.* 10, pp. 1–82, 1968.

McIntosh, J. R., and S. C. Landis: The Distribution of Spindle Microtubules During Mitosis in Cultured Human Cells. *Journal of Cell Biology,* vol. 49, pp. 468–497, 1971.

Markovics, J., J. Glass, and G. G. Maul: Pore Patterns on Nuclear Membranes. *Experimental Cell Research,* vol. 85, pp. 443–451, 1974.

Mathews, J. L., and J. H. Martin: *Atlas of Human Histology and Ultrastructure.* Lea & Febiger, Philadelphia, 1971.

Mazia, D.: The Cell Cycle. *Scientific American,* vol. 230, no. 1, pp. 55–64, January, 1974.

Miller, O. L., Jr.: The Visualization of Genes in Action. *Scientific American,* vol. 228, no. 3, pp. 34–42, March, 1973.

Neutra, M., and C. P. Leblond: The Golgi Apparatus. *Scientific American,* vol. 220, no. 2, pp. 100–107, February, 1969.

Northcote, D. H.: The Golgi Apparatus. *Endeavour,* vol. 30, pp. 26–33, 1971.

Olmsted, J. B., and G. G. Borisy: Microtubules. *Annual Review of Biochemistry,* vol. 42, pp. 507–540, 1973.

Porter, K. R., and M. A. Bonneville: *Fine Structure of Cells and Tissues,* 4th ed. Lea & Febiger, Philadelphia, 1973.

Rhodin, J. A. G.: *Histology. A Text and Atlas.* Oxford University Press, New York, 1974.

Robertson, J. D.: The Structure of Biological Membranes. *Archives of Internal Medicine,* vol. 129, pp. 202–228, 1972.

Roos, U. P.: Light and Electron Microscopy of Rat Kangaroo Cells in Mitosis. *Chromosoma,* vol. 40, pp. 43–82, 1973.

Weisiger, R., and I. Fridovich: Superoxide Dismutase: Organelle Specificity. *Journal of Biological Chemistry,* vol. 218, pp. 3582–3592, 1973.

Wessells, N. K.: How Living Cells Change Shape. *Scientific American,* vol. 225, no. 4, pp. 76–82, October, 1971.

Wilkins, M. H. F.: Molecular Configuration of Nucleic Acids. *Science,* vol. 140, pp. 941–950, 1963.

Wischnitzer, S.: The Nuclear Envelope: Its Ultrastructure and Functional Significance. *Endeavour,* vol. 33, pp. 137–142, September, 1974.

Epithelial Tissue

Epithelium covers surfaces, lines cavities, and takes part in the formation of glands. It forms the outer layer of the skin, the hair, nails, front of the eyeballs, and, in fact, all that is ordinarily seen of any healthy living being. Furthermore, epithelium lines all the body cavities, the nose, mouth, and hollow visceral organs. It is the most cellular tissue of the body, and the cells are always in close proximity to one another, varying in appearance according to location and function.

The thinnest epithelium forms partitions between the fluid compartments. Thick multilayered epithelium is concerned mainly with protection of the deeper tissues, the cells commonly having to adapt to changing conditions of the external environment. Others manufacture and secrete substances, such as enzymes, or are involved in absorption or excretion. Cells of some epithelia have become specialized in other ways, for example, as transducers of energy in sensory end organs.

TYPES OF EPITHELIUM

It is customary to classify epithelia into **simple** and **stratified** types, according to whether they consist of one or more than one layer of cells. It is also customary to designate them according to the shape of their component cells. The shape of the outermost cells of a stratified epithelium gives it its name. These are the cells that are most mature, specialized, or differentiated. Flat cells impart the name **squamous**, and tall cells, **columnar**, to epithelia. One finds simple squamous and simple columnar epithelia as well as stratified squamous and stratified columnar epithelia. Furthermore, there are two special categories of epithelia: pseudostratified and the so-called transitional type. Principal features of epithelia are listed in Table 3.1.

Simple Squamous Epithelium Sheets of flat cells make up simple squamous epithelium. Figure 3.1 illustrates several varieties, some thinner than others. Functional partitions formed by this type of epithelium vary with the firmness of contact of the individual cells. In some locations these thin cells are fenestrated.

Table 3.1 Principal Features of Epithelia

	Squamous		Columnar		
	Simple	**Stratified**	**Simple**	**Stratified and pseudo-stratified**	**Transitional (urinary)**
Shape of cells	All flat cells	Surface cells flat; others, polyhedral or columnar	Various heights (low and tall)	Surface cells tall; basal cells low (in pseudostratified epithelium, all cells rest on basal lamina)	Surface cells wide, with irregular lower surface
Number of layers	One	Many	One	Two to six	Variable
Free surface	Plasma membrane	Often cornified layer of cells	Specialized borders	Specialized borders; commonly ciliated	Plasma membrane
Main function	Permeable lining	Protection	Absorption; secretion	Secretion; protection	Protection, adapting to distention
Examples	Endothelium of vessels; mesothelium of body cavities	Epidermis; mucous membrane of oral cavity	Mucous membrane of stomach and intestines; glands and ducts	Mucous membranes of respiratory tract and certain genital ducts; other large ducts	Mucous membrane of urinary ducts and bladder

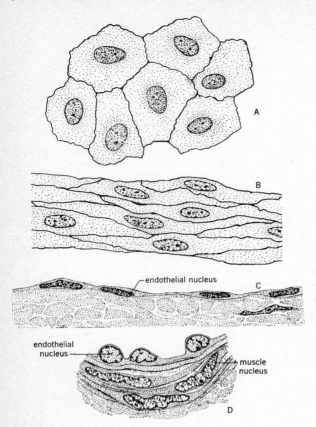

Figure 3-1 Simple squamous epithelium: *A*, mesothelium on the surface of the mesentery; and *B*, endothelium lining a venule; the cell boundaries of both were marked by deposition of silver between the cells. *C*, a section through mesothelium and subjacent connective tissue on the surface of the gallbladder of a monkey. *D*, a section through a contracted arteriole of the same animal; endothelial cell nuclei bulge into the lumen. ×900. *(JFN)*

Simple squamous epithelium is never found in an exposed place where protection is needed. It is the epithelium of the blood-tissue-fluid and the tissue-fluid-lymph interfaces. Under the name **endothelium** it forms linings of capillaries and then continues into the larger blood vessels and the heart. It goes by the name **mesothelium** in peritoneal, pleural, and pericardial cavities. A single layer of flat cells resembling mesothelium lines the spaces containing the special tissue fluids, such as the aqueous humor of the eye, fluids of the internal ear, synovial fluid of joints, and cerebrospinal fluid. That lining the lung alveoli is an exceedingly thin variety of simple squamous epithelium.

Simple Columnar Epithelium   The cells of simple columnar epithelium are at least as high as they are wide. The facets by which each cell joins its neighbors have an area as great as, or greater than, the area of the outer or inner cell surface. Basal laminae are well defined.

Low simple columnar epithelium is usually designated as "simple cuboidal epithelium" (Fig. 3.2). Its cells are not cubes but polyhedrons of eight sides, or actually even more complex shapes. This type of epithelium is prevalent in

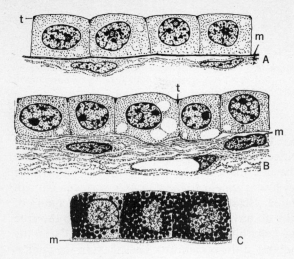

Figure 3-2 Low simple columnar (cuboidal) epithelium: *A*, small renal collecting tubule of a monkey; *B*, thyroid follicle of a monkey; *C*, pigmented epithelium of ciliary process of rabbit eye. Terminal bars, *t*, are shown as black patches at cell junctions. Basement membrane, *m*, is present between the epithelium and connective tissue. ×1,200. *(JFN)*

glands and glandlike organs. Examples of it are found in the thyroid gland, tubules of the kidney, and the pigmented layer of the retina. A modified form of low columnar epithelium makes up the parenchyma of the liver. In most of the endocrine glands, cells resembling low columnar epithelium are arrayed in cords and designated as "epithelioid cells," although even some of these may have a free border.

High simple columnar epithelium is the prevalent type found in the gastrointestinal tract and illustrated in the gallbladder in Fig. 3.3. That lining the intestines consists of absorptive cells alternating with mucus-secreting cells, as shown in Fig. 3.17*A*. The epithelium found in many glands (Fig. 3.17*B*) and glandular ducts is simple columnar epithelium in which the cells assume the shape of truncated pyramids. Columnar cells in some places are ciliated (Fig. 3.4). In glands they may contain specialized secretory precursors.

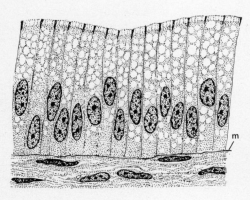

Figure 3-3 Tall simple columnar epithelium lining the monkey gallbladder. Prominent terminal bars and faintly striated border are present; a basement membrane, *m*, is seen above connective tissue. × 900. *(JFN)*

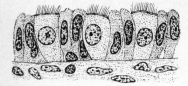

Figure 3-4 Simple columnar epithelium of cat uterine tube. Ciliated cells alternate with groups of nonciliated cells. × 900. *(JFN)*

Pseudostratified Epithelium   The type of columnar epithelium illustrated in Fig. 3.5 is called pseudostratified. The tallest cells of this type of epithelium extend from the well-defined basal lamina to the free surface. Cells whose nuclei lie at intermediate and low levels appear to have no free surfaces but can be seen to rest on the basal lamina. Electron micrographs show that many of these intermediate and basal cells do have narrow necks extending to the free surface. Mucus-secreting goblet cells alternate with tall ciliated cells in the pseudostratified columnar epithelium of the respiratory passages. In the genital ducts of the male, the tall columnar cells possess cilialike surface projections that are actually tall microvilli, though often referred to as "stereocilia" (Fig. 25.15). Nonciliated pseudostratified epithelium is found in a few places, notably in large excretory ducts of glands.

Stratified Columnar Epithelium   Truly stratified columnar epithelium is of rare occurrence. It is encountered in a few large excretory ducts, such as those of the salivary glands.

Stratified Squamous Epithelium   The body surfaces and orifices are covered and lined with stratified squamous epithelium. Figure 3.6 illustrates a variety of this type of epithelium occurring in the esophagus. The cells of the outer layers are squamous, but the deeper layers consist of polyhedral and, at the base of the epithelium, columnar cells. Cells of the intermediate layers vary in height as they move toward the surface during growth. They adhere tightly to one another.

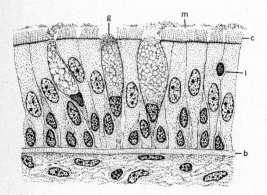

Figure 3-5 Pseudostratified epithelium with motile cilia, *c*, lining monkey trachea. Goblet cells, *g*, are secreting mucus, *m*, onto the epithelial surface; a prominent basal lamina, *b*, is present above loose fibrous connective tissue; a lymphocyte, *l*, is migrating through the epithelium. × 900. *(JFN)*

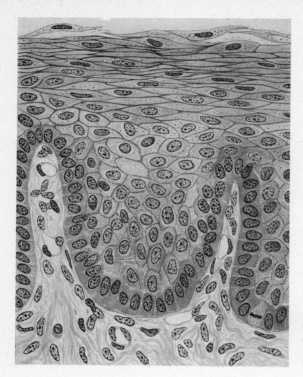

Figure 3-6 Stratified squamous epithelium lining the esophagus of a human infant. Papillae of connective tissue indent the epithelium from below. × 900. *(JFN)*

The cytoplasmic matrix of cells of epidermal stratified squamous epithelium contains a dense web of microfilaments. These are protein precursors of keratin, the main constituent of such epithelial derivatives as hair and nails. They tend to converge upon attachment points along the cell borders, especially at desmosomes. Their clumping renders them visible with light microscopy, the visible clumps of filaments being called "tonofibrils" (Fig. 3.7).

The stratified squamous epithelium of the esophagus is an example of the noncornified epithelium. Other locations are the mouth, oral pharynx, upper part of the larynx, lower part of the anus, vagina, and outer part of the urethra. A simpler variety of stratified squamous epithelium covers the transparent cornea of the eyeball (Fig. 17.3).

Glands, associated with noncornified stratified squamous epithelium, provide secretions that lubricate its surface. Drying and unusual abrasion of a noncornified surface may result in its cornification. Other types of epithelium occasionally are transformed to stratified squamous epithelium when they are subjected to drying or abrasion.

Stratified squamous epithelium of the cornified variety (Figs. 3.8 and 3.9) covers the entire external surface of the body, giving way to the noncornified variety at all the body orifices. With its appendages—the hair, nails, sweat glands, and sebaceous glands—it presents special features (see Chap. 18).

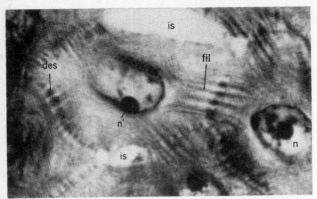

Figure 3-7 Tonofibrils are clumps of filaments, *fil,* converging on desmosomes, *des,* of adjacent cells of human stratified squamous epithelium. Other abbreviations are: *is,* interstitial space; *n,* nucleus, *n',* nucleolus. *(Photomicrograph from Turtox News. With permission of the General Biological Supply House, Chicago.)*

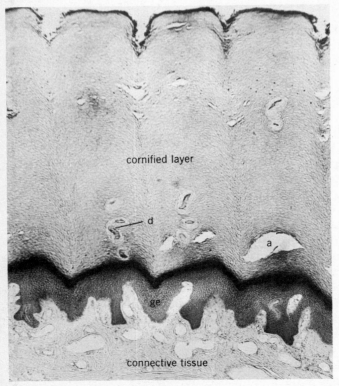

Figure 3-8 Thick cornified epithelium of stratified squamous variety from human finger tip. Living cells of the germinative layer, *ge,* lie beneath the cornified layer; *a,* artifact; *d,* duct of sweat gland. Connective tissue beneath the epithelium contains tactile corpuscles and blood vessels. Photomicrograph at low magnification, about ×75.

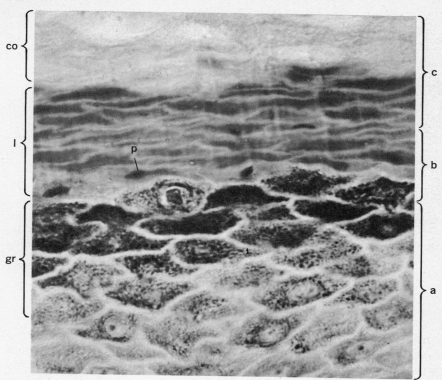

Figure 3-9 Stratified squamous epithelium of human finger tip. On the right: *a*, zone of living cells, the upper layer filled with granules; *b*, zone of dying cells with dark nuclei, *p; c,* zone of dead cells. On the left: *gr*, stratum granulosum; *l*, stratum lucidum; *co*, stratum corneum. Photomicrograph, ×900.

Transitional Epithelium   The lining of most of the urinary passages consists of an epithelium traditionally called transitional. This is structurally and functionally similar to noncornified stratified squamous epithelium; however, the cells of the free surface appear flat in the urinary bladder only during distention. In the empty bladder and in the urinary ducts, the superficial cells form polyhedrons with convex free borders. Other facets of these cells are deeply indented by pear-shaped cells which lie beneath the superficial layer (Fig. 3.10). The cells change shape over one another during filling and emptying of the bladder.

CELL INTERRELATIONS

Many epithelia have a free surface. Simple squamous cells have a relatively smooth surface, or one indented by microvesicular pits; in moist environments they have microvilli. The free surface of stratified squamous epithelium of the skin is covered with dead, cornified cells (Fig. 3.9). Their cytoplasm is packed with fibrils of keratin. On the other hand, highly specialized free surfaces are encountered on simple columnar epithelia in a number of organs.

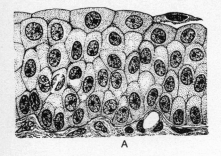

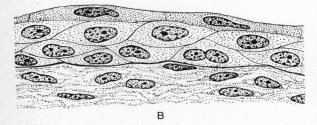

Figure 3-10 Transitional epithelium: *A*, contracted urinary bladder of a dog; *B*, distended urinary bladder of a rabbit. ×900. *(JFN)*

Striated borders, made up of brush processes, are associated with absorptive cells of the intestinal tract and in renal tubules (Fig. 3.11). Elsewhere, notably in the lining of the respiratory tract and some of the genital ducts, the free surfaces of epithelial cells are sometimes **ciliated.** Surface projections are covered by the plasmolemma of their cells. The cores of these projections may contain microfilaments and microtubules, attaining marked complexity in cilia and flagellae (Chap. 2).

Epithelial cells ordinarily adjoin without protoplasmic continuity. Mutual cohesion holds them together. In places where special junctional complexes are not found, some movement of cells over one another can occur.

The cells of columnar epithelia commonly display interdigitating folds along their lateral borders. Figure 3.12 illustrates an unusually complex arrangement which serves to greatly increase the lateral cell surfaces.

The amount of space between epithelial cells varies in width in different locations depending to some extent on how actively the movement of fluid substances into and out of the cells is progressing. The space is part of the interstitial-fluid compartment of the body. Most intercellular spaces in epithelial tissue are 200 to 300 Å wide and contain an amorphous glycoprotein ground substance produced by the cells.[1]

Intercellular spaces provide not only avenues for transporting various nutrients, metabolic products, and hormones throughout the epithelium, but also routes of entrance for leucocytes and for nerve-fiber terminals.

---

[1]This material can be rendered visible by appropriate technical procedures and has long been designated "intercellular cement."

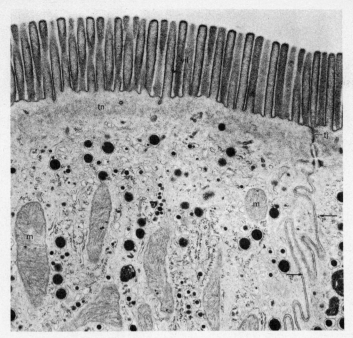

Figure 3-11   Parts of two absorptive cells from an intestinal villus of a rat. Arrows mark cell boundaries. Abbreviations: *vil*, microvilli on free border; *tn*, terminal net or web of microfilaments just beneath the microvilli; *m*, mitochomdrion; *t_j*, tight junction. Black bodies are lipid. Electron micrograph×15,000. *(Contributed by S. L. Palay.)*

The basal surface of columnar epithelial cells is extensively folded in some organs (Fig. 23.12). There, too, the plasma membranes of the folds are separated by interstitial spaces.

Epithelium, with few exceptions, lies on a **basal lamina** of ground substance about 300 to 700 Å thick (Fig. 3.13). This usually presents a homogenous appearance, although high-resolution electron micrographs reveal a finely granular or filamentous structure in its central portion (Fig. 23.8). The basal lamina is a product of the epithelial cells. Its outer portion is continuous with the amorphous ground substance of intercellular spaces. Its inner border contains fine reticular fibrils of the subepithelial connective tissue.

The term **basement membrane** is applied to the combined homogenous substance of the basal lamina and subjacent reticular tissue network. The two components are inseparable by light microscopy (Chap. 4).

A barrier function is performed by epithelia in a number of locations. The cells lining brain capillaries, for example, are securely locked together, thus preventing large molecules and lymphocytes from entering the brain parenchyma from the blood. Similarly, the tall simple columnar absorptive cells of the intestines are firmly united, thus preventing contents of the intestinal lumen from gaining direct access to the interstitial fluid compartment. The epidermis

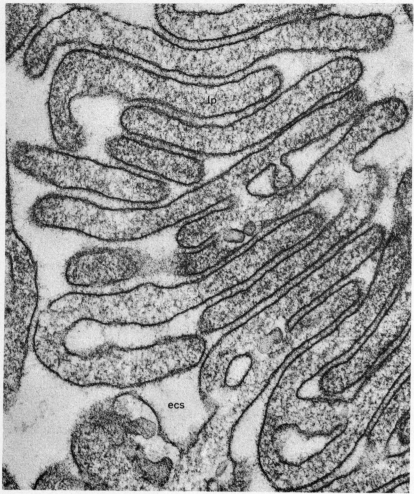

Figure 3-12   Lateral processes of complex form on adjacent epithelial cells of the gallbladder (toad). Considerable extracellular space, *ecs,* is present. Processes show a surface coating. Electron micrograph × 75,000. *(Contributed by J. Rosenbluth.)*

provides the barrier against the external environment, and its cells, too, are tightly attached to one another.

Specializations of the plasma membranes of epithelial cells provide several types of junctional structures. The most intimate cell union is appropriately called a **tight junction** ("zonula occludens"). The outermost components of adjacent unit membranes fuse to form a single leaflet, as shown in Figs. 3.14 and 20.13, with the result that no intercellular space exists at that site. Tight

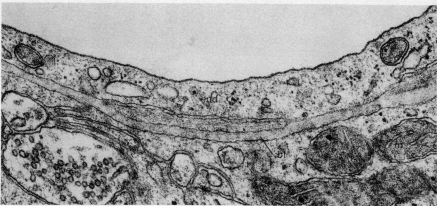

Figure 3-13 Basal lamina, *bl*, beneath endothelium, *end*, of a blood vessel in the cerebral cortex (rat). Other abbreviations: mitochondrion, *m*; synaptic vesicles, *ves*. Compare with those in the lung (Fig. 22-13) and kidney (Fig. 23-8). Electron micrograph, × 43,400. *(Contributed by D. S. Maxwell.)*

junctions occur between endothelial cells of brain capillaries. They are found encircling the free borders of columnar epithelial cells of the intestines.[2]

An **intermediate junctional** specialization of the plasma membranes of columnar epithelial cells may be seen just below the tight junction in Fig. 3.14. Space between the components is about 200 Å wide and contains some electron-dense substance. This type of junction (also called "zonula adherens") is characterized by condensations of filamentous elements of the terminal net along a thickened plasmolemma.

A third type of junction is known as a **desmosome** ("macula adherens"). One of these structures appears in Fig. 3.14. It presents electron-dense thickenings of the plasma membranes to which loops of microfilaments are attached (Fig. 3.15). The intercellular space is about 250 Å wide and contains some substance visible in electron micrographs. Desmosomes are the principal junctional structures in stratified squamous epithelium. There they assume such prominence that adjoining cells appear to be connected by "intercellular bridges" (Fig. 3.7).

A fourth type of junction between epithelial cells is known as the **gap junction** or nexus (Fig. 3.16). In it the plasma membranes are separated by a space only about 20 Å wide, containing an array of macromolecules. The gap junctions are believed to provide points of electronic coupling between cells, permitting information to pass from one to another. They are prominent features of cells in some other tissues, notably smooth muscle.

[2]In the latter place, the light microscope reveals a dense structure known as the "terminal bar." This is probably composed of the junctional complex structures (Figs. 3.2 and 3.3). Terminal bars are found elsewhere also, as in ependymal lining of the neural tube.

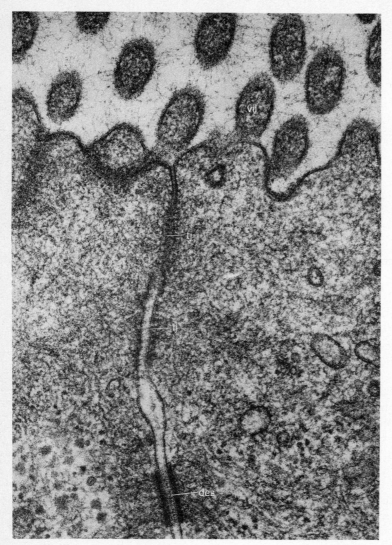

Figure 3-14 Junctional complex between two columnar epithelial cells of the gallbladder (toad), consisting of three main components: tight junction, *tj;* intermediate junction, *ij;* and a desmosome, *des.* Tonofilaments converge on the latter two (Fig. 3-15). Microvilli, *vil,* are sectioned obliquely; their surface is coated with a delicate coagulum called "glycocalyx." Electron micrograph, ×75,000. *(Contributed by J. Rosenbluth.)*

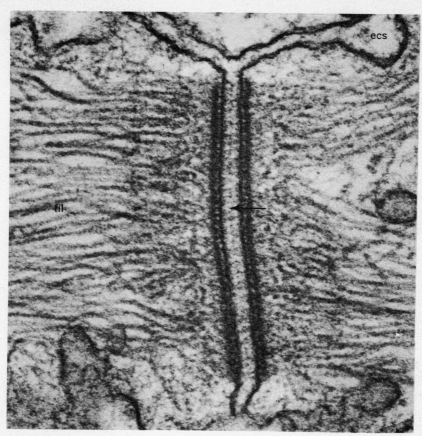

Figure 3-15 Tonofilaments, *fil,* forming loops on the border of a prominent desmosome in the epidermis (newt). The thickened plasma membranes are separated at the desmosome by some electron-dense material *(arrow).* Extracellular spaces, *ecs,* are prominent in the epidermis. Osmic acid fixation. Electron micrograph, × 157,500. *(Contributed by D. E. Kelly.)*

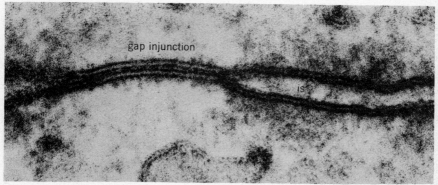

Figure 3-16 Gap junction or nexus between two ependymal cells (mouse). The interstitial space, *is,* is greatly diminished at the junction. Electron micrograph, ×300,000. *(Contributed by M. W. Brightman and T. S. Reese).*

Regeneration The body surfaces and orifices and the linings of respiratory and digestive tracts are exposed to trauma and to action of noxious agents leading to damage of epithelial cells. Ordinary wear and tear result in the loss of superficial cells of stratified epithelia. Cells of the deep layers of stratified epithelia are mitotic and provide replacements.

Cells of epithelia ordinarily are relatively static and exhibit minimal migratory tendencies, but when a stratified epithelium is damaged, some of its cells adjacent to the wound acquire the ability to migrate. They form a slowly moving layer which tends to cover the damaged area. This process plays a part in healing of small, uncomplicated surface wounds. Regeneration of simple columnar and pseudostratified epithelia takes place in a similar manner, often starting at the places where ducts of glands open onto the epithelial surface.

SECRETORY EPITHELIUM, GLANDS

Cells of columnar epithelia are involved in secretion, absorption, and excretion. The latter two functions are discussed in Chaps. 20 and 23. Secretion is one of the principal functions of epithelial cells, notably in alimentary, respiratory, urogenital, and integumental organs. It is vested in sheets of cells lining organs, in clusters or cords of cells, or in tubules and saccules constituting glands of various types. In some places the processes of secretion and absorption are carried out by different cells of the same epithelium.

Secretion involves synthesis, storage, and release of protein, nucleic acid, carbohydrate, and lipid substances. The main intracellular organelles involved in the process are ribosomes, granular endoplasmic reticulum, golgi complex, and agranular endoplasmic reticulum.

Synthesis of proteins and nucleic acids, whether for the cell's own use or for the organism as a whole, is a function of polysomes. The granular endoplasmic reticulum is involved in storing and transporting substances designed for export. The synthesized products are transferred to cisternae of the golgi complex, where they are concentrated or altered and passed on into the more peripheral cytoplasm in prosecretion vesicles. There the secretion products can be stored in tubules of the agranular endoplasmic reticulum or formed into membrane-bounded secretion granules for release at the plasma membrane of the epithelial cell by exocytosis.

Secretion of mucus of various types involves combination of proteins with carbohydrates in the golgi complex to form glycoproteins. Fatty acids, cholesterols, and other lipid substances are synthesized in the golgi complex. Methods of release of secretion products differ in various epithelial secretory cells and glands.

Secretions are delivered directly onto surfaces, into tissue spaces, or indirectly through ducts. Groups of cells secreting into ducts form the common **exocrine glands**, such as the salivary glands. Cells passing their secretions into the tissue spaces and thence to the blood stream constitute **endocrine glands**, or glands of internal secretion.

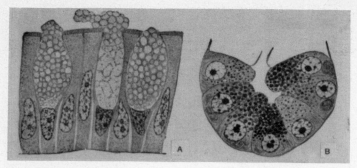

Figure 3-17 Glandular epithelium: *A*, unicellular glands are represented by mucus-secreting goblet cells on the surface of an intestinal villus; *B*, part of a multicellular serous acinus of the pancreas; dark zymogen granules are shown. × 900. *(JFN)*

In most glandular epithelia, watery secretions pass out the free surface of the cell by the process of exocytosis without producing visible changes in the surface. Glands secreting in this manner are classified as **merocrine;** some of their cells are illustrated in Fig. 3.17*B*. In other epithelia, the surface is altered, and a small portion of the cytoplasm beneath it appears to be extruded with the secretion. Such a process, illustrated in Fig. 3.18, occurs in **apocrine glands.** Cells of a few glands produce lipid secretions and die in the process; the sebaceous glands are of this **holocrine** type. They are formed by stratified squamous epithelium. Their degenerating, secretion-filled cells are replaced as rapidly as they are destroyed (Fig. 18.14).

Unicellular glands are represented in mammals by "goblet cells," found in the epithelium of the intestines and respiratory tract. They secrete mucin, which forms the lubricating substance mucus upon hydration. There are several varieties of mucin. That in goblet cells first appears as minute droplets that run together and produce a swelling in the cytoplasm, deforming the basally placed nucleus and compressing the adjacent cells. Goblet cells are shown in Fig. 3.17*A*.

Multicellular glands of the simplest type are represented by the simple columnar secreting epithelia, such as those of the gastric and uterine mucosae.

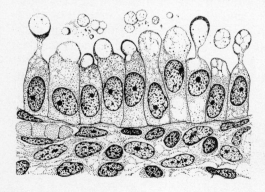

Figure 3-18 Apocrine secretion in the simple columnar epithelium of a human uterine gland. × 900.*(JFN)*

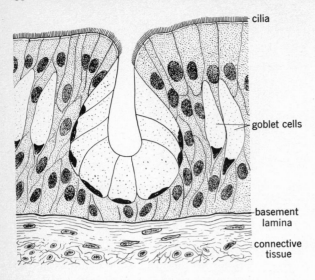

cilia

goblet cells

basement lamina

connective tissue

Figure 3-19 Simple acinous intraepithelial gland from the mucous membrane of the upper respiratory tract. Redrawn from O. Bucher. *(WEL)*

Intraepithelial glands are found in a few places, though they are uncommon in mammals. Figure 3.19 illustrates one in pseudostratified columnar epithelium. Other multicellular glands are extraepithelial. Some glands are of microscopic size, like the tiny ones in the walls of the mouth, trachea, stomach, and intestines. Others are so large that they may weigh hundreds of grams. The liver is in the latter category.

Multicellular glands may be simple tubes which are relatively short depressions of an epithelial layer, such as intestinal glands, or they may be long coiled tubes, like those of the sweat glands. In some locations, several **tubular glands** open into one duct, forming a branched tubular gland.

The next step in increasing glandular complexity is produced by lateral outpocketing from the simple tube, which thus becomes branched. The blind ends of the branches may be dilated, and secretory cells may be confined to these dilatations. The thinner tubular portions become the ducts, and the actively secretory dilatations are called acini or alveoli. A gland constructed in this manner is called an **acinous gland**. Several acini openings along the course of one duct or forming a cluster at the end of a duct build a simple branched acinous gland. Such a gland resembles a bunch of grapes, with the main duct representing the stem. Glands combining the structure of tubular and acinous glands are called tubuloacinous; they are compound glands. The parotid gland is an example. Figure 3.20 illustrates diagrammatically the various types of gland.

Large exocrine glands are located in connective tissue beneath the surface of an epithelium. Their secretions traverse a system of ducts and are poured out onto the epithelial surface. The complexity of the duct system is partly related to the size of the gland. In the largest glands, secretion is carried considerable

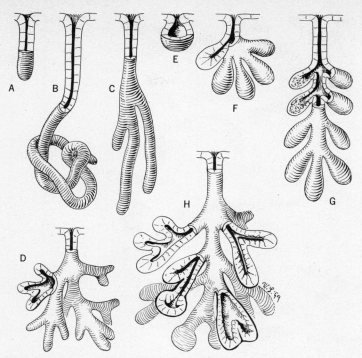

Figure 3-20 Types of glands: *A*, simple tubular; *B*, coiled tubular; *C, D*, branched tubular; *E*, simple acinous; *F, G*, branched acinous; *H*, compound tubuloacinous glands. *(WEL)*

distances, and the glands may be placed far away from the epithelium onto which the secretion is emptied.

The large glands are subdivided into lobes and lobules, and they are elaborately supplied with blood vessels, lymphatic vessels, and nerves which reach them through the encapsulating and partitioning connective tissue.

Some endocrine glands arise embryologically as simple outpocketings from epithelium, but they lose this connection. Occasionally a remnant of the duct, such as the thyroglossal duct of the thyroid gland, may persist.

Cells of exocrine glands are not always of a uniform type. Some acinous and tubuloacinous glands have two varieties of cells: **serous** and **mucous**. These may be intermingled in one acinus or may occupy different acini. The submandibular salivary gland is an example of one with components producing a thin, watery, serous fluid and a thicker mucus (Fig. 3.21).

In sections stained with hematoxylin and eosin, serous cells are apt to be unstained or are stained an acidophilic pink, and mucous cells usually stain a basophilic blue. However, some mucous cells are pale, and some serous cells contain blue chromophil substance; so one should not depend on color to identify the type of gland. Serous cells have elliptic nuclei, whereas the mucous-cell

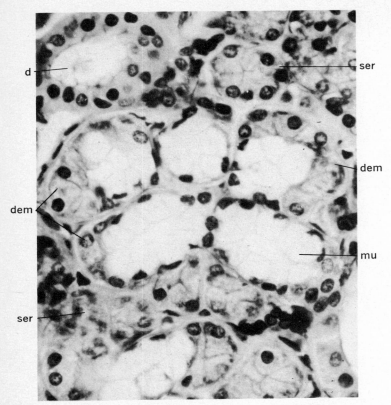

Figure 3-21 Compound tubuloacinous gland (submandibular), serous, *ser*, and mucous, *mu*, acini, some of the latter with serous demilunes, *dem*. A duct, *d*, is visible. Photomicrograph, ×600.

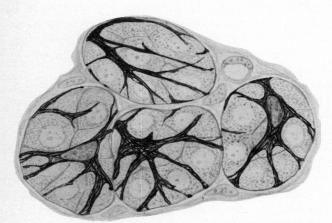

Figure 3-22 Branching myoepithelial cells of serous acini of salivary gland (pig). ×600. *(JFN)*

nuclei may be flattened and pressed against the base of the cell during storage phases of the secretory cycle. Crescentic groups of serous cells are often pushed aside by swollen mucous cells, forming caps for mucous acini. These serous end-complexes are called "demilunes" in the submandibular and sublingual salivary glands.

Secretion in many exocrine glands is under neural control. One way by which the flow of secretions from acini into the duct system is enhanced is by contraction of certain basketlike cells that clasp the acini. These **myoepithelial cells** possess some filaments of contractile protein and resemble primitive muscle cells. Some of these elements in a salivary gland are shown in Fig. 3.22.

SUGGESTED READING

Barridge, M. J., and J. L. Oschman: *Transporting Epithelium.* Academic Press, Inc., New York, 1972.

Bell, M.: A Comparative Study of Sebaceous Gland Ultrastructure in Subhuman Primates. *Anatomical Record*, vol. 170, pp. 331–342, 1971.

Dodson, J. W., and E. D. Hay: Secretion of Collagenous Stroma by Isolated Epithelium Grown In Vitro. *Experimental Cell Research*, vol. 65, pp. 215–220, 1971.

Farquhar, M. G., and G. E. Palade: Junctional Complexes in Various Epithelia. *Journal of Cell Biology*, vol. 17, pp. 375–412, 1963.

Fawcett, D. W., and K. R. Porter: A Study of the Fine Structure of Ciliated Epithelia. *Journal of Morphology*, vol. 94, pp. 221–281, 1954.

Friend, D. S., and N. B. Giluda: Variations in Tight and Gap Junctions in Mammalian Tissues. *Journal of Cell Biology*, vol. 53, pp. 758–776, 1972.

Hollman, K. H.: The Fine Structure of the Goblet Cells in the Rat Intestine. *Annals of the New York Academy of Sciences*, vol. 106, pp. 545–554, 1963.

Kaye, G. I., H. O. Wheeler, R. T. Whitlock, and N. Lane: Fluid Transport in Rabbit Gall Bladder. A Combined Physiological and Electron Microscopic Study. *Journal of Cell Biology*, vol. 30, pp. 237–268, 1966.

Ross, R.: Wound Healing. *Scientific American*, vol. 220, no. 6, pp. 40–50, June, 1969.

Fibrous Connective Tissue

Connective tissue, unlike epithelium, has only a small proportion of cells. The interstitial ground substance and especially the fibers in the ground substance are the components that characterize it.

Several types of connective tissue, including adipose tissue, cartilage, bone, and blood, will be considered in succeeding chapters. Fibrous connective tissue is described in the present one. It is found in almost all regions of the body, connecting one part with another and, equally important, separating one group of cells from another. When it is encountered in the dissecting laboratory, it is called "fascia." It is the padding material underneath the skin, between the muscles, and along the nerves and blood vessels.

All connective tissue is derived from the mesenchyme of the fetus. Gradually this simple type (Fig. 4.1) differentiates into mature forms, and there are few places in the adult where remnants of it persist. However, throughout the loose fibrous connective tissue of the body there are undifferentiated or "indifferent" cells with potentialities of mesenchymal cells.[1] These primitive cells can provide replacements for the adult types.

[1] We arbitrarily employ the term "mesenchymal cell" in reference to developmental cells, and the term "indifferent cell" for those with similar potentials in the body after the formative period.

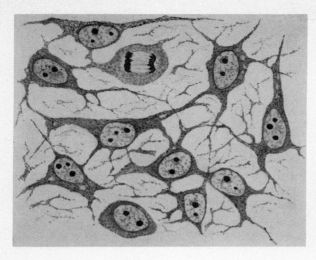

Figure 4-1 Cells of mesenchyme in a dog fetus. The branching processes, overlapping, give an illusion of syncytial continuity. Silver stain. ×900. *(JFN)*

COMPONENTS

Connective tissue has three basic components, its fibers, interstitial ground substance, and cells, but there are marked regional differences in amount and arrangement of fibers and variety of cells. There are also distinct functional differences.

Fibers Three types of fiber are encountered, but the one most prevalent and easiest to demonstrate is the **collagenous fiber**. Tissue consisting of collagenous fibers looks white in the fresh state, and the term "white fibrous connective tissue" is often used for it. Collagenous fibers resist stretching and impart strength to structures formed by them. They vary in diameter from 1 to 10 μm or more and are thick and compactly arranged where tensile strength is needed, but thin and irregularly arranged in the loose tissue through which blood vessels and nerves run. Collagenous fibers varying in thickness are illustrated in Figs. 4.2 and 4.3.

Each fiber is made up of bundles of fine collagenous fibrils 0.5 μm or less in diameter. The fibrils, in turn, are composed of many microfibrils less than 1000 Å in diameter and invisible with the light microscope. Collagenous fibrils show cross striations in electron micrographs (Fig. 4.4). These transverse bands occur at intervals of approximately 640 Å, due to a staggered arrangement of macromolecules of tropocollagen in their filaments.

Reticular fibers are associated with the cells of reticular connective tissue (Fig. 4.5) and are encountered in small quantities elsewhere in the adult. They can be demonstrated with special stains in the walls of blood vessels and form mattings beneath basal laminae. Reticular fibers stain intensely with silver, and, for that reason, are often called "argyrophilic" fibers. They are composed of

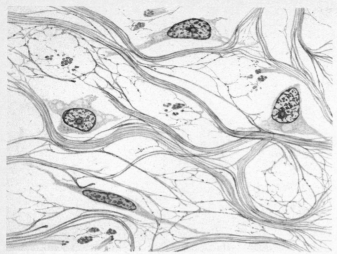

Figure 4-2 Young collagenous fibers and fibroblasts in the jaw of a 7-month human fetus. ×900. *(JFN)*

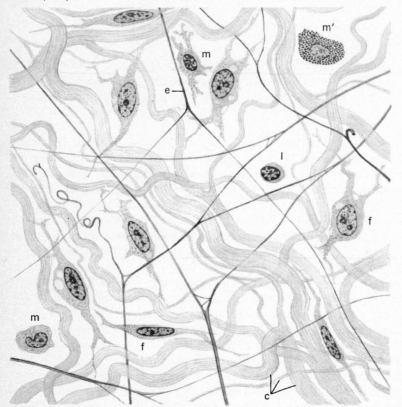

Figure 4-3 Teased preparation of supravitally stained areolar connective tissue of a kitten: *c*, collagenous fibers; *e*, elastic fiber; *f*, fibrocytes; *l*, lymphocyte; *m*, macrophages; *m'*, labrocyte (mast cell). ×900. *(JFN)*

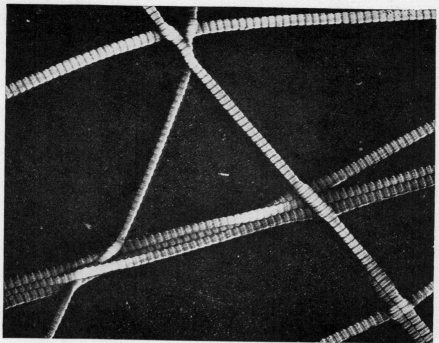

Figure 4-4 Collagen unit fibrils from the dermis of human skin, showing crossbanding at intervals of 640 Å. Electron micrograph of metallic-shadowed tissue, × 32,000. *(Reproduced from R. O. Greep, Histology, McGraw-Hill Book Company, New York, 1954.)*

fibrils similar to collagenous fibrils but thinner. They have the same periodicity although fewer adjacent units (less polymerized) and more surface carbohydrates. Reticular fibers can be seen to merge with collagenous fibers in some places. Most connective-tissue fibers of young individuals, being smaller than adult collagenous fibers, are argyrophilic, probably because of the negative-charge groups of the more abundant carbohydrates.

A third type of fiber in connective tissue, the **elastic fiber**, differs chemically from the preceding two types. It shows no cross striations in electron micrographs. When elastic fibers are arranged in large bundles, they appear yellow in the fresh state. They occur as isolated branching threads among collagenous fibers in loose connective tissue (Fig. 4.3) or in prominent layers encircling large arteries (Fig. 11.12). The neck ligament of grazing animals is composed of large elastic fibers. Special stains are required to differentiate elastic from collagenous fibers. As their name implies, these fibers can be stretched, and in this respect they are unlike collagenous and reticular fibers.

Connective-tissue fibers are produced by cells derived from mesenchymal cells or indifferent cells. Reticular cells engage in forming reticular fibers; fibroblasts produce the other types. The cytoplasm of fibroblasts contains the organelles associated with the process of protein synthesis, namely ribosomes,

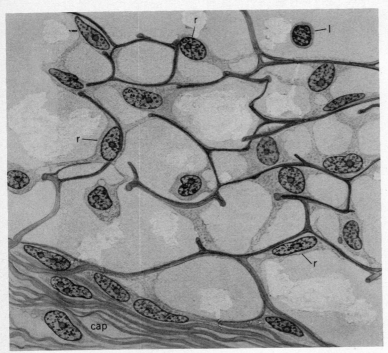

Figure 4-5 Reticular tissue adjacent to the capsule, *cap*, of lymph node from a cat. Most lymphocytes, *l*, have been washed out of the peripheral lymph sinus, leaving only reticular cells, *r*, and reticular fibers which are the branching linear elements darkly stained with silver carbonate. ×1,200. *(JFN)*

arrays of granular endoplasmic reticulum, and a distinct golgi complex (Fig. 4.6). The granular endoplasmic reticulum is the site of synthesis of the initial collagen precursor molecules. These are transferred to spherical parts of the golgi complex where they first appear as tangled fine filaments that soon become aligned in parallel arrays of procollagen molecules. Prosecretion vesicles, containing the latter, bud from the golgi cisternae, move toward the cell surface and release their contents at the plasmolemma by the process of exocytosis. **Procollagen** molecules become **tropocollagen** and the latter is polymerized into **collagen**.

Production of collagen is a continuing process, accelerating when healing of wounds is called for. The amount of collagen in the body increases with aging. For example, collagenous fibers tend to replace the parenchyma of organs undergoing age involution.

Elastic fibers consist of two structural entities: peripherally arranged microfilaments 30 to 150 Å in diameter and a central mass of amorphous substance. They are formed by fibroblasts in connective tissue proper that are indistinguishable microscopically from those synthesizing collagen. In blood-ves-

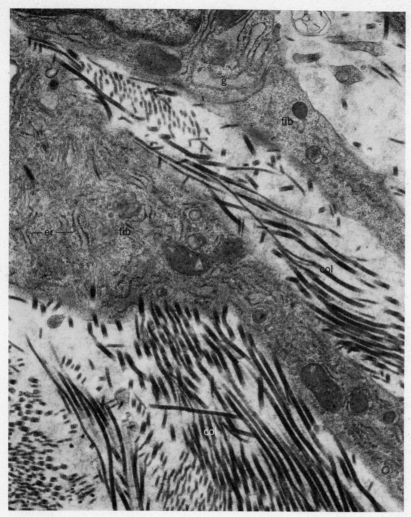

Figure 4-6 Portions of two fibroblasts, *fib,* with associated collagen, *col,* from subcutaneous tissue of a rat. Note the endoplasmic reticulum, *er,* and golgi complex, *g.* Electron micrograph, × 18,000. *(Contributed by K. R. Porter.)*

sel walls, elastic fibers are formed by smooth-muscle cells. The basic protein, **elastin,** differs chemically from tropocollagen, but is synthesized in a similar manner and released by exocytosis at the plasmolemma.

Ground Substance The interstitium of fibrous connective tissue contains **ground substance**, a usually inconspicuous amorphous material. Although it is invisible in routinely prepared histologic sections, it can be demonstrated by special histochemical methods. It is easier to see in some regions than in others.

A readily observed ground substance is that in the umbilical cord of the fetus.[2] Ground substance in young individuals forms a continuous jellylike matrix permeating the fiber bundles of connective tissue.

Preservation of tissues for histologic study coagulates or dissolves the ground substance, leaving artifactitious spaces here and there. Normally in the healthy individual there are no fluid-filled spaces in the ground substance of fibrous connective tissue. However, tissue injury can result in leakage of fluid from damaged blood vessels, causing regions of displacement of the homogenous ground substance.

The gelatinous matrix of ground substance is composed of mucoproteins and mucopolysaccharides, notably hyaluronic acid and chondroitin sulfuric acid. It is produced by cells of connective tissue, presumably by the fibroblasts. The ground substance in synovial cavities of joints, primarily hyaluronic acid, has a less gel-like consistency than that in some other connective-tissue spaces. That of cartilage is rich in chondroitin sulfuric acid and is a firm substance.

A homogenous substance, less amorphous than connective-tissue ground substance, is that composing the **basal laminae** (Chap. 3). It is a product, not of connective-tissue cells, but of the cells with which it is found closely associated, notably epithelial cells, but also neurolemma cells of peripheral nerves, lipocytes of adipose tissue, and muscle cells. The basal lamina lies upon a network of reticular connective tissue and is continuous with the ground substance of the latter. Basal lamina and subjacent reticular fibers in some places form **basement membranes.**

The ground substance of connective tissue contains a considerable amount of chemically bound water. Diffusion of oxygen and other metabolic materials takes place through it, but there is no flow of fluid in the usual sense. The ground substance offers the means of communication between the blood stream and parenchymal cells of various organs of the body through their connective-tissue stroma.

Cells   The cells of connective tissue are relatively few in number and inconspicuous in many histologic sections. Some of them, in healthy adults, appear to be in a quiescent state. Although pluripotential cells, known as **indifferent cells**, are believed to exist in the adult, they cannot be identified in ordinary histologic sections.

The most characteristic cell of adult fibrous connective tissue is the **fibrocyte**. Its appearance varies with its location (Figs. 4.3 and 4.7). Fibrocytes generally are spindle-shaped cells with branching processes. In the usual histologic preparation of adult connective tissue, the nucleus, often the only part visible, can be differentiated from that of most other cells. It is somewhat elongated and contains finely divided chromatin, staining lightly. However, the nuclei of endothelial cells in capillaries coursing through loose fibrous connective tissue have a similar appearance.

[2]There it is known as "Wharton's jelly."

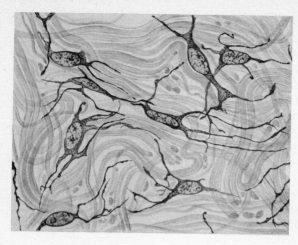

Figure 4-7 Fibrocytes in connective tissue from the tongue (dog). Silver stain ×900. *(JFN)*

Fibrocytes are related to chondrocytes and osteocytes, which are cells associated with cartilage and bone. Special names are given to fibrocytes in some other locations.

The term **fibroblast** is used by some histologists synonymously with fibrocyte. It is an appropriate name for the cells actively engaged in production of extracellular matrix (Fig. 4.2). The fibroblast is an active cell, as is evident from the prevalence of granular endoplasmic reticulum and well-formed golgi complex in its cytoplasm (Fig. 4.6). Fibrocytes, on the other hand, are relatively inactive cells. Their cytoplasm contains fewer arrays of granular endoplasmic reticulum. Thus fibrocytes and fibroblasts represent different phases of activity in the same cell.

Fibroblasts are numerous in wound healing and young connective tissue and decrease in number as development proceeds, eventually becoming fibrocytes. The latter can resume synthesis of collagen and ground substance when the occasion arises.

Reticular cells[3] engaging in fiber formation are related to fibroblasts (Fig. 4.5). They produce the fine reticular structural network of organs such as lymph nodes. Some have phagocytic potentials, but it is uncertain that those producing reticular fibers do.

The **phagocyte** of connective tissue is called a **macrophage** (synonym: histiocyte[4]) to distinguish it from the blood neutrophil (microphage). Macrophages are numerous in loose fibrous connective tissue but are seldom found in the dense variety. Two principal forms are recognized. Some with outstretched processes that seem to hold the cell in place among fibers are called "fixed" macrophages; they represent a relatively inactive stage. When responding to

---

[3]Note that the term "reticulocyte" has been preempted by hematologists for an erythrocyte that contains a stainable reticulum.

[4]Use of the name "histiocyte" is declining. Its meaning, tissue cell, is too vague.

inflammation, these cells become ameboid and are then designated "free" macrophages.

The macrophages in histologic sections can be recognized as different from fibrocytes by their darker and appreciably smaller nuclei. However, their cytoplasm is hardly visible with the usual staining. When, on the other hand, loose connective tissue from an animal is examined after vital staining, it is possible to make out the contours of macrophages because the cytoplasm has become filled with dye particles.

The fine structure of the cytoplasm of free macrophages is characterized by numerous membrane-bounded dark bodies, identified as phagosomes. The cell surface is irregular owing to presence of pseudopodial processes. Material being phagocytized may be seen between the processes where it is engulfed by the plasmolemma. The cytoplasm of free macrophages in tissue cultures often appears frothy (Fig. 4.8). Engulfed materials of various kinds are shown in the macrophages illustrated in Fig. 4.9.

Phagocytes have been designated by special names in different locations. For example, they are called "littoral cells" in lymphatic organs and bone marrow; "splenocytes" in the spleen; "Kupffer cells" in the liver; "dust cells" in lung alveoli; and "monocytes" in the blood. All these cells are similar to macrophages of loose fibrous connective tissue.

Some of the endotheliumlike cells in the sinusoids and many of the reticular cells in the delicate stroma of the bone marrow and lymphatic organs are strongly phagocytic. They, too, belong to the macrophage system. They do not differ greatly from other macrophages, and there is little reason to continue to grace them with specific names. The term **reticuloendothelial system** is often applied to the entire collection of macrophages and cells with macrophage potentialities.

Although macrophages in loose connective tissue seem to be inactive dur-

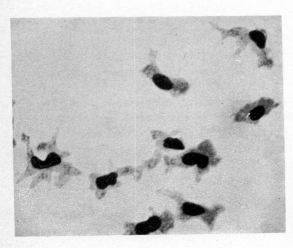

Figure 4-8 Macrophages in a tissue culture of mouse lung. Photomicrograph, about ×600. *(Reproduced from R. O. Greep,* Histology, *McGraw-Hill Book Company, New York, 1954.)*

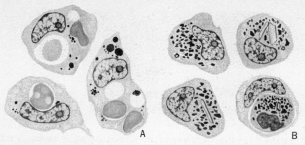

Figure 4-9 Macrophages exhibiting engulfed material: *A,* erythrocytes and granules of blood pigment in liver macrophages; *B,* carbon and silica particles in the cytoplasm of lung macrophages (one has engulfed another carbon-laden degenerating macrophage). ×900. *(JFN)*

ing normal healthy conditions, those in a few locations constantly phagocytize the products of physiologic degeneration. To the macrophages of the bone marrow, liver, and spleen falls the task of disposing of worn-out blood corpuscles and fragments of corpuscles. It is remarkable that they never attack healthy cells but only those whose functional lives are spent.

The origin of macrophages is noteworthy. There is an occasional need for large numbers of them in defending the body against invading microorganisms. Free macrophages in loose fibrous connective tissue arise from monocytes of the blood. These blood cells migrate out of small vessels at sites of infection and become macrophages. A humoral factor from the liver activates formation of macrophages.

Macrophages are called into action more slowly than are the neutrophils of the blood. The latter reach the scene first; macrophages come in later. Foreign particles too large for a single macrophage are handled by large cells formed by combination of two or more macrophages (multinucleated giant cells). Phagocytosis and subsequent treatment of the engulfed material by enzymes of lysosomes results in the foreign proteins and polysaccharides being rendered incapable of acting as antigens.

Another cell frequently encountered in loose fibrous connective tissue is the **lipocyte**, or "fat cell." It is conspicuous because of its large size. Both the nucleus and cytoplasm are displaced by a single large drop of lipid material. Lipocytes ordinarily occur in groups along small blood vessels in connective tissue, notably those in the omentum. In large aggregates they constitute "adipose tissue" which is described in the next chapter.

Labrocytes constitute another class of connective-tissue cell, likewise often encountered along the course of small blood vessels. These cells are usually called **mast cells.**[5] It is unfortunate that they cannot be visualized in the usual histologic preparation. The large specific cytoplasmic granules, up to

[5]Early German histologists noted their robust, almost satiated, appearance; hence the name (mast = food).

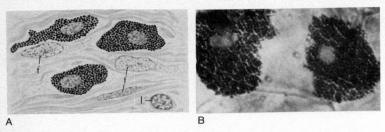

A   B

Figure 4-10 Labrocytes (mast cells). *A,* in the capsule of a human palatine tonsil; one lymphocyte, *l,* and three fibrocytes, *f,* are lightly stained. ×900. *(JFN) B,* in the skin of a mouse; nuclei are light spots in the masses of dark granules. Photomicrograph, ×900.

1.5 μm in diameter, are their characteristic feature. Like those of blood basophils, they disappear after treatment of tissues with aqueous fixing solutions, leaving the cells inconspicuous and indistinguishable from other connective-tissue cells. When alcohol-fixed preparations are stained with certain basic dyes, such as toluidine blue, they are clearly visible, as shown in Fig. 4.10. Their basophilic granules exhibit metachromasia; i. e., they take on a tint that is different from the characteristic color of the dye used. The rest of the cytoplasm is lightly basophilic and does not normally stain at all with acid dyes. The nucleus presents a pale vacuolated appearance in the midst of the intensely stained cytoplasmic granules. As a rule, one can judge the outer boundary of a labrocyte only by the pattern of its granules. Frequently the granules are observed extending in thin streamers and giving the cell a ruptured appearance. Their contents are released into interstitial spaces.

Labrocytes are found in abundance in most species of animal, the rabbit being an exception. The number of these cells in the human being increases after birth and decreases markedly in old age, at which time the cells are apt to show more metachromasia than they had earlier.

The granules of labrocytes contain heparin, an anticoagulant first observed in the liver of dogs, where these cells are numerous. Histamine and serotonin (in rodents) are also associated with labrocytes. These secretion products may be released under conditions of shock, causing vasodilation.

Melanocytes occur in the fibrous connective tissue of certain regions. Examples of these pigmented cells are shown in Fig. 4.11. They occur in such places as the iris and choroid of the eye and beneath the epidermis, where they are especially numerous in dark-skinned persons.

There are several other types of cell that are often encountered in loose fibrous connective tissue but are more commonly associated with reticular connective tissue. **Lymphocytes** are in this category (Fig. 4.12). These are small cells with a darkly staining nucleus and scanty cytoplasm; they are ameboid in loose connective tissue. Examples appear in several illustrations of this chapter. Lymphocytes play an essential role in immunity and are considered further in Chaps. 7 and 13.

Tissue **eosinophils** resemble those of the blood. They are not numerous in connective tissue of normal human beings, but are plentiful in that of some

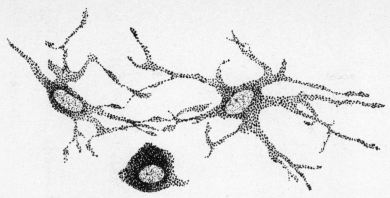

Figure 4-11 Melanocytes in the stroma of the iris of a rabbit eye. × 900. *(JFN)*

other species, such as the rat. More are found beneath mucous membranes of digestive and respiratory tracts, and in the human lactating mammary gland, than elsewhere. They become more prevalent in persons with allergic disease and parasitic infections and are capable of phagocytosis.

Plasmocytes bear some resemblance to large lymphocytes. They are, indeed, derived from the latter under certain conditions. None is present in the fetus or newborn infant; they appear in response to the need for specific antibodies.

The plasmocyte nucleus contains blocks of chromatin giving it an irregular checkered appearance. The basophilic cytoplasm is more plentiful than that of the lymphocyte. It has a rather prominent pale region near the nucleus which is the negative image of a large golgi complex. The plasmocyte cytoplasm is filled with cisternae of granular endoplasmic reticulum; ribosomes are numerous. These points reflect the intense activity of plasmocytes in synthesis of pro-

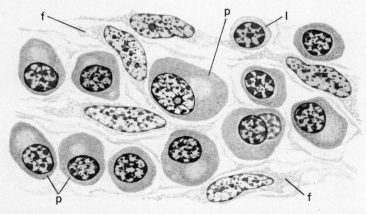

Figure 4-12 Plasmocytes, *p*, fibrocytes, *f*, and a lymphocyte, *l*, in the lamina propria of the intestine of a cat. × 900. *(JFN)*

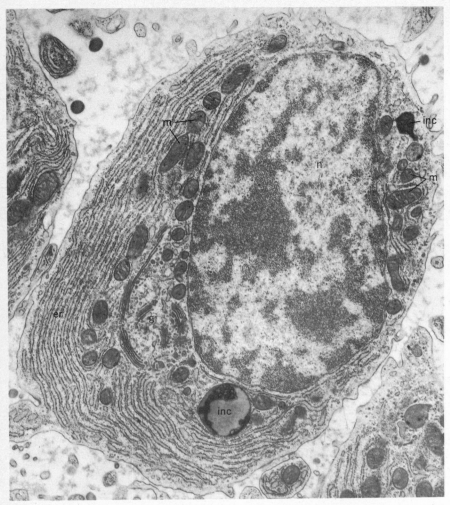

Figure 4-13 Plasmocyte from human bone marrow. Note the compact arrays of granular endoplasmic reticulum, *er,* and the golgi complex, *g.* Mitochondria, *m,* surround the nucleus, *n,* and two inclusion bodies, *inc,* (possibly lysosomes), are present in this section. Electron micrograph, ×14,000. *(Contributed by J. A. Freeman.)*

teins—the globulins of antibodies. Prominence of centrosomes correlates with the cell's ability to divide.

Plasmocytes are not found normally in circulating blood and lymph. They are confined largely to the lymphatic organs and the diffuse lymphatic tissue beneath epithelia of the digestive and upper respiratory systems. Figure 4.12 illustrates and compares plasmocytes, lymphocytes, and fibrocytes. Figure 4.13 shows the fine structure of a plasmocyte. Further consideration of these vitally important cells is found in Chap. 13.

CLASSIFICATION

The appearance and characteristics of fibrous connective tissue vary considerably in different locations. It is possible to classify this tissue according to fiber type and density and, to a lesser extent, according to its cellular organization.

Mesenchymal Connective Tissue   The source of all connective-tissue cells is **mesenchyme**, the cellular tissue filling spaces between epithelial layers in embryos. Mesenchyme consists of irregularly shaped cells with branching processes that form a network, the spaces of which are filled with ground substance (Fig. 4.1). The surfaces of these unspecialized cells are difficult to distinguish with light microscopy because they blend with their surroundings. Mesenchymal connective tissue changes in appearance as development proceeds. Fibroblasts and other connective-tissue cells arise in the mesenchyme in the latter part of gestation. However, not all the cells of adult connective tissue are present at birth. Noteworthy in this regard is the dearth of cells concerned with antibody production.

Reticular Connective Tissue   The stroma of certain organs is formed largely by reticular fibers and associated cells, which together are designated reticular connective tissue. The fibers are arranged in delicate latticelike frameworks, supporting such cells as lymphocytes and colonies of hemopoietic cells.

When lymphocytes of a lymph node are washed away artificially, the cells of reticular tissue present a primitive appearance similar to those of mesenchyme (Fig. 4.5). Their processes extend along the reticular fibers. In some places, reticular cells line blood and lymph sinuses and resemble endothelium. Some serve only as lining cells or supporting cells, but many have developed phagocytic characteristics and have become macrophages. Thus, there are nonphagocytic cells associated with reticular fibers, not unlike the fibrocytes of collagenous fibers; and there are phagocytic cells, indistinguishable from other macrophages, in this rather simple form of connective tissue.

Loose Fibrous Connective Tissue   Loose fibrous connective tissue is usually called **areolar tissue**. In it are a few elastic fibers, but the collagenous fibers abound. The fibers are arranged in no particular pattern but run in all directions and form a loose meshwork in the ground substance.

Areolar tissue is the most widely distributed connective tissue. It accompanies blood vessels and nerves, which course almost everywhere. It extends in and out among the components of most organs. It is found beneath mucous and serous membranes. A description of its components would only duplicate the general description of fibers, ground substance, and cells of fibrous connective tissue. Figure 4.3 illustrates the appearance of a spread preparation of areolar tissue.

Dense Fibrous Connective Tissue   In many places, the collagenous fibers

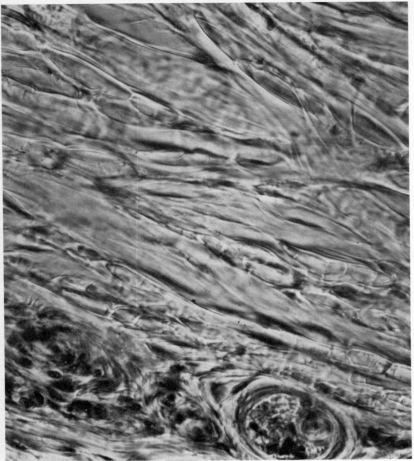

Figure 4-14 Collagenous fibers of dense connective tissue in the dermis of thick human skin. Note blood vessels at the bottom. Photomicrograph, × 600.

of connective tissue increase in size and number and tend to crowd out the ground substance and cells. The role of elastic fibers in dense fibrous connective tissue is usually secondary (Fig. 4.15). The cells are mainly fibrocytes, although macrophages can be found. Other varieties are rarely seen.

Fibrous connective tissue forming the dermis of the skin is densely arranged in most regions (Fig. 4.14). The fibrous capsules of some organs, such as the spleen and testicle, are examples of this tissue. Some rather heavy fibrous membranes, notably the dura mater of the brain, the periosteum of bone, and perineurium surrounding bundles of nerve fibers, are similarly composed of dense fibrous connective tissue. The heart valves and the rings of the cardiac orifices likewise are constructed of dense fibrous connective tissue. The transition from areolar tissue to dense fibrous connective tissue is gradual.

A special kind of dense fibrous connective tissue occurs in the cornea of the eye, where transparency of early embryonic tissues has been maintained. The stroma of the ovary is made up of another special variety, in which cells are extraordinarily numerous. In other locations, collagenous fibers are lamellated, as in some of the sensory end organs.

The densest form of fibrous connective tissue is found in **tendons** and **ligaments**. Tendons join muscle to bone, and ligaments join bone to bone. Tendons are constructed of parallel collagenous fibers bundled together compactly and clasped by winglike cytoplasmic projections of the tendon cells. These cells, related to fibrocytes, form longitudinal rows as indicated in Fig. 4.16. They are compressed by the surrounding tendon-fiber bundles so that they resemble thin rods in profile view but are stellate in cross section (Fig. 4.17).

Tendons are sheathed by dense fibrous connective tissue of the less organized type. Septa, as seen in Fig. 4.17, subdivide tendons. The sheaths and septa of tendons are continuous with the sheaths and septa of muscles at the myotendinal junctions. Blood vessels and nerves traverse them to enter the ten-

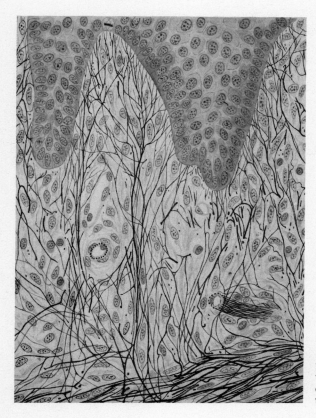

Figure 4-15 Elastic fiber network in the lamina propria of the lingual mucous membrane of a rabbit. Stained for elastic fibers. × 600 *(JFN)*

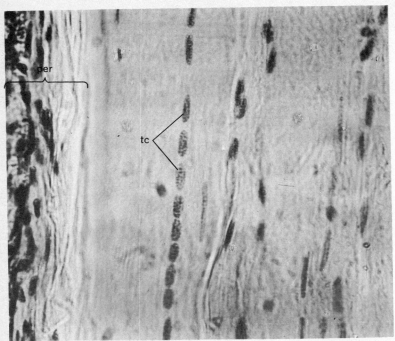

Figure 4-16   Rows of tendon-cell nuclei, *tc*, in a longitudinal section of tendon. Less compact connective tissue of the peritendineum, *per*, with blood vessels is seen. Photomicrograph, × 600.

don. However, the blood supply of tendons is not rich, and healing after injury is accomplished slowly.

Aponeuroses and **ligaments** are constructed like tendons but are of different shapes, and their fibers are less compactly arranged. Most are collagenous, but an elastic ligament occurs in the neck of large grazing animals (Fig. 4.18).

SEROUS MEMBRANES

Both of the fundamental tissues thus far considered enter into the formation of serous membranes lining peritoneal, pleural, and pericardial cavities and covering the abdominal viscera, lungs, and heart.

The **peritoneum** is structurally similar to the other serous membranes. It consists of fibrous connective tissue supporting a simple squamous epithelium, known as mesothelium. The free surfaces of the epithelial cells are richly supplied with microvilli and a glycocalyx coating, the probable function of which is to ease movement of one membrane upon another.

The peritoneum forms a closed cavity and may be divided into a parietal portion, on the body wall, and a visceral portion, reflected over most of the abdominal organs. It forms a thin double layer, the **mesentery**, which is attached

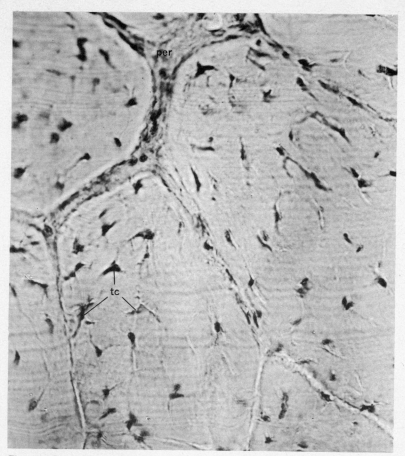

Figure 4-17 Tendon in cross section, showing cells, *tc*, with wing-shaped projections. Note the peritendinal septa, *per*. Photomicrograph, × 600.

to the intestine and conveys the many blood vessels, lymphatic vessels, and nerves of this organ. The peritoneum doubles back upon itself below the stomach to form the **omentum**.

Fibrous connective tissue of the loose variety containing many cells occurs in the mesenteries and omentum. The omentum also contains much adipose tissue, especially in obese persons. The visceral peritoneum on the surfaces of some organs, such as the spleen, consists of dense fibrous connective tissue forming a capsule. The peritoneum is supplied by blood vessels for its own nutrition, besides those traversing it to supply the viscera.

The omentum presents features of special interest. The parts of it not loaded with adipose tissue are thin and fenestrated. There the scanty areolar

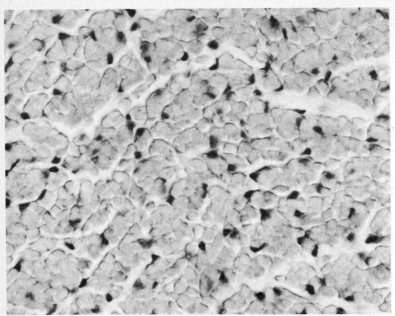

Figure 4-18 Elastic neck ligament of an ox, sectioned transversely. Compare with tendon in Fig. 4-17. Photomicrograph × 600.

tissue is richly supplied with capillaries surrounded by many connective-tissue cells. Macrophages and lymphocytes are numerous and may even be found in large clumps, called "milk spots," which are visible to the naked eye. The omentum may play a role in defense of the abdominal cavity against disease.

The peritoneal cavity is ordinarily only a potential space containing just enough fluid to lubricate the membrane surfaces and permit the viscera to slide freely over one another. The quantity of this fluid is small in healthy individuals, but disease conditions, which change the permeability of the capillary walls and the peritoneum itself, often lead to accumulation of a considerable amount of "peritoneal exudate." Normally there are a few free cells in the peritoneal fluid, derived from the mesothelium, from the areolar tissue of the membranes, and from the blood, but the exudate may contain great numbers of leucocytes during inflammation of the abdomen.

The peritoneal membrane is readily traversed by a number of substances in solution. For example, a fluid can be injected into the abdominal cavity to "absorb" toxic substances from the blood of uremic patients, after which the fluid is withdrawn and the procedure repeated.

A small portion of the peritoneal cavity has become detached in the male and occupies a position in the scrotum. There it forms the **tunica vaginalis testis**. Its structure is similar to that of the abdominal peritoneum.

The **pleura** is a membrane of the thoracic cavity similar to the peritoneum of the abdomen. The visceral pleura covers the lungs. It is formed by connective tissue containing numerous elastic fibers, especially in the deeper portion. Its surface is paved with mesothelium. Parietal pleura lines compartments of the thoracic cage. As in the abdomen, visceral and parietal surfaces are lubricated by a small amount of fluid which increases during certain disease conditions and is then known as "pleural exudate."

The **pericardium** is a similar membrane in the mediastinum between pleural cavities. Its outer parietal layer forms a strong fibrous sac for the heart, the serous pericardium being backed by fibrous connective tissue denser than that found in the pleura and peritoneum. The serous layer is reflected onto the great veins and arteries which pierce the dense fibrous coat to enter and leave the heart. The fibrous coat fuses with the adventitia of the great blood vessels and with the central tendons of the diaphragm. Visceral pericardium constitutes the epicardium.

SUGGESTED READING

Alpert, E. N.: Developing Elastic Tissue. *American Journal of Pathology*, vol. 69, pp. 89–102, 1972.

Andrews, P. M., and K. R. Porter: The Ultrastructural Morphology and Possible Functional Significance of Mesothelial Microvilli. *Anatomical Record*, vol. 177, pp. 409–426, 1973.

Briggaman, R. A., F. S. Dalldorf, and C. E. Wheeler, Jr.: Formation and Origin of Basal Lamina and Anchoring Fibrils in Adult Human Skin. *Journal of Cell Biology*, vol. 51, pp. 384–395, 1971.

Gersh, I., and H. R. Catchpole: The Organization of the Ground Substance and Basement Membrane and Its Significance in Tissue Injury, Disease, and Growth. *American Journal of Anatomy*, vol. 85, pp. 457–521, 1949.

Morse, D. E., and F. N. Low: The Fine Structure of Developing Unit Collagenous Fibrils in the Chick. *American Journal of Anatomy* vol. 140, pp. 237–261, 1974.

Myer, K.: Nature and Function of Mucopolysaccharides of Connective Tissue, pp. 69–76, in D. Nachmansohn (ed.), *Molecular Biology*. Academic Press, Inc., New York, 1960.

Pearsall, N. N., and R. S. Weiser: *The Macrophage*. Lea & Febiger, Philadelphia, 1970.

Porter, K. R., and G. D. Pappas: Collagen Formation by Fibroblasts of the Chick Embryo Dermis. *Journal of Biophysical and Biochemical Cytology*, vol. 5, pp. 153–156, 1959.

Ross, R., and P. Bornstein: Elastic Fibers in the Body. *Scientific American*, vol. 224, no. 6, pp. 44–52, June, 1971.

Smith, D. E.: The Tissue Mast Cell. *International Review of Cytology*, vol. 14, pp. 327–386, 1963.

Van Winkle, W., Jr.: The Fibroblast in Wound Healing, *Surgery, Gynecology & Obstetrics*, vol. 124, pp. 368–369, 1967.

Weinstock, M., and C. P. Leblond: Formation of Collagen. *Federation Proceedings*, vol. 33, pp. 1205–1218, May, 1974.

Chapter 5

Adipose Tissue

Adipose tissue is a special type of connective tissue of widespread occurrence in normal human beings. Except in emaciated and obese persons, it forms 10 to 15 percent of the body weight and, in effect, composes an organ of considerable functional significance. Once considered to be a rather static tissue primarily concerned with insulation and padding, adipose tissue is now known to be highly labile. The turnover of its fat content is rapid and continuous. A major function of this tissue in most regions is provision of a ready source of fuel for metabolic processes.

There are two varieties of adipose tissue, differing both structurally and functionally. The more prevalent univesicular form, known as "white fat,"[1] makes its appearance in late fetal life as a rather evenly distributed subcutaneous layer, the **panniculus adiposus,** at which time it forms an energy store that will be useful in the early postnatal period. Another variety of adipose tissue, the so-called "brown fat," is also present in the fetus, but there is less of it, and it has a more limited distribution. It is concerned with heat production; in newborn animals subjected to a cold environment, it is quickly depleted.

[1]Its color is yellow in human beings.

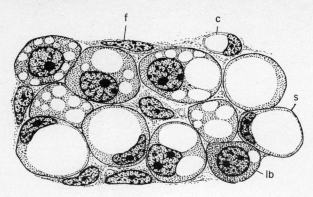

Figure 5-1 Development of univesicular adipose tissue in a newborn kitten: *lb,* cell designated by some histologists as "lipoblast"; *c,* blood capillaries; *f,* fibrocyte nucleus; *s,* "signet-ring" cell. ×900. *(JFN)*

Univesicular Adipose Tissue   Lipocytes are among the major cellular components of connective tissue. In many localities they occur so closely packed that the tissue appears to be composed exclusively of them. A few places, notably the eyelids, areola and nipple, scrotum and penis, lack them.

The bulk of univesicular adipose tissue is found in subcutaneous layers, especially those of the abdomen, breasts, thighs, and buttocks, and in the omentum and posterior abdominal wall. Variations in distribution associated with age, sex, and nutritional state are reflected as differences in body contour.

The structure of adipose tissue can be appreciated by considering the development of lipocytes; stages are illustrated in Fig. 5.1. Mesenchymal cells along fetal capillaries withdraw their cytoplasmic processes to become ovoid in shape. Soon lipid droplets appear in the cytoplasm, merging into larger droplets until a single large drop fills the cell. This results in displacement of the nucleus to the periphery. Univesicular cells of this kind represent the final stage in development, and when they are sectioned through the nucleus they present a "signet-ring" appearance. Development is not confined to prenatal stages, but continues throughout life, responding to changing nutritional states.

The precursors of lipocytes appear to be among the indifferent cells of mature connective tissue, and are indistinguishable from precursors of such elements as fibrocytes. Figure 5.2 illustrates this concept of their origin. It is believed that fibroblasts and lipoblasts possess separate specificities, and that cells derived from one can not change into the other.

Preparation of univesicular adipose tissue for histologic study usually alters its appearance because the chemicals used disolve the fat contents of the cells, leaving only empty spaces and often permitting the walls to become wrinkled. A section of well-preserved human subcutaneous adipose tissue is

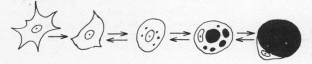

Figure 5-2 Schematic derivation of a lipocyte from an indifferent cell. *(CHP)*

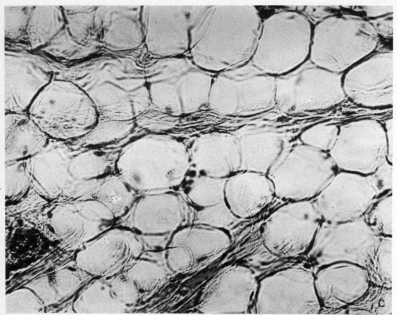

Figure 5-3 Section of human univesicular adipose tissue, subcutaneous region. Photomicrograph, × 300.

shown in Fig. 5.3. Lipocytes are large cells, often measuring 0.1 mm or more in diameter, and thin histologic sections seldom pass through the region of the nucleus. A preparation of compact adipose tissue may bear little resemblance to the adipose tissue of a living subject. Figure 5.4 shows a small cluster of lipocytes in a fresh preparation. Figure 5.5 illustrates a preparation in which the fat was stained black.

The fine structure of univesicular lipocytes presents few unusual characteristics. Small rod-shaped mitochondria, a few ribosomes, a golgi complex,

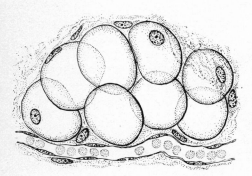

Figure 5-4 Small clusters of lipocytes in a fresh preparation of loose fibrous connective tissue (kitten), showing unstained appearance. A blood capillary is visible below the lipocytes. × 300. *(JFN)*

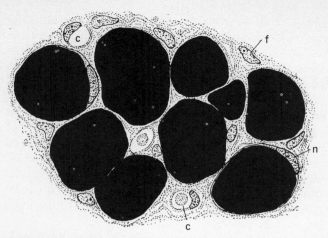

Figure 5-5 Small cluster of lipocytes in loose fibrous connective tissue (kitten), blackened with osmic acid. Note capillaries, *c;* fibrocyte nuclei, *f;* and lipocyte nuclei, *n.* × 300. *(JFN)*

and elements of agranular endoplasmic reticulum are encountered in the attenuated cytoplasm, especially around the nucleus. Micropinocytotic vesicles may be seen at the cell surface. Outside the plasmolemma there is a thin basal lamina[2] and a meshwork of reticular connective tissue fibers (Fig. 5.6) through which capillaries make their way.

[2]Other cells of connective tissue lack an external layer of ground substance comparable to the basal lamina of epithelia.

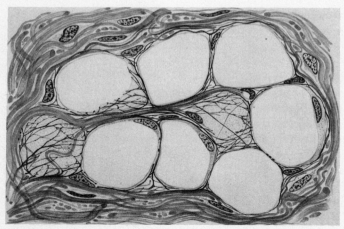

Figure 5-6 A small cluster of lipocytes in loose fibrous connective tissue of a dog. Reticular fibers (fine black lines) form a network around individual cells. × 300. *(JFN)*

Adipose tissue is organized into lobes and lobules, varying in size and definition, and separated from one another by septa of fibrous connective tissue. Blood vessels and nerves course through the septa. The blood supply of univesicular adipose tissue is about as rich as that of skeletal muscle, although it is not easy to visualize it in ordinary histologic sections. Each individual lipocyte at some point is in contact with at least one capillary.

The primary function of most univesicular adipose tissue is storage and release of metabolic fuel. The vesicular material of lipocytes consists largely of triglyceride. Neutral fat does not enter and leave the cell as such. It is derived from several sources. The lipocytes themselves can synthesize it from carbohydrate, i.e., from blood glucose. Chylomicrons in blood plasma, derived from intestinal digestion of fat, provide a major source of fatty acids that can be incorporated by the lipocyte. Other materials, including lipoproteins from liver, contribute to the formation of lipocyte triglyceride.

The processes of fat storage and release are regulated hormonally. Transport out of the cell involves lipolysis, i.e., hydrolysis of triglyceride by an enzyme to form soluble fatty acid and glycerol. Lipolysis abates during food intake and accelerates under fasting conditions. The adipose tissue in some regions of the body is more actively involved in the cyclic processes of storage and release than that in other regions. This is especially true of abdominal and omental adipose tissue. In some other locations, the orbital adipose tissue for example, there is little or no indication of turnover of triglyceride.

Storage of fat in conspicuous places will continue unabated in persons who consume "three square meals a day" laden with fatty and carbohydrate-rich foods, when they exceed the requirements of ongoing metabolism. Since the excess cannot be disposed of in other ways, the lipocytes add fat to their already burgeoning stores, and more lipoblasts take up the task.

A purely structural and protective function is assigned to lobules of adipose tissue in a few locations, such as the soles of the feet and certain structures in joints, where heavy connective tissue encapsulates the groups of adipose-tissue cells.

Multivesicular Adipose Tissue   This type of adipose tissue, commonly designated as "brown fat," occurs in the human fetus and infant but soon regresses and has not been identified definitely in the normal adult, perhaps because both varieties of adipose tissue are colored. It is located mainly in the posterior wall near the kidneys and suprarenal glands, and beneath the sternum. It is abundant in a number of other species, notably in hibernating animals.

The color of multivesicular adipose tissue—tan when full of lipid, turning to red-brown as the contents of the cells are depleted—is due to mitochondrial cytochrome in the cells and to a high vascularity.

The histologic appearance of this type of adipose tissue is illustrated in Fig. 5.7. Cells are smaller than those in univesicular adipose tissue, and the cy-

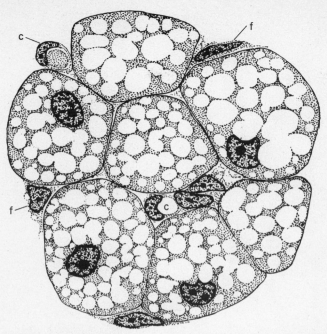

Figure 5-7 Multivesicular adipose–tissue cells filled with lipid droplets; blood capillaries, *c;* fibrocyte nucleus, *f.* From neck of infant rhesus monkey. Compare with Fig. 5-1. × 900. *(JFN)*

toplasm contains multiple droplets of lipid that do not coalesce as in univesicular adipose tissue. Mitochrondria are large, ovoid, and more numerous than in univesicular lipocytes. Compare the two types in Fig. 5.8. They pack the interstices between fat droplets. Multivesicular adipose tissue has an exceptionally rich blood supply. A network of reticular fibers separates the cells, and capillaries and unmyelinated nerve fibers are present in it.

Multivesicular adipose tissue differs functionally from the more common univesicular type. It is not primarily a source of fuel to be called forth and metabolized elsewhere in the body. It is, per se, a site of heat production, a function that is particularly important to newborn infants, especially those of animals subjected to a cold environment at birth. The lipid droplets of the cells of multivesicular adipose tissue are quickly depleted in such conditions. While lipocytes of univesicular adipose tissue are depleted by starvation, those of brown adipose tissue are depleted by cold exposure (Fig. 5.9).

Although human brown adipose tissue is gradually replaced by the univesicular variety during the first year of life, it may reappear under certain abnormal conditions. Adult persons who are chronically hypoxemic tend to reconstitute their brown fat. Victims of the sudden infant death (crib death) syndrome have been found to retain this type of adipose tissue, possibly in response to a state of hypoxemia.

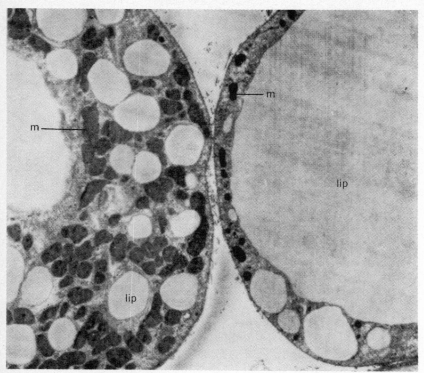

Figure 5-8 Right: Developing white adipose-tissue cell; small mitochondria, *m*, are scattered among lipid inclusions, *lip*. Left: Developing brown adipose-tissue cell; many large mitochondria, *m*, newborn rabbit. Electron micrograph, about ×6,000. *(From D. Hull, British Medical Bulletin, vol. 22, pp. 92–96, 1966. By permission of the publishers.)*

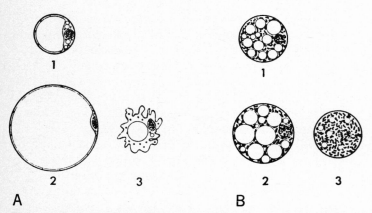

Figure 5-9 Cells of white (*A*) and brown (*B*) adipose tissue. Developing cell (1); mature cells (2); and lipid-depleted cells (3). Clear areas are lipid; black elements are mitochondria. Modified from D. Hull.

SUGGESTED READING

Barnard, T.: The Ultrastructural Differentiation of Brown Adipose Tissue in the Rat. *Journal of Ultrastructral Research*, vol. 29, pp. 311–332, 1969.

Cushman, S. W.: Structure-Function Relationship in the Adipose Cell. I. Ultrastructure of the Isolated Adipose Cell. *Journal of Cell Biology*, vol. 46, pp. 326–341, 1970.

Hull, D.: The Structure and Function of Brown Adipose Tissue. *British Medical Bulletin*, vol. 22, pp. 92–96 January, 1966.

Merklin, R. J.: Growth and Distribution of Human Fetal Brown Fat. *Anatomical Record*, vol. 178, pp. 637–645, 1974.

Naeye, R. L.: Hypoxemia and the Sudden Infant Death Syndrome. *Science*, vol. 106, pp. 837–838, 1974.

Slavin, B. G.: The Cytophysiolgy of Mammalian Adipose Cells. *International Review of Cytology*, vol. 33, pp. 297–334, 1972.

Teplitz, C., and Y. Lim: The Diagnostic Significance of Brown Adipose Tissue (BAT). Transformation of Adult Human Periadrenal Fat: A Morphologic Indicator of Severe Chronic Hypoxemia. *Laboratory Investigation*, vol. 30, p. 390, 1974.

Supporting Tissues

Supporting tissues are the special types of connective tissue forming the skeleton and its articulations, i.e., cartilage and bone. Both are composed of cells and matrix. The matrix consists of ground substance containing fibers. Cartilage and bone are different chemically as well as structurally. The one is practically avascular; the other has a rich blood supply. Table 6.1 presents a comparison of four types of connective tissue.

CARTILAGE

Although the adult role of cartilage as a skeletal component is a minor one, its function in body growth is of major importance. It forms the skeleton of early mammalian fetuses, but it is gradually replaced in the growing individual by bone, and only remnants of it are encountered in the skeleton after maturity. At that time cartilage is one of the least prevalent constituents of the human body.

Hyaline Cartilage This, the principal type, is illustrated in Figs. 6.1 and 6.2. The common name of it is "gristle." It has a blue-white, translucent appearance in the fresh state. Nearly all bones except some of the flat bones of the skull at first are cast in this material. How they become reconstructed and as-

Table 6.1 Comparison of Connective Tissues

	Fibrous	Adipose	Cartilage	Bone
Tissue fluid	Considerable	Negligible	Negligible	Negligible
Matrix	Ground substance	Basal lamina	Cartilage matrix	Bone matrix
Collagenous fibers	Main component	In septa	Invisible in matrix; numerous in fibrocartilage	Invisible in matrix; perforating fibers
Reticular fibers	Prominent component in many locations	Present around cells	Negligible	Negligible
Elastic fibers	Absent in some membranes; sparse in most loose and dense connective tissue; rich in walls of elastic arteries	Negligible	Prominent in elastic cartilage of ear, epiglottis, etc.	Negligible
Cells	Fibrocytes; labrocytes; macrophages; etc.	Lipocytes of two types	Chondrocytes	Osteoblasts; osteoclasts; osteocytes

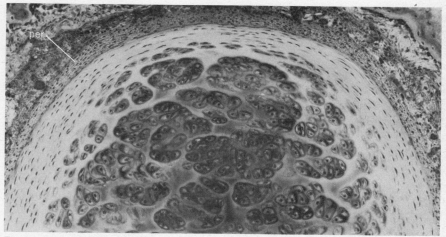

Figure 6-1 Hyaline cartilage from the nose of a young animal. Two types of growth are seen. The dark central region contains groups of dividing chondrocytes in lacunae, illustrating endogenous growth. Cells from the perichondrium, *per,* give rise to new chondrocytes in the peripheral zone, illustrating appositional growth. Photomicrograph, about × 150.

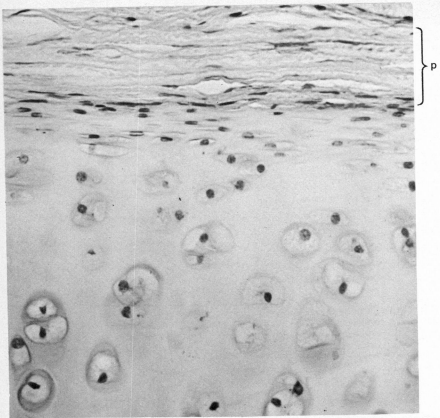

Figure 6-2 Perichondrium, *p*, on hyaline cartilage of the trachea of a young individual. The transition from indifferent connective tissue cells of the perichondrium to chondrocytes illustrates appositional cartilage growth. Photomicrograph, ×300.

sume their permanent characteristics is described later in this chapter. Hyaline cartilage also forms parts of the ribs, nose, larynx, trachea, and bronchi of the adult body. With advancing age, even some of these few cartilages tend to become ossified (Fig. 22.4), and their fibrous extracellular component becomes more prominent. One of the earliest signs of aging is said to be a transformation of hyaline cartilage into fibrocartilage, accompanied by a change in color from blue-white to a yellowish hue in the fresh state. Hyaline cartilage is simpler than fibrous connective tissue. For instance, its cells, **chondrocytes,** are of one kind. On the surface of growing cartilage, they are called **chondroblasts.**

Collagen constitutes about 40 percent, dry weight, of cartilage. The collagenous fibers are formed by chondrocytes in the cartilage **matrix.** They are fine fibers, invisible in ordinary histologic preparations, but they can be demonstrated with special stains (Fig. 6.3). They are unlike mature collagenous fibers in other connective tissues, for the characteristic 640-Å periodicity of crossbanding is lacking in simple hyaline cartilage. Articular cartilages do contain some larger fibers in which crossbands can be demonstrated.

The ground substance of cartilage matrix is formed by protein-polysaccharide complexes containing chondroitin sulfuric acid. It differs from ground substance of areolar tissue by being a firm gel. The capsular zones surrounding mature chondrocytes in the central regions of hyaline cartilage appear to be denser than those near the periphery (Fig. 6.1). They stain readily with basic dyes. This is especially so in the **capsules** surrounding single and groups of mature chondrocytes. By virtue of its acid-mucopolysaccharide content, the matrix exhibits metachromasia.

Chondrocytes show few noteworthy features in the usual histologic preparation. Their fine structure during active growth of cartilage is illustrated in Fig. 6.4. The cytoplasmic organelles resemble those of some other protein-synthesizing cells. The cytoplasm also often contains clumps of glycogen particles and occasional lipid inclusions. The cell surface has many small processes, which are invisible in well-preserved chondrocytes viewed under the light microscope. Poor fixation of tissue commonly results in shrinkage of chondrocytes, which then seem to be stellate.

Fibrous connective tissue adjacent to cartilage constitutes the **perichondrium,** forming a compact layer except at articular surfaces. Vessels and nerves enter the perichondrium from the surrounding loose fibrous connective tissue. The outer layer of the perichondrium consists of bundles of collagenous fibers among which are fibroblasts and indifferent cells. The inner layer of perichondrium is a region of transition where the collagenous fibers merge with those of the cartilage matrix and chondroblasts appear (Figs. 6.1 and 6.2).

Cartilage develops from mesenchyme in the embryo. The mesenchymal cells multiply rapidly, withdrawing their processes to become rounded. These

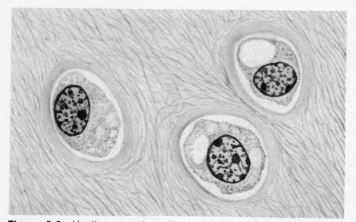

Figure 6-3 Hyaline costal cartilage (monkey) showing collagenous fibers in the matrix. Three chondrocytes are encapsulated in separate lacunae; shrinkage from the lacunar walls is artifact. About × 900. *(JFN)*

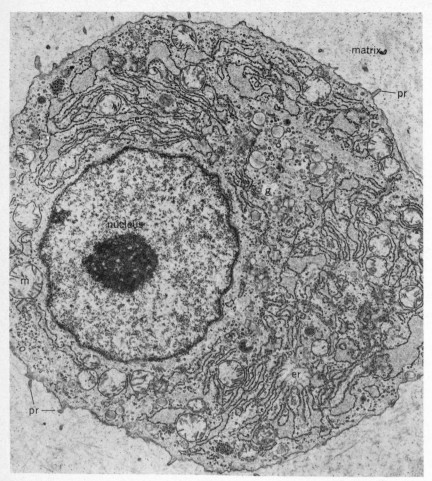

Figure 6-4 Chondrocyte surrounded by hyaline matrix into which thin processes, *pr*, extend. Note granular endoplasmic reticulum, *er*, golgi complex, *g*, and numerous mitochondria, *m*, as well as the nucleus and a distinct nucleolus. Electron micrograph. About × 15,000. *(Contributed by H. C. Anderson, Journal of Cell Biology, vol. 41, p. 59, 1965. By permission of the publishers.)*

transformed mesenchymal cells, or chondroblasts, are crowded into masses, known as centers of chondrification. The more centrally placed chondroblasts increase in size, and droplets appear in their cytoplasm. At this early stage, they form **precartilage** in which there is as yet little matrix, and cells are rather evenly spaced. The matrix has less density than that of true cartilage. Chondroblasts surrounded by matrix continue to divide and give rise to clusters or nests of chondrocytes separated from one another by matrix.

Further growth of cartilage is accomplished in two ways. So long as the cartilaginous matrix is soft and yielding, as it is in the young individual, nests of chondrocytes can continue to expand by cell division. Each cell in the nest surrounds itself with more matrix. The result is endogenous or interstitial growth. At the same time, more chondroblasts are derived from indifferent cells in the perichondrium. These divide and form chondrocytes at the periphery of the cartilage mass, a process called exogenous or appositional growth. It is almost the only type of growth occurring in adult cartilage. Both types of growth are illustrated in Fig. 6.1.

As compact matrix forms in cartilage, the chondrocytes find themselves lodged in separate little compartments, known as **lacunae.** The walls of the lacunae of adult cartilage are more refractive than the surrounding matrix, and stain more intensely with basic dyes because of the high concentration of chondroitin sulfuric acid in their matrix. They form capsules for the chondrocytes. During life, chondrocytes fill their lacunae, but their cytoplasm shrinks away from the walls during histologic fixation of cartilage. With increasing density of the matrix, chondrocytes that have undergone one or two final cell divisions become locked in their lacunae and can no longer move apart by deposition of new matrix. Young chondrocytes in the region of appositional growth are elongated and have little visible cytoplasm. Older cells, deeper in the cartilage mass, are larger and rounded.

Since cartilage is avascular, all nutriments, oxygen, and products of metabolism must diffuse through the interstitial matrix. This occurs in the same manner as in the ground substance of areolar tissue. There is a limit to the distance a cell can live away from its source of supply, the perichondrial capillaries. Large masses of cartilage sometimes develop in such a way that channels of vascular connective tissue, called **cartilage canals,** extend into the matrix and increase the surface of the mass, which facilitates nutrition. In the large masses of cartilage at the ends of long bones of the young individual, the problem is solved in another way. The older, larger chondrocytes die and, during this process, tear down their walls of matrix, whereupon connective tissue and blood vessels invade the region and build bone in the place of cartilage.

Hyaline cartilage is not easily repaired after it has been injured. A fracture may be healed by invasion of vascular connective tissue which forms a scar. New cartilage cells can develop at the junction of the scar tissue with the cartilage, but healing is slow. After injury or disease, fragments of articular cartilages in a joint cavity continue to live and often must be removed because, in the absence of a perichondrium, there is no chance for them to be reunited.

Elastic Cartilage   The least common type is elastic cartilage. It is found only in the auricle of the ear, external auditory meatus, auditory tube, epiglottis, and some minor cartilages of the larynx. Elastic cartilage differs from the hyaline variety mainly by the presence of elastic connective-tissue fibers in the matrix. Collagenous fibers are present beneath the perichondrium, but are inconspicuous. The chondrocytes in their capsules are isolated as shown in Fig. 6.5. Photomicrographs of elastic cartilage are seen in Figs. 6.6 and 22.3.

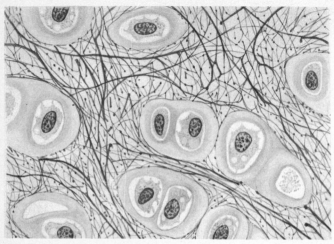

Figure 6-5 Elastic fibers especially stained in cartilage from the ear of a pig. Compare with Fig. 6-3. About × 900. *(JFN)*

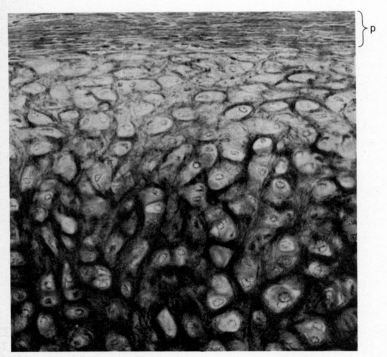

Figure 6-6 Elastic cartilage from a human ear stained especially for the fibers. Perichondrium, *p.* Compare with Fig. 6-2. Photomicrograph, × 300.

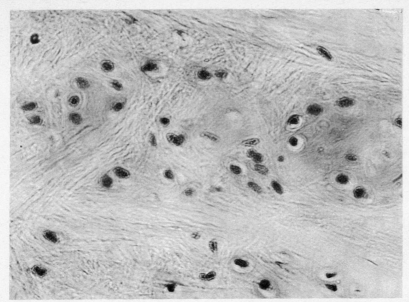

Figure 6-7 Fibrocartilage in a human intervertebral disc. Islands of hyaline cartilage are seen in a dense mat of collagenous fibers. Photomicrograph, × 300.

Fibrocartilage This is a type transitional between hyaline cartilage and dense fibrous connective tissue of tendons and ligaments. Its cells tend to be grouped in capsules, separated from each other by thick bundles of collagenous fibers, as shown in Fig. 6.7. The cells are enclosed in capsules of matrix. There is no true perichondrium.

Fibrocartilage in young individuals occurs mainly in the intervertebral discs, the knee joint, and the symphysis pubis. These are places where ligamentous bands are required to unite the bones. Later in life it may be seen in tendons at their junction with articular cartilages and at other places where tendons are subjected to friction.

A small body of tissue bearing slight resemblance to degenerating cartilage, and known as the **nucleus pulposus,** is found in the center of the intervertebral disc. Its position corresponds to that of the notochord of the embryo.

BONE

Bone, a type of rigid supporting connective tissue made up of fibers, ground substance, and cells, forms the skeleton and occurs in a few other places.[1] Living bone does not lend itself readily to classroom study by light microscopy. Students ordinarily must content themselves with stained sections cut from

---

[1]Examples are the sesamoid bones in certain tendons, the bone in the interventricular septum of the heart in large ungulates, and the os penis in a number of mammals.

fixed decalcified bone tissue and with tiny pieces of dry bone ground and polished until translucent. The latter type of preparation is instructive, although it goes without saying that cytologic details are lacking.

In beginning the study, it is well to start with a gross longitudinal section through a long bone (Fig. 6.8). Two types of bony tissue, one compact and the other spongy, will be seen. They are continuous with one another and are actually different arrangements of the same histologic elements. **Spongy bone** consists of a framework of anastomosing bars or "trabeculae" of various sizes and shapes. Their directions and points of contact are so arranged as to give each bone a maximum rigidity and resistance to changes in shape. The spaces among trabeculae are filled with marrow.

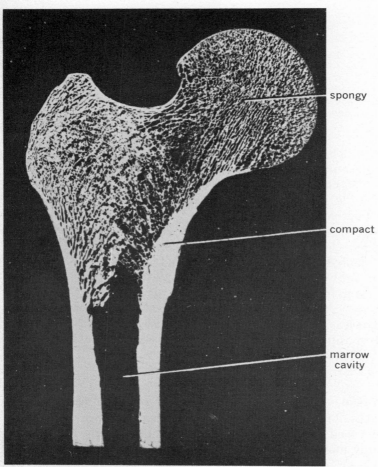

spongy

compact

marrow cavity

Figure 6-8 Human femur; a saw cut through the upper end; natural size. *(Reproduced from R. O. Greep,* Histology, *McGraw-Hill Book Company, New York, 1954.)*

Compact bone occurs at the bone surface. In the larger long bones, the shaft or **diaphysis** consists of compact bone and has in its center a marrow cavity. The dilated extremities or **epiphysis** of long bones consist of spongy bone covered with a thin layer of compact bone. Compact bone is actually less dense than it appears, for it is traversed by innumerable vascular channels.

Matrix   The matrix of bone differs from that of cartilage by its high mineral content. Its primary organic component, collagenous fibers, forms a strengthening framework, invisible in preparations by the usual methods, but demonstrable with special stains, as illustrated in Fig. 6.9. The fibrous elements of bone matrix are produced by cells just as they are in cartilage. Collagen is the principal organic structure in bone, but when the matrix becomes impregnated with mineral salts, it is no longer visible.

The ground substance of bone matrix consists of protein-polysaccharides with considerably less chondroitin sulfuric acid than that of cartilage. It is a product of bone-forming cells. Through it course the collagenous fibers. Bone mineral, the composition of which is mainly hydroxyapatite, forms in bone matrix within "matrix vescicles" from osteoblasts, and then is found within collagenous fibrils as apatite crystals. The crystals are of submicroscopic size, the largest measuring only about 400 Å in length and 30 Å in thickness. They are illustrated in an electron micrograph of a collagenous fibril in Fig. 6.10. The mineral content of bone increases in the course of development, reaching about 65 percent of bone, dry weight, in adult human beings.

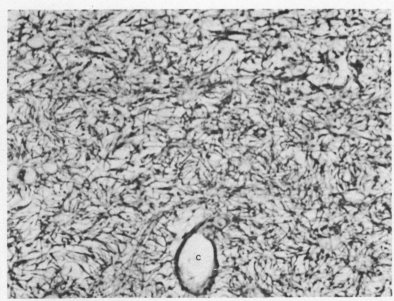

Figure 6-9   Compact bone, showing collagenous fibers stained by a silver method. A communicating canal, c, is seen at the bottom of the illustration. Photomicrograph, about × 600.

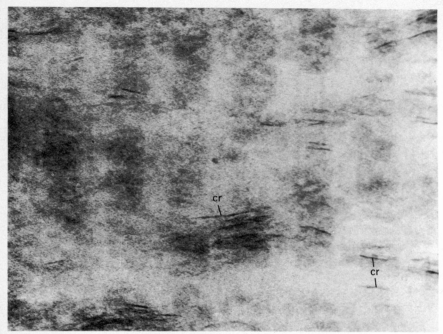

Figure 6-10 Inorganic crystals, *cr,* deposited in a collagen fibril of embryonic bone (chick). The periodic banding of collagen appears in the background. Unstained, nondecalcified section. Electron micrograph, ×240,000. *(Contributed by M. J. Glimcher.)*

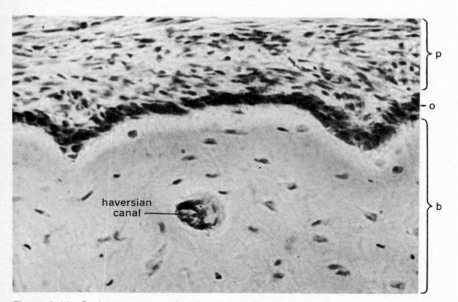

Figure 6-11 Periosteum, *p,* on developing maxilla of a kitten. Osteoblasts, *o,* form a layer on the new bone, *b.* One haversian canal can be seen. Photomicrograph, × 300.

Periosteum and Endosteum   Bone, like cartilage, is covered by a connective-tissue layer, the **periosteum** (Fig. 6.11). This forms a dense fibrous investment, structurally resembling perichondrium, in the outer layer of which run blood vessels to and from the bone. Flattened cells occupy the inner portion of the periosteum and can give rise to bone-forming cells, under appropriate conditions. They are tall and so numerous along the inner layer of the periosteum of young, growing bone that they form a layer resembling epithelium. The capacity of the periosteum to produce new bone is remarkable. If a large part of the shaft of a long bone is shelled out from the periosteum, it may be replaced completely. The periosteum provides the mechanism for knitting fractured bones.

The junction of periosteum and bone is marked, in some places, by visible collagenous fibers extending inward from the fibrous tissue of the periosteum. These **perforating fibers** hold the periosteum firmly onto the bone, and are seen best at the sites where ligaments or tendons attach to bone.

Extensions of connective tissue accompany blood vessels from the periosteum into canals in compact bone. This scanty areolar tissue contains cells that can give rise to new bone cells when called upon to do so. Thin layers of connective tissue form the **endosteum,** lining the marrow cavities in bone. This is most evident in large spaces filled with yellow marrow after bone formation ceases, and is scarcely perceptible in spongy bone where hemopoietic tissue occurs.

Cells   There are three main types of bone cell: osteocytes, osteoblasts, and osteoclasts. They are interrelated, and one can change to another under appropriate conditions.

Osteocytes are not easily studied in ordinary histologic preparations of decalcified bone. They occupy **lacunae** in the bone matrix, as illustrated in Fig. 6.12. Unlike chondrocytes, which appear spheroidal, they are stellate, sending out long branching processes. The lacunae in which they lie are interconnected

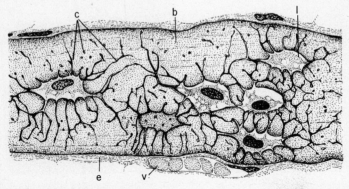

Figure 6-12   Bone trabecula of a human femur, showing canaliculi, c, bone matrix, b, and osteocytes in lacunae, l. It is covered by endosteum, e, containing a capillary, v, filled with erythrocytes. About ×600. (JFN)

and communicate with the bony vascular canals by means of innumerable **canaliculi.** In young living bone, the osteocytes fill the lacunae and extend processes into the canaliculi, in some instances making contact with the processes of their neighbors. The extensive system of intercommunicating lacunae, canaliculi, and vascular canals in the bone matrix permits materials in solution to permeate through all parts of the bone, enabling osteocytes to live in a medium that is otherwise solidified by mineral salts.

Osteocytes have small, ovoid, highly chromatic nuclei. The cytoplasm contains an inconspicuous golgi complex and a few components of endoplasmic reticulum. Ribosomes are not numerous. These features suggest that osteocytes are less active than osteoblasts (Fig. 6.13).

Osteoblasts are the precursors of osteocytes and are derived from mesenchyme or, later, from indifferent connective-tissue cells of the periosteum, endosteum, or osteogenic buds of loose fibrous connective tissue, as is

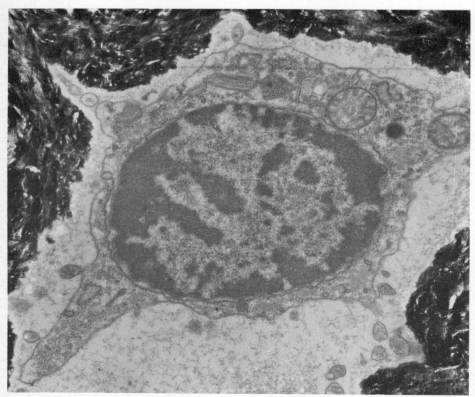

Figure 6-13 Osteocyte in lacuna surrounded by bone matrix (black masses of crystals). Electron micrograph, about × 15,000. *(Contributed by R. R. Cooper with permission of Journal of Bone and Joint Surgery.)*

described below. They are found wherever new bone is being built. As new matrix is laid down, osteoblasts are captured in the matrix and become osteocytes.

Osteoclasts are giant cells with several or many darkly staining nuclei and lightly eosinophilic cytoplasm. They, too, are associated with the processes of growth and remodeling of bone. It is thought that they can arise by fusion of several osteoblasts or from osteocytes and chondrocytes liberated in the process of resorption of bone and cartilage matrix. The structures of osteoblasts and osteoclasts are described later in this chapter.

Structural Organization A freely anastomosing system of small blood vessels influences the arrangement of bone cells and the organization of the matrix in which they are embedded. The blood supply of long bones is represented by a **nutrient artery** that passes directly to the marrow and by numerous smaller vessels arising from arteries in the outer layer of periosteum. The periosteal vessels perforate the external layer of compact bone in small horizontal **communicating canals**[2] that connect with an anastomosing network of other canals running parallel to the long axis of the compact bone. The latter are designated **haversian canals.** This arrangement of blood vessels in canals reaching all parts of the bone provides ready access to the body's mineral stores.

In a thin, polished piece of compact bone cut at right angles to the long axis, the haversian canals appear as black spots. They vary in diameter but average roughly 50 μm. Around each of these canals is a variable number (4 to 20 or more) of thin plates or **lamellae** of matrix. Between lamellae are seen the lacunae, containing the osteocytes during life, from each of which emerge many fine canaliculi. The series of lamellae, lacunae, and canaliculi surrounding one haversian canal is called a **haversian system** (Figs. 6.14 and 6.15). Forming the outer boundary of such a system and separating it from adjacent ones, a bright thin line, the "cementing line," is often noticed. The haversian system is not only the structural unit of bone but is also the functional unit and, as such, goes by the name of **osteon.**

The bone matrix of **haversian lamellae** has collagenous fibers arranged in a radial fashion, those of one lammella at approximately a right angle to those of the neighboring lamella. Thus the haversian system has a helical framework in which the pitch of the adjacent spirals alternates. When viewed with polarized light, the successive lamellae appear alternately dark and light.

The bone between haversian systems is arranged in parallel lamellae with different orientation. These are known as **interstitial lamellae,** representing remnants of haversian systems that were partly absorbed in the rebuilding process accompanying growth of bone.

The cortex, or most external layer of compact bone, consists of a series of thin concentrically arranged lamellae produced by the periosteum. These are circumferential or **periosteal lamellae**; they impart a smooth appearance to the bone surface. Similar lamellae, fewer in number, line the wall of the marrow

[2]Formerly called "Volkmann's canals."

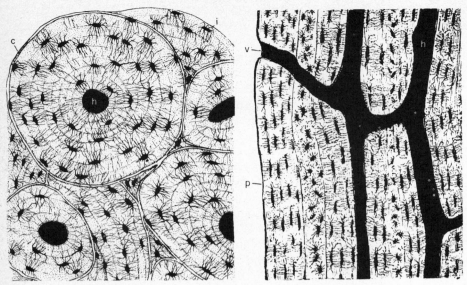

Figure 6-14 Compact bone. Cross section (left) and longitudinal section (right) of dry preparations ground thin and polished. Haversian canals, *h*, and communicating canals, *v*, as well as many lacunae, are black because they were filled with the polishing powder. Several haversian systems show concentric lamellae; interstitial lamellae, *i*, lie between them. Periosteal lamellae, *p*. Cementing lines, *c*, are visible in the cross section. About × 300. *(JFN)*

cavity. They are related to the thin layer of fibrous connective tissue of the endosteum and are called **endosteal lamellae.** The periosteal lamellae are pierced by the communicating canals, which in life conduct blood vessels into the haversian canals. The communicating canals are not surrounded by concentric lamellae.

The structure of trabeculae of spongy bone is simpler than that of compact bone. The small trabeculae lack haversian systems, for they are not penetrated by blood vessels but are surrounded by vascular marrow spaces.

Functions   Bone tissue has an important metabolic function. It constitutes the principal mineral depot of the body. Hormone of the parathyroid glands either directly or indirectly exerts control over the mechanism of calcium metabolism and therefore over the mineral of bone. The inorganic salts are not permanently bound in the bone matrix. When compounds containing radioactive calcium or phosphorus are administered to animals, radioactivity can be demonstrated in their bones within a few hours. Experiments of this type have shown that about one-third of the phosphorus in the skeleton of an adult rat is replaced in 3 weeks. There is a continuous turnover of the inorganic constituents of bone, which are completely removed and replaced many times during life. Just as sodium and chloride are banked in the ground substance of fibrous connective tissue, so calcium and phosphorus are banked in the matrix of bone.

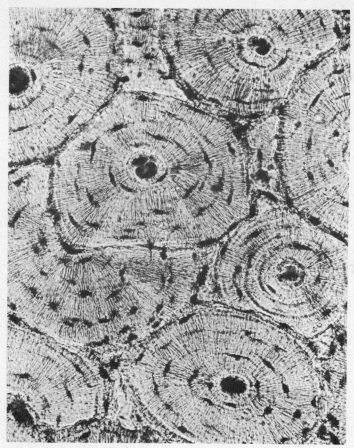

Figure 6-15 Compact bone from the tarsus of a giraffe; a cross section ground and polished. Parts of nine haversian systems and seven canals can be seen. The apparent overlapping is due to partial replacement of older by newer systems. Interstitial lamellae occur between the two upper haversian systems. Cementing lines appear as narrow bright bands at the periphery of some of the systems. Photomicrograph, about × 300.

Bone is constantly changing—rapidly in the early years of life, more slowly in later years. With increasing demands for support, it can undergo some hypertrophy and, with disuse, some atrophy. Considerable molding can be effected surgically.

Development, Growth, and Remodeling At the time of birth, half of the centers of ossification have not appeared, and less than one twenty-fifth of the bone of the adult has been produced. Bone size increases over a considerable fraction of the life-span, and, since bone never completely loses its ability to undergo changes and repair, it is necessary to know how its growth and reconstruction take place. Bone is not simply laid on and on until adult size is reached, but growth is accomplished by a twofold process of construction and destruction.

Before a discussion of development, growth, and reorganization of bone, it is well to consider the roles of the cells that have much to do with these processes. The osteoblasts are easy to identify in sections of growing bone, where they occur in single rows on the surface of bone trabeculae (Fig. 6.16). They resemble plasmocytes because they have dark eccentric nuclei, basophilic cytoplasm, and sometimes a pale region near the nucleus, which is the negative image of a prominent golgi complex. The basophilic cytoplasm is rich in ribosomes on cisternae of the endoplasmic reticulum, as is the case of other cells engaged in protein synthesis. The first material formed by osteoblasts lacks the inorganic bone salt, deposition of which lags behind formation of organic components. This substance is called "osteoid" by some writers. When osteoblasts are caught up in the matrix and are transformed into osteocytes, they become relatively inactive.

Osteoclasts are less numerous than osteoblasts. They can be identified by their giant size, the presence of multiple darkly staining nuclei, and their acidophilic cytoplasm (Fig. 6.17). One often finds them in small indentations or lacunae in the bone trabeculae.[3] Osteoclasts are present in regions where bone resorption is in progress, and their number is said to be indicative of the rate of resorption; however, the part they play is not clear. Some resorption of bone may take place in the absence of osteoclasts. Nevertheless, there is considerable evidence that they do assist in the process of remodeling bone. Osteoclast cytoplasm contains vacuoles and dense bodies, some of which are lysosomes. The cell surface adjacent to bone is thrown into irregular folds, giving it a striated appearance called the "rippled border" (Fig. 6.18).

The ground substance of newly forming bone is less firm than that of older established bone. Furthermore, in regions of bone resorption, the state of polymerization of the ground substance changes, with the result that it becomes more permeable, allowing greater chemical reactivity of the inorganic compounds of the matrix. The processes of bone formation and resorption are regulated by a number of factors, endocrine and metabolic.

The simplest picture of bone formation will be seen in studying **intramembraneous ossification** of bones arising in embryonic connective tissue. The bones involved are the flat bones at the vault of the skull, the face, and the jaw. In fetal centers of ossification, numerous mesenchymal cells appear in a loose layer of fine collagenous **osteogenic fibers.** The mesenchymal cells are about to become osteoblasts. As they assume the characteristics of osteoblasts, they line up on fibers, and some matrix—the precursor of bone, although not yet containing bone salts—appears along one side of the row of cells. This is soon built into irregular bars or trabeculae with osteoblasts covering their surfaces. Shortly thereafter, the matrix begins to be infiltrated with fine apatite

---

[3]These have been called "Howship's lacunae."

mesenchymal cells   osteoblasts

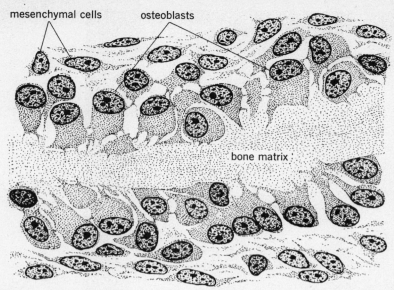

bone matrix

Figure 6-16 Intramembranous bone formation in the maxilla of a cat fetus. Osteoblasts are aligned along a trabecula of new bone. ×1,200. *(JFN)*

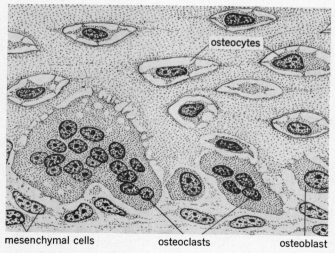

osteocytes

mesenchymal cells   osteoclasts   osteoblast

Figure 6-17 Osteoclasts, the larger one in an indentation on a trabecula of fetal jaw bone. ×900. *(JFN)*

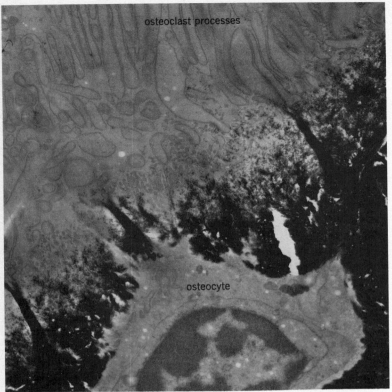

Figure 6-18 Border of an osteoclast (above) with multiple processes and folds next to mineralized bone matrix (black) in which there is an osteocyte. Electron micrograph, about × 15,000. *(Contributed by R. R. Cooper; reproduced with permission of Journal of Bone and Joint Surgery.)*

crystals, and the first bone has been formed. This process extends in three dimensions.

The bars first laid down grow in thickness by deposition of new matrix at the osteoblast-matrix junction. Growth in length is accomplished by transformation of additional mesenchymal cells into osteoblasts that appear in strands along the osteogenic fibers. Here, too, as matrix is deposited, some of the osteoblasts become imprisoned in the new bone by deposition of matrix all around them. The spaces between trabeculae contain mesenchyme and small blood vessels. Later some of the mesenchymal cells become the hemopoietic elements of bone marrow.

All the time bone is being built in the manner just described, the fetus is growing apace. Bones of the proper head or jaw size for one stage of development are quickly outgrown and are redesigned from day to day. Resorption in one place goes on simultaneously with production of new bone at an immediately adjacent site, so subtle is the transformation and so delicate the response to changing need.

While the membrane bones of the cranium are forming, a similar phenomenon occurs in the miniature cartilaginous models of the bones of the appendicular skeleton. The process by which most of the cartilaginous skeleton is transformed into bone is known as **endochondral ossification.** It is illustrated diagrammatically in Fig. 6.19. For long bones, it begins at and around the center and proceeds in an orderly manner toward the ends until the definitive bone has been completed. A curious feature is that bone formation never quite

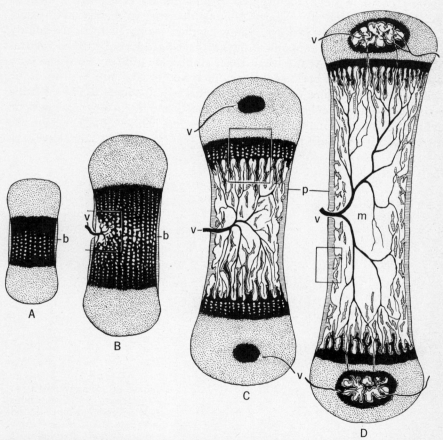

Figure 6-19 Diagrams of the ossification of a long bone: *A*, early cartilaginous stage; *B*, stage of eruption of the periosteal bone collar by an osteogenic bud of vessels; *C* and *D*, older stages with a primary marrow cavity and early centers of calcification in the epiphyseal centers of ossification. Calcified cartilage in all diagrams is black; *b*, periosteal bone collar; *m*, marrow cavity; *p*, periosteal bone; *v*, blood vessels entering the centers of ossification. *(JFN)*

overtakes the growth of cartilage, and in many bones of the body, more than a trace of cartilage remains on articular surfaces long after the process of ossification has been completed.

Endochondral ossification is accompanied by **periosteal bone formation**. In long bones, this starts around the center of the shaft where a ring of osteoblasts forms in the fibrous perichondrium. This membrane is appropriately renamed periosteum as soon as the first matrix appears between osteoblasts and cartilage. The process involves deposition of matrix on osteogenic fibers and its subsequent calcification—exactly as in membrane bones. Figures 6.20 and 6.21 illustrate stages in development of periosteal bone.

While this goes on, or just preceding it, cartilage cells in the center of the fetal bones begin to align themselves in longitudinal rows. Their lacunae enlarge (Fig. 6.19 *A* and *B*). A corresponding decrease in matrix takes place. With continuation of this process, many lacunae merge to form irregularly elongated cavities, while remnants of the cartilage become calcified by infiltration with calcium salts. At the same time, embryonic connective tissue with blood vessels erodes the periosteal bone collar and breaks into cavities in the calcifying cartilage, forming **osteogenic buds** (Figs. 6.20 and 6.22). These bring in the connective-tissue cells that form osteoblasts and the osteogenic fibers on which to build bone. Bone then proceeds to develop, just as it does beneath the periosteum and in the skull membranes of the embryo. The bits and slivers of

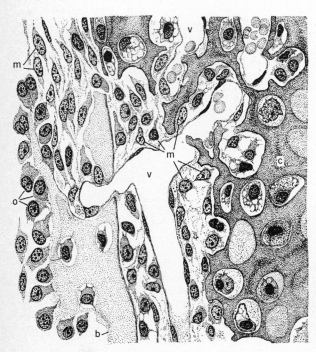

Figure 6-20 Diaphysis of a metacarpal bone of a cat fetus, showing penetration of vessels and osteogenic mesenchyme into calcified cartilage: *b*, periosteal bone collar; *c*, calcified cartilage; *m*, osteogenic mesenchyme; *o*, osteoblasts; *v*, blood vessels of an osteogenic bud. This figure corresponds to the region outlined in Fig. 6-19*B*. ×600. *(JFN)*

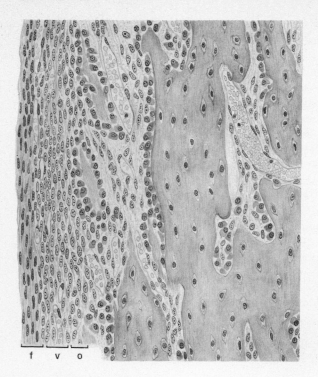

Figure 6-21 Periosteal bone in the humeral diaphysis of a 2-week-old kitten; *f,* young fibrous ligament lying on the surface of *v,* the vascular layer of periosteum; *o,* osteoblastic layer of periosteum. This figure corresponds to the region outlined in Fig. 6-19*D.* × 300.

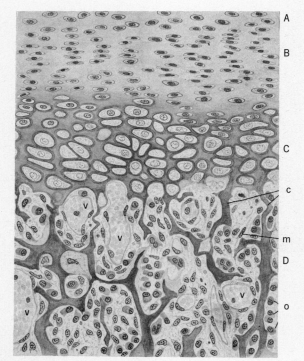

Figure 6-22 Endochondral bone formation in the ulna of a guinea pig fetus: *A,* cartilage; *B,* zone of proliferating cartilage cells; *C,* zone of calcification of cartilage and hypertrophy of lacunae; *D,* zone of ossification; osteoblasts, *o,* appear on trabeculae of calcified cartilage, *c;* other cells of the osteogenic buds, *m,* may be seen; blood vessels, *v,* are present in the buds. The region corresponds to that outlined in Fig. 6-19*C.* × 300. *(JFN)*

the calcified cartilage that were left over after erosion of the cartilage matrix offer convenient foundations for deposition of bone matrix. Consequently, trabeculae of bone, in the centers of which are deeply basophilic calcified cartilage remnants, are encountered (Figs. 6.23 and 6.24).

The process of endochondral ossification extends toward the ends of the bones, preceded by rapid growth of the cartilage. Much later, after birth in almost all bones, secondary centers of ossification arise in the cartilage at the ends of the bone, exactly as the primary ossification centers were formed (Fig. 6.19 *C* and *D*). As this process spreads out toward the oncoming primary ossification center, a band of cartilage marks the junction of diaphysis and epiphysis. This is the **epiphyseal cartilage.** Its continuing growth makes possible the lengthening of the bone. Length is acquired by active endochondral bone formation on the diaphyseal side of the epiphyseal cartilage. The epiphyseal side is inactive. The cartilaginous layer gradually narrows, and when ossification overtakes the cartilage after puberty, it is finally obliterated. The diaphysis and epiphysis fuse, and no further lengthening can occur. Throughout the

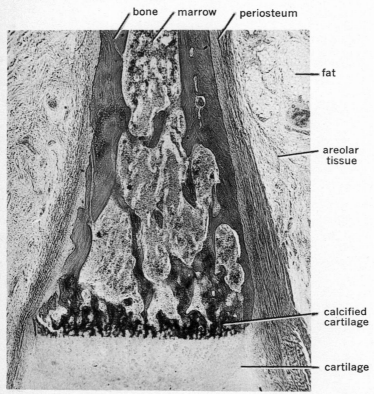

Figure 6-23 Ossification in the terminal phalanx of a human infant's finger. A dark zone of calcifying cartilage borders the hyaline cartilage. Photomicrograph, × 30.

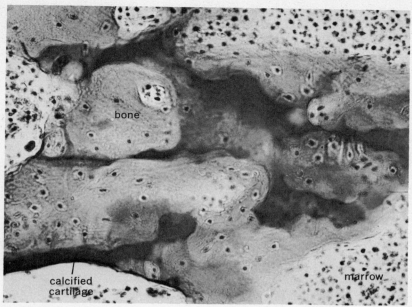

Figure 6-24 Trabecula of bone, showing cores of darkly stained calcified cartilage. Same specimen as in Fig. 6-23. Photomicrograph, × 300.

course of growth, the bone increases in thickness by periosteal ossification. As growth in length and diameter proceeds, resorption and reconstruction take place to keep pace with the ever-changing needs.

Here it would be well to take up the human femur that was sawed longitudinally at the beginning of this study and, while contemplating it, to bear in mind that it was smaller than a paper safety match at the time ossification began in its center during the third fetal month.

ARTICULATIONS

The histology of joints introduces no new tissues. Bone, cartilage, and fibrous connective tissue are the main elements involved in their construction. The immovable or only slightly movable unions of cartilage to bone (synchondroses) and bone to bone (sutures and syndesmoses) compose one category, the **synarthroses.** Their components are united without an intervening cavity, being held together firmly by dense fibrous connective tissue, some of which is in the form of ligaments. Figure 6.25 *A* and *B* illustrates two types of synarthroses.

In movable joints, or **diarthroses,** the ends of the bones are separated by a cavity containing some fluid (Fig. 6.25 *C*). The articular surfaces are covered by a layer of cartilage—usually hyaline cartilage, although the fibrous form occurs in some places, notably the intervertebral discs and symphysis pubis. The outer surface of the articular cartilage lacks perichondrium and possesses

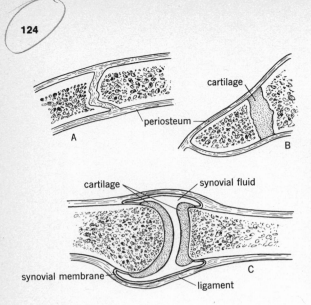

Figure 6-25 Diagram to illustrate three types of joints. *A,* suture of bones of the skull, dense fibrous connective tissue uniting the bones; *B,* synchondrosis from the base of the skull, cartilage uniting the bones; *C,* diarthrosis, represented by a finger joint, in which cartilages at the ends of bones are separated by a cavity filled with synovial fluid. Periosteum and ligaments encapsulate the joints. *(WEL)*

rows of flattened chondrocytes. The deep cartilage is calcified. A dense fibrous-connective-tissue **capsule,** ligamentous in nature, surrounds the joint and blends with the periosteum of the bones.

Within the ligamentous capsule of the joint is a layer of connective tissue, varying from dense fibrous to areolar or even adipose tissue. This layer may be thrown into folds projecting into the articular cavity and forming the **synovial membrane** of the joint. Its folds are the **synovial villi** which may bear secondary villi. The villi are made of areolar or adipose tissue and are partly covered by flattened connective-tissue cells resembling mesothelium. Some are vascular folds, as shown in Fig. 6.26. The connective tissue of the synovial membrane

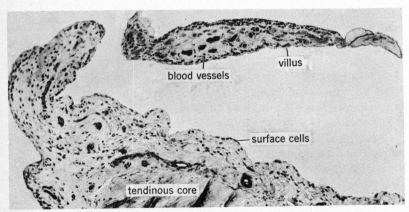

Figure 6-26 Synovial fold and villus from a diarthrosis. A tortuosity of the villus accounts for the apparent break in continuity. Surface cells resemble endothelium. The main part of the fold is formed by fibrous connective tissue containing small blood vessels; it has a tendinous core. Photomicrograph, × 100.

becomes continuous with the perichondrium at the edges of the articular cartilages. **Articular discs** or plates of dense fibrous connective tissue or fibrocartilage, continuous with the synovial membrane, are wedged into the space between the articular cartilages of some of the large joints, such as the knee.

Joint cavities are connective-tissue spaces containing special tissue fluid, the mucoid **synovial fluid**, which serves as a lubricant for smooth action of the joint. Free cells, mostly monocytes and other macrophages in small numbers, are found in it.

Joint cavities sometimes communicate with **bursae** outside the articulation. These are connective-tissue spaces around tendons or between muscles. They, too, permit easy movement of one structure upon another. They are formed by connective-tissue membranes lined with flattened cells and containing fluid similar to that in the cavities of joints.

The articular capsules are supplied with blood vessels and lymphatic vessels, but dense fibrous and fibrocartilaginous components of the synovial membrane contain relatively few vessels. Afferent end organs, such as lamellated corpuscles, are found in and around the capsules of joints. These are pressure receptors.

SUGGESTED READING

Anderson, D. R.: Ultrastructure of Elastic and Hyaline Cartilage of the Rat. *American Journal of Anatomy*, vol. 114, pp. 403–439, 1964.

Bernard, G. W., and D. C. Pease: An Electron Microscopic Study of Initial Intramembranous Osteogenesis. *American Journal of Anatomy*, vol. 125, pp. 271–290, 1969.

Brookes, M.: *The Blood Supply of Bone. An Approach to Bone Biology*. Appleton-Century-Crofts, Inc., New York, 1971.

Cooper, R. R., J. W. Milgram, and R. A. Robinson: Morphology of the Osteon. An Electron Microscopic Study. *Journal of Bone and Joint Surgery*, vol. 48A, pp. 1239–1291, 1966.

Enlow, D. H.: *Principles of Bone Remodeling*. Charles C Thomas, Publisher, Springfield, Ill., 1963.

Goel, S. C.: Electron Microscopic Studies on Developing Cartilage. *Journal of Embryology and Experimental Morphology*, vol. 23, pp. 169–184, 1970.

Ham, A. W.: Bone, Chap. 15, pp. 378–447, in *Histology*, 7th ed. J. B. Lippincott Company, Philadelphia, 1974.

Owen, M.: The Origin of Bone Cells. *International Review of Cytology*, vol. 28, pp. 213–238, 1970.

Scherft, J. P.: The Lamina Limitans of the Organic Matrix of Calcified Cartilage and Bone. *Journal of Ultrastructure Research*, vol. 38, pp. 318–331, 1972.

Thyberg, J.: Ultrastructural Localization of Aryl Sulfate Activity in Epiphyseal Plate. *Journal of Ultrastructure Research*, vol. 38, pp. 332–342, 1972.

Vaughan, J. M.: *The Physiology of Bone*. Oxford University Press, London, 1970.

Wilsman, N. J., and D. C. Van Sickle: Cartilage Canals, their Morphology and Distribution. *Anatomical Record*, vol. 173, pp. 79–94, 1972.

Chapter 7

Blood and Lymph

Blood is a simple form of connective tissue, first formed in mesenchymal vascular spaces of human embryos at early somite stages. In the adult it composes 7 to 8 percent of the body weight—roughly 6 liters. About 55 percent of this is fluid. All the rest is made up by cellular elements, there being no fibrous component under normal conditions.

Blood is a circulating tissue, integrating one region of the body with another. It is the vehicle for transporting respiratory gases, nutritional materials, metabolic wastes, and various substances produced by cells; and it distributes body heat. Pervading all organs, it provides a means of mobilizing defenses against tissue damage and disease.

BLOOD PLASMA

The fluid interstitial ground substance of blood is called **plasma**. Cells and other formed elements, unattached to one another, are suspended in it. It is a pale yellowish, slightly alkaline fluid, invisible in histologic sections. Plasma contains inorganic salts in ionized form (mainly sodium, calcium, potassium, bicarbonate, chloride, and phosphate) as well as proteins (notably, globulins and albumins). Constant levels of these constituents are maintained. Plasma contains varying amounts of substances that are involved in nutrition (e.g., glucose, amino acids, and lipids), waste products of metabolism (such as urea), and a number of substances produced by cells (hormones, for example). The volume of the blood plasma is held at a constant level, even, when necessary, at the expense of the volume of fluid in the interstitial and intracellular compartments.

When vessels are opened and blood is exposed to the air, coagulation occurs, and a globulin (fibrinogen) of the plasma precipitates in the form of delicate fibrils of **fibrin**. The formed elements are enmeshed in the clot. The remaining clear fluid is known as **serum**. This should not be confused with plasma, the fluid part of unclotted blood. Fibrin bears some resemblance to collagen. The fibrils have cross striations, but their periodicity is about 250 Å instead of 640 Å.

FORMED ELEMENTS

The formed elements of the blood are erythrocytes, leucocytes, and platelets. Only the leucocytes are complete cells with nuclei. Mature erythrocytes lack nuclei and are appropriately called red blood corpuscles (RBC). The platelets are cytoplasmic pieces of certain large cells in bone marrow. The formed elements of blood are illustrated in Fig. 7.1.

Erythrocytes Red blood corpuscles are minute circular biconcave discs. They are highly differentiated cells that have lost their nuclei during the last stage of their development in the bone marrow. Mature erythrocytes have lost not only their nuclei but also their mitochondria. Electron micrographs show no golgi complex, endoplasmic reticulum, nor ribosomes—just a dark, finely granular mass enclosed by the plasmolemma.

Erythrocytes of adult human beings vary only slightly in size. They are about 1.9 μm thick and 8.5 μm in diameter in fresh blood. The diameter is 7.5 μm or less in blood films and only about 7.2 μm in fixed tissues. The corpuscle is a handy measuring stick for estimating size of adjacent structures in histologic sections; for this purpose, it is considered to be 7 μm in diameter.

The shape of the erythrocyte is particularly well suited to the function it performs. Transport of oxygen and carbon dioxide is effected by the iron-containing pigment, **hemoglobin,** in its cytoplasm. Biconcavity and small size place all the hemoglobin of the erythrocyte in close proximity to its surface. The total surface area of all the erythrocytes of an adult person is about 2,000 times that of the body, or nearly an acre.

The substance of the erythrocyte is about two-thirds water and one-third solids, of which almost 95 percent is hemoglobin. This pigment imparts a pale greenish-yellow hue to the individual corpuscle, but in mass it reflects red light, which accounts for the color of blood. Hemoglobin is denser near the surface than in deeper parts of the cytoplasm. The amount of this pigment in each 100 ml of blood is about 15 g, slightly less in women than in men. There is about 1 mg of iron in each milliliter of packed corpuscles.

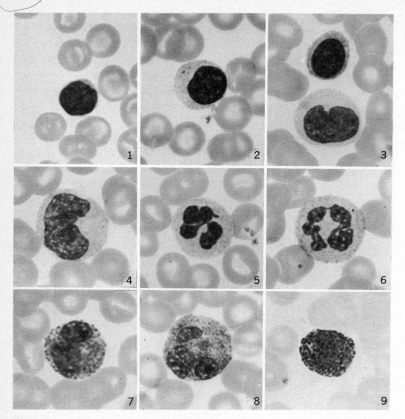

Figure 7-1 Formed elements of human blood: *1*, small lymphocyte; *2*, medium-sized lymphocyte with azurophilic granules in the cytoplasm; *3*, lymphocyte and monocyte; *4*, monocyte; *5* and *6*, neutrophils; *7* and *8*, eosinophils; *9*, basophil; platelets are present in *2* and *5*. Wright's stain. Photomicrographs, ×1,200.

Erythrocytes appear as flexible and elastic bodies when examined in the capillary circulation of living animal. They bend in adjusting to the lumen of the smallest blood vessels as they pass through.

Erythrocytes are the most numerous formed elements, and it is usual to express their number per cubic millimeter of blood. Some normal variation occurs, but the mean values are about 4.5 million per cubic millimeter in adult women and 5 million in men. The total number of erythrocytes in the body has been estimated at 25×10^{12}. The number of corpuscles per cubic millimeter of blood increases at high altitudes and may reach 6 or 7 million. The number in the newborn infant is about the same as that in the adult.

There is usually little time in histology courses to devote to techniques of hematology, but much can be gained by looking at fresh blood under the microscope. If a drop of blood is placed on a slide under a cover slip, dispersed corpuscles, presenting front and profile views, revealing their characteristic shape, will be seen. In thick films of fresh blood, corpuscles sticking together and resembling stacks of coins may be observed. These, known as "rouleaux," are shown in Fig. 7.2 as they appear in a scanning electron micrograph. If a little of the fluid is allowed to evaporate from a fresh preparation, the surfaces of erythrocytes will be found beset with conical and knoblike projections. They are said to have become "crenated." Crenation occurs in consequence of an increase in density of the plasma, causing it to become slightly hypertonic. If its density is decreased by allowing water to diffuse into it, the plasma becomes hypotonic, and the corpuscles appear swollen, assume globoidal shape, and finally burst. This phenomenon is known as "hemolysis." The shadowy remains of erythrocytes consist mainly of their delicate membranes.

Erythrocytes are constantly undergoing destruction, and new ones are added to the blood stream. Their life-span is about 120 days. Their immediate predecessors are hemoglobin-containing cells with darkly staining nuclei, found in the bone marrow but seen in circulating blood of healthy human beings only during early infancy. At birth, about 1 percent of the erythrocytes are these nucleated cells. After appropriate supravital staining, a few of the nonnucleated

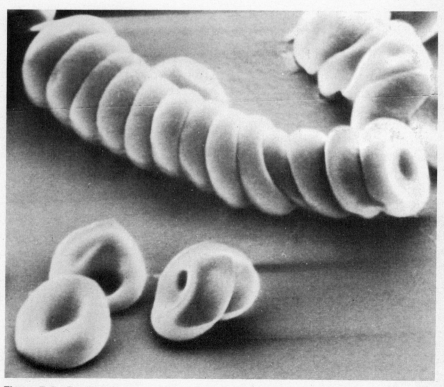

Figure 7-2 Erythrocytes in rouleaux formation. Scanning electron micrograph by the late Sarah Luce. About ×3,400. *(Contributed by E. W. Dempsey.)*

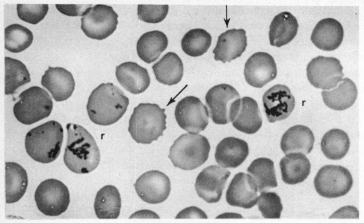

Figure 7-3 Reticulated erythrocytes, *r*, in a blood film from a newborn human infant. Note the variation in size among the corpuscles and a tendency toward crenation in some indicated by *arrows*. Photomicrograph, ×1,200.

erythrocytes—about 1 percent in adults and 6 percent in the newborn infant—exhibit a blue network, seen in Fig. 7.3. This is a remnant of polysomes. These cells are called reticulated erythrocytes, or **reticulocytes**. An increase in their number in the adult is indicative of acceleration of erythrocyte production. Few erythrocytes in blood films depart from the 7.5 μm average diameter, but some larger and smaller than average are encountered in the blood of the newborn infant (Fig. 7.9).

Erythrocyte metabolism is anaerobic; glucose is oxidized to lactic acid to provide energy. Hemoglobin combines loosely with oxygen in the lungs to form oxyhemoglobin. Upon arrival in tissues where the oxygen tension is lower than that in the lungs, oxygen is given up, and the contents of the erythrocytes become slightly less acidic, making it possible for carbon dioxide to be accepted. Returning to the lungs, the process is reversed; carbon dioxide leaves, the hemoglobin becomes a little more acidic, oxygen is taken up again.

The plasma membrane of the erythrocyte is not simply an inert encasement for the contents. Its molecular structure is such that binding sites for specific antibodies are provided.

Leucocytes Colorless "white" blood corpuscles are called leucocytes. They are much less numerous than erythrocytes, numbering only about 7,000 to 8,000 per cubic millimeter of human blood. These cells are relatively inactive while being transported in the blood or lymph streams, but are able to move out and occupy interstitial spaces. More than one kind of leucocyte can be identified in microscopic preparations of fresh blood, but these can be studied most advantageously in stained blood films. Table 7.1 presents a comparison of leucocytes.

Two categories of leucocyte are based on the presence or absence of specific membrane-bounded granules in the cytoplasm. Those with granules are designated **granular leucocytes**; those without them, **agranular leucocytes**. The two differ also in respect to other structural features. Granular leucocytes have oddly shaped nuclei, often multilobulated, while agranular leucocytes have relatively large spherical or indented nuclei and lightly basophilic cytoplasm.

Granular leucocytes, erythrocytes, and blood platelets are formed and go through maturation in the bone marrow; therefore, they have been designated the **myeloid series** of blood elements. The agranular leucocytes arise from bone-marrow stem cells that pass into lymphatic organs where they continue to multiply and mature; therefore, they have been designated the **lymphoid series** of cells.

Human granular leucocytes are of three kinds, differing from one another in respect to the staining reaction of their specific cytoplasmic granules. Those with large granules that stain intensely pink with the acid dye eosin are called acidophilic or eosinophilic granulocytes, or simply "eosinophils." Those with large granules colored just as brilliantly with the basic dye polychrome methylene blue are known as basophilic granulocytes, or simply "basophils." The third, and much the most numerous variety, have smaller granules, most of which are only faintly visible with the usual stains. Their specific granules are

Table 7.1 Comparison of Leucocytes

	Neutrophils	Eosinophils	Basophils	Lympho-cytes	Monocytes
Percentage	65 to 75	2 to 5	0.5	20 to 25	2 to 6
Size, μm	10 to 12	10 to 14	9 to 12	6 to 12	12 to 15
Nucleus	Dark; two to five lobes	Light; two to three lobes	Light; two to three lobes	Dark; slightly indented in large cells	Light; indented or curved
Specific granules	Small neutrophilic	Coarse eosinophilic	Few coarse basophilic	Nongranular (occasionally azurophilic granules)	Nongranular (few azurophilic granules)
Cytoplasmic background	Unstained	Unstained	Unstained	Basophilic	Less basophilic
Relative amount of cytoplasm	Great	Great	Great	Small	Great
Phagocytosis	Marked	Negligible	Negligible	Negligible	Marked
Motility	Marked	Less marked	Marked	Marked	Marked

neither bright pink nor dark blue, but a pale intermediate neutral shade. Consequently, these leucocytes have been designated as neutrophilic granulocytes, or simply "neutrophils." Structural differences among the three types of granular leucocytes are seen in Fig. 7.1.

Neutrophils compose 65 to 75 percent of all leucocytes. They are larger than erythrocytes, usually measuring 10 to 12 μm in diameter. The cytoplasm is characterized mainly by the membrane-bounded specific granules. A golgi complex, some mitochondria, glycogen inclusions, but few ribosomes are seen in electron micrographs (Fig. 7.4).

The granules vary in size. A few electron-dense primary granules, about 0.4 μm in diameter, contain hydrolyzing enzymes like those in lysosomes. These are azurophilic granules, visible in stained preparations. More numerous secondary granules are lighter, measure only about 0.3 μm in diameter, and contain antibacterial enzymes. In stained preparations these "neutral" specific granules are barely visible.

The nuclei of neutrophils are variously shaped but most often consist of long, twisted or bent masses of darkly staining chromatin, constricted into two

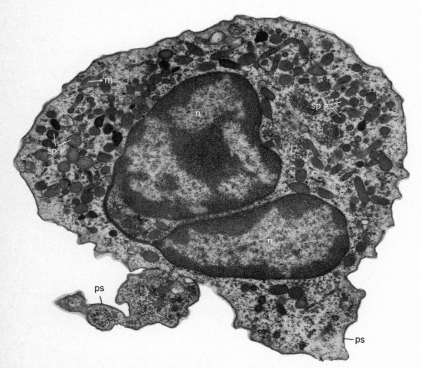

Figure 7-4 Part of a neutrophil (human). Two connected lobes of the nucleus, *n*, mitochondria, *m*, many specific granules, *sp g*, and a few ribosomes, *r*, are visible. Pseudopodia, *ps*, are extended. Electron micrograph, ×14,000 *(Contributed by J. A. Freeman.)*

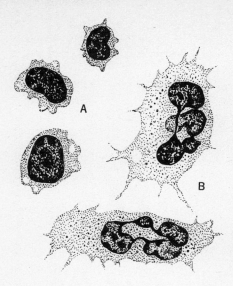

Figure 7-5 Lymphocytes, *A,* and neutrophils, *B,* in supravitally stained preparation of fresh blood on a warm stage, showing pseudopodia extended. ×1,200. *(JFN)*

to five lobules. For this reason, some writers call them "polymorphonuclear" leucocytes. Multilobulation of the nucleus characterizes the older neutrophils. Young neutrophils, with a simpler nucleus, shaped like a U or V, compose about 3 to 5 percent of the leucocytes. The sex chromatin body is visible in some of the neutrophils of females. An increase in number of young neutrophils indicates increased leucopoietic activity.

Neutrophils are migratory and phagocytic. They excel among all forms of leucocytes in ameboid movement (Fig. 7.5). It is probable that neutrophils do not perform any function within the blood stream, but they are not confined there. They can make their way out between the endothelial cells of the capillaries. They respond to the presence of certain substances in tissues by migration toward or away from them; i.e., they exhibit positive and negative chemotaxis. The lives of all granulocytes in the blood are short; indeed, they live only about 8 hours after leaving the bone marrow.

Neutrophils may be thought of as forming a large standing army, constantly mobilized and ever ready for body defense, for they are the first on the scene in case of infections. Infections call out reserves from the bone marrow. A marked rise in their number in the blood constitutes inflammatory "leucocytosis." Once out in the tissues, neutrophils can engulf small particles and bacteria. They appear to have a predilection for the pyogenic organisms. Neutrophils differ from other phagocytes, which are not mobilized so quickly and often engulf bacteria without killing them. Neutrophils are sometimes called "microphages" in contrast to the slower macrophages.

Eosinophils are more spectacular in appearance, although less numerous, than neutrophils (Fig. 7.6). They constitute 2 to 5 percent of all leucocytes, and are slightly larger than neutrophils (up to 14 μm in diameter). The nucleus is usually less polymorphous, often appearing as two lobes connected with a nar-

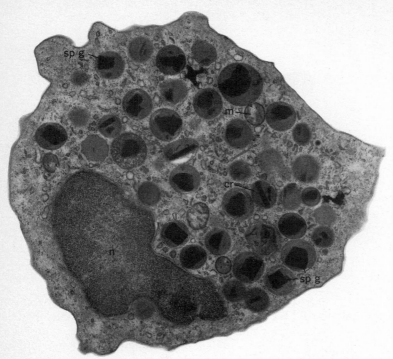

Figure 7-6 Part of an eosinophil (human). One lobe of the nucleus, *n*, mitochondria, *m*, and numerous specific granules, *sp g*, some containing rectangular electron-dense crystalloid bodies, *cr*, are visible. Electron micrograph, ×14,000. *(Contributed by J. A. Freeman.)*

row bridge. Their characteristic feature is the prominent acidophilic granules in their cytoplasm. No one with normal color vision can miss these, yet it is common experience for students to mistake neutrophils for eosinophils. In blood films, there will be one leucocyte to every 600 erythrocytes, but only one eosinophil to 20,000 erythrocytes.

The granules of eosinophils are larger than those of neutrophils, measuring up to 1 μm in diameter (compare them in Figs. 7.4 and 7.6). Many of them contain lamellated crystalloid bodies. The cytoplasm of eosinophils contains a few mitochondria, and a distinct golgi complex is often seen.

Eosinophils perform no noteworthy functions while circulating, but they are migratory cells that are more easily found outside the blood stream in loose connective tissue. There they exhibit antibacterial activities and phagocytosis of antigen-antibody complexes. Increased numbers of eosinophils appear in the blood and tissues of patients with certain parasitic and allergic diseases.

Basophils are the rarest of all cells in human blood. They constitute only about 0.5 percent of the leucocytes, or one basophil to 120,000 erythrocytes. Therefore, the student should not be surprised if he fails to find one in the first hour or so. Should one be found, there will be no question about its identity, because basophils are fully as spectacular as eosinophils. The chief difference is that their large granules are stained dark blue with the usual blood stains. Granules are so striking that one often overlooks the rather large, lightly stained nucleus, less polymorphous than that of other granular leucocytes and often bilobed or kidney-shaped. The granules of basophils are water-soluble. For this reason, the cells do not show up in routine histologic sections. The blood basophils appear to be phagocytic, and their granules contain some lysosomal enzymes. An anticoagulant substance, heparin, and another substance, histamine, which causes muscle contraction and increased capillary permeability, are components of basophil granules. An immunoglobulin (IgE), produced by plasmocytes, binds to sites on the surface of basophils. Reentry to the body of the antigen that induced secretion of the immunoglobulin results in release of the basophilic granules with their heparin and histamine. A severe allergic reaction, as in bronchial asthma, or an anaphylactic response may follow. These functions are shared by the basophils of connective tissue, known as labrocytes or "mast cells."

The agranular leucocytes are lymphocytes and monocytes, both of which are noticeably different from the leucocytes of the myeloid series. Both are involved in immunity mechanisms.

Lymphocytes, the smallest leucocytes, are illustrated in Figs. 7.1 and 7.5. Most of them measure 6 to 8 μm in diameter in blood films, about the same size as erythrocytes, although some are 8 to 10 μm, and a few as large as 12 μm in diameter will be encountered. They are nearly one-third as numerous as neutrophils, constituting 20 to 25 percent of all leucocytes under healthy conditions. In the smaller members of this class, the cytoplasm is scanty and forms just the slightest pale blue crescent around a spherical, darkly stained, and blotched nucleus. The cytoplasm is a little more plentiful, and the nucleus is slightly indented in the larger circulating lymphocytes. The nucleus of the small lymphocyte is dark, and the nucleolus rarely visible except in thin sections (Fig. 7.7). Lymphocytes, especially large ones, may have a few azurophilic granules in the cytoplasm. Mitochondria are not numerous, and a golgi complex is present but not often conspicuous. The ribosomes are scantily represented.

Lymphocytes are actively ameboid cells and make their way through the endothelium of capillaries. They are found in great numbers in the surrounding loose fibrous connective tissue and, especially, the reticular tissue of lymphatic organs, where they arise. They even pass through the mucous membranes lining digestive, respiratory, and urogenital passages of the body. Lymphocytes in the blood and lymph streams are inactive cells.

Although it seems from inspection of lymphocytes in stained blood films that they are of one kind, varying only in size and amount of cytoplasm, we know that there are at least two types, each with very different functions. Lymphocytes of one functional type circulate for many years, even for life. Those of the other type have short lives. Both types play important roles in the mechanisms of immunity and are discussed further in this regard in Chap. 13.

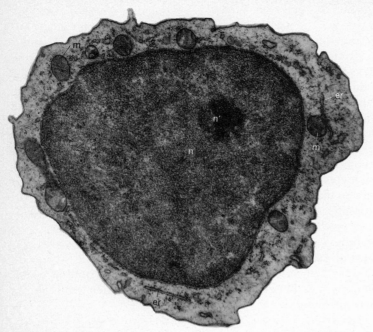

Figure 7-7 Lymphocyte (dog). Note the small amount of cytoplasm as compared with the amount of it in granulocytes. The nucleus, *n*, has a distinct nucleolus, *n'*. The cytoplasm has mitochondria, *m*, and scanty endoplasmic reticulum, *er*. Electron micrograph, ×14,000 *(Contributed by J. A. Freeman.)*

Monocytes are less numerous than lymphocytes and are larger, measuring 12 to 15 μm in diameter, or even more. The larger, older monocytes have a characteristic structure, but the smaller, younger ones are practically indistinguishable from large blood lymphocytes. The cytoplasm may be a little less basophilic, commonly containing a few azurophilic granules. The nucleus is eccentrically placed and is more or less deeply indented; it may be kidney-shaped or even horseshoe-shaped in the larger monocytes (Figs. 7.1 and 7.8). Golgi complex, centrioles, mitochondria, and other organelles are represented in the cytoplasm.

Monocytes constitute only 2 to 6 percent of all leucocytes in the blood stream. As with other agranular leucocytes, the blood stream is not their natural habitat. They are more important cells than their small number seems to signify. They are marshaled into the tissues during inflammation more slowly than the neutrophils. They are more commonly encountered in such a disease as tuberculosis than they are in the acute infectious processes that attract neutrophils. Once monocytes reach the connective tissue, they are indistinguishable from tissue macrophages. They can become distended with tissue detritus and bacteria in regions of degeneration or infection.

Lymphocytes and monocytes are related to each other, and both are related to other connective-tissue cells. They are only slightly differentiated

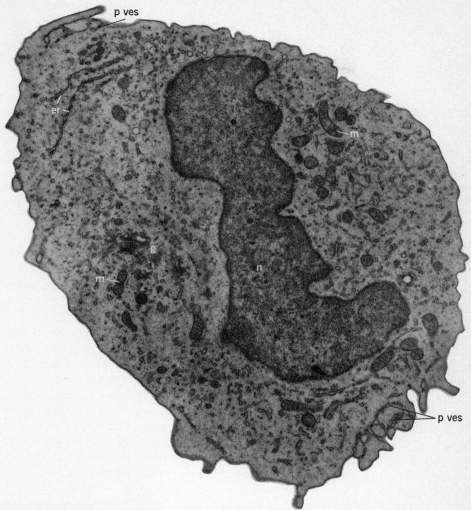

Figure 7-8 Monocyte (dog). Note the nucleus, *n*, mitochondria, *m*, and pinocytotic vesicles, *p ves*. Endoplasmic reticulum, *er*, and golgi complex, *g*, are visible. Electron micrograph, ×10,000. *(Contributed by J. A. Freeman.)*

cells and can undergo further differentiation. The interrelationship among lymphocytes, monocytes, plasmocytes, tissue macrophages, fibrocytes, reticular cells, and some endothelial cells appears to be quite close. Both lymphocytes and monocytes can become neoplastic.

Stained blood films commonly contain leucocytes that were deformed in preparation. A crushed neutrophil nucleus can be mistaken for a basophil, for example. On the other hand, blood may contain basophilic particles from nuclei

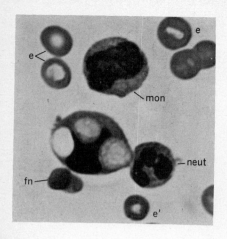

Figure 7-9 Unusual forms of blood corpuscles in an infant. A large agranular leucocyte appears in the center; its nucleus is deformed by three inclusions. Just below it is a free nucleus, *fn*, from a normoblast. Other leucocytes are monocyte, *mon*, and young neutrophilic granulocyte, *neut*. Several erythrocytes, *e*, are seen, one of which is microcytic, *e'*. Photomicrograph, ×1,200.

of cells that have died and disintegrated. These particles are called "hemoconia." An abnormally vacuolated agranular leucocyte is shown among other blood cells of a human infant in Fig. 7.9.

Blood Platelets   Other formed elements of the blood are tiny ovoid, biconvex bodies measuring only about 2 to 4 μm in diameter. There are about 250,000 of these blood platelets in each cubic millimeter of human blood. Their life-span is about 10 days. They are not always easily observed in stained blood films. When blood is drawn, they tend to stick to one another and to anything else with which they come in contact. Careful scrutiny reveals a central, more basophilic, region and a peripheral, clear, hyaline zone. Electron micrographs show specific granules, lamellae of endoplasmic reticulum, microvesicles, and scattered ribosomes in the protoplasm (Fig. 7.10). Platelets are not cells,[1] but simply bits of the cytoplasm of certain giant cells of the bone marrow, known as megakaryocytes. Their formation is described in Chap. 8.

Blood platelets participate in the formation of blood clots. Their numbers are decreased in certain blood disorders including various forms of anemia. They tend to disintegrate when hemorrhaging blood makes contact with other tissues.

Normal hemostasis appears to depend on synthesis of platelet prostaglandins.[2] Inhibition of synthesis by administration of aspirin prolongs bleeding time. Experimental administration of a fatty-acid precursor of platelet prostaglandins (arachidonic acid) has been shown to cause aggregation of platelets of rabbits, forming platelet thrombi in the lungs. A sudden release of this pecur-

---

[1]They are sometimes erroneously referred to as "thrombocytes," a term that is more appropriately applied to true cells of similar function in the fowl, but not limited in occurrence to birds.
[2]See Chap. 24.

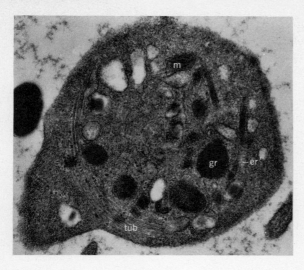

Figure 7-10 Platelet in human blood. Note specific (alpha) granules, *gr*, tubular agranular endoplasmic reticulum, *er*; a mitochondrion, *m*; and peripheral bundle of microtubules, *tub*. Electron micrograph, ×30,000. *(Contributed by J. Rosenbluth.)*

sor substance may help explain the basis for such thrombotic diseases as pulmonary embolism, myocardial infarction, and stroke.

LYMPH

Lymph is a fluid collected from most parts of the body. It has limited clotting ability. Tissue fluid enters lymph capillaries of the periphery to become peripheral lymph. Whatever cells are contained in the lymph—large and small lymphocytes only, under healthy conditions—are added during its passage through lymph nodes (Fig. 11.1*E*). The composition of lymph varies according to the organ in which it arises. Thus, lymph from the liver is unusually rich in proteins. That from the small intestines contains lipids during digestion. Fatty lymph is known as "chyle." The milky appearance of this fluid has imparted the name "lacteals" to the lymph capillaries of the mesenteries. Lymph joins the blood stream by way of the thoracic and right lymphatic ducts. Dark-field examination of fresh blood, drawn after the subject has eaten a meal containing fat, reveals the presence of innumerable tiny lipid particles known as **chylomicrons**. These are contributed to the blood by the lymph of the thoracic duct.

BLOOD GROUPS

Human blood can be classified on an immunologic basis into groups A, B, O, and AB. Everyone's blood is of one of these four types. Although no visible structural differences exist, erythrocytes of some individuals have on their membranes molecules of antigen A, while those of some others carry on their surface antigen B. These antigens can react with anti-A and anti-B serum antibodies (immunoglobulins), often disastrously. Safety in transfusing blood from one person to another depends on matching erythrocytes of one against serum of the other beforehand.[3]

Another antigen, the Rh factor, is found on erythrocyte membranes of about 85 percent of individuals, and is responsible for certain transfusion reactions. A person is Rh-compatible with another when his or her erythrocytes do not induce an immune reaction in another person whose blood carries anti-Rh antibodies.

SUGGESTED READING

Bainton, D. F., and M. G. Farquhar: Segregation and Packaging of Granule Enzymes in Eosinophilic Leukocytes. *Journal of Cell Biology*, vol. 45, pp. 54–73, 1970.

Berlin, N. I., T. A. Waldmann, and S. M. Weissman: Life Span of Red Blood Cell. *Physiological Reviews*, vol. 39, pp. 577–616, 1959.

Harris, J. W.: *The Red Cell, Production, Metabolism, Destruction: Normal and Abnormal*. Harvard University Press, Cambridge, Mass. 1963.

Malawista, S. E., and K. G. Bensch: Human Polymorphonuclear Leukocytes: Demonstration of Microtubules and Effect of Colchicine. *Science*, vol. 156, pp. 521–522, 1967.

Pirkle, H., and P. Carstens: Pulmonary Platelet Aggregates Associated with Sudden Death in Man. *Science*, vol. 185, pp. 1062–1064, 1974.

Silver, M. J., W. Hoch, J. J. Kocsis, S. M. Ingerman, and J. B. Smith: Arachidonic Acid Causes Sudden Death in Rabbits. *Science*, vol. 183, pp. 1085–1087, 1974.

Tanaka, Y., and J. R. Goodman: *Electron Microcopy of Human Blood Cells*. Harper & Row, Publishers, Incorporated, New York, 1972.

Whitelaw, D. M.: The Intravascular Lifespan of Monocytes. *Blood*, vol. 28, pp. 455–464, 1966.

[3]Blood of group A is compatible with blood of other persons of group A and of persons with group AB blood, but is not compatible with blood groups B or O. Blood of group-B individuals can be given to subjects with blood of groups B or AB, but not to those with blood of groups A or O. Blood of group-O persons can be transfused to those with blood of any group (universal donor), but a group-O individual cannot receive blood of any type except group O. Group-AB blood can be given only to individuals with group-AB blood, but a person with this type of blood can receive transfusions of any other group (universal recipient).

Bone Marrow

Bone marrow is a simple, diffuse organ consisting of a special form of connective tissue related to blood. Its stroma is reticular connective tissue; its parenchyma, various marrow cells, some engaged in formation of blood elements and others storing fat.

Bone marrow is a vital organ, well protected by encasement in the bones. It is one of the largest organs of the body, constituting altogether nearly 5 percent of the body weight; this makes it more than twice the size of the liver.

Bone marrow is essential not only for production of blood corpuscles and platelets throughout life but also for bone formation and reconstruction (particularly in the young individual), erythrocyte destruction, and lipid storage. Moreover, it is an important component of the immune system.

Two types of bone marrow are described in the adult, yellow and red, according to the predominance or lack of predominance of lipocytes, found to some extent in all bony spaces. The two varieties are compared in Fig. 8.1. Red marrow, or **myeloid tissue**, is most abundant in young individuals and is the only type present in prenatal life. During postnatal growth, the warmer cavities of the more centrally located bones retain more of the red marrow than the cooler cavities of the peripheral long bones, which become filled with yellow marrow. Bones of the extremities contain much yellow marrow. The proportion of the two types can change in the bone with fluctuation in metabolic conditions and temperature. Yellow marrow can be made to give way to red marrow experi-

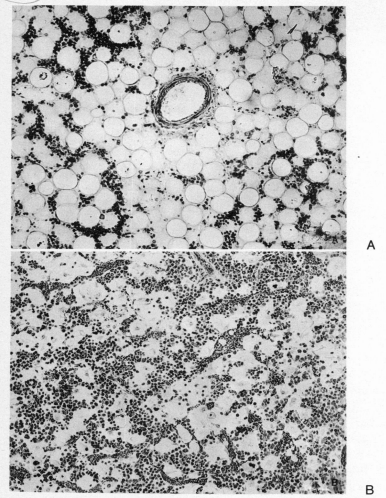

Figure 8-1 Bone marrow (monkey). *A*, yellow marrow showing many lipocytes, an arteriole, and a few groups of hemopoietic cells; *B*, red marrow containing few lipocytes and many hemopoietic elements. Photomicrograph, ×150.

mentally by locally increasing temperatures and maintaining them at the higher level.

Yellow Marrow The structure of yellow marrow is simple. It is formed mainly by lipocytes in a fine network of reticular fibers. The lipocytes appear to be somewhat less compactly arranged than those in the adipose tissue beneath the skin. They crowd out the hemopoietic red marrow, leaving only a small island of it here and there. Yellow marrow is of less concern at present than the red variety. The term "bone marrow" henceforth will be used for red marrow unless the other type is specifically designated.

Red Marrow The tissue of bone marrow is so soft that it can be aspirated through a sternal-puncture needle. Its cells, like those of blood, can be spread and examined in stained films. The organization of bone marrow, however, is best determined in histologic sections.

The stroma of bone marrow is difficult to see in sections stained by the usual methods. It is heavily overlaid with the marrow cells. Although it appears to be quite delicate, the stroma does lend some support to the blood vessels that enter and leave the marrow, especially the intrinsic sinusoidal vessels. There are no lymphatic vessels in bone marrow.

The marrow sinusoids, as shown in Fig. 8.2, are wide, thin-walled blood vessels. Their walls are formed by flattened cells that differ from endothelial cells by their phagocytic property. They are actually fixed macrophages, sometimes called "littoral cells," belonging in the reticuloendothelial category. These lining cells of the sinusoids detach themselves from the walls with ease and then make their way, as free macrophages, through the blood stream of the marrow sinusoids. Both the fixed and free macrophages serve an important function: They engulf and digest particulate matter, including the remains of worn-out erythrocytes as they circulate slowly through the bone marrow and brush against the sinusoid walls.

The thin sinusoidal walls are readily penetrated by cells formed in the bone marrow. Erythrocytes, leucocytes, and the other formed elements reach the

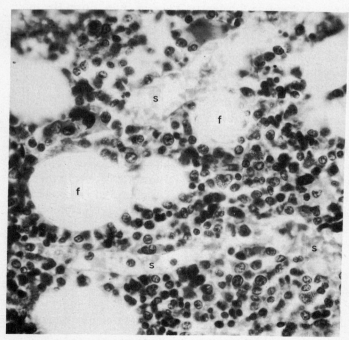

Figure 8-2 Human red bone marrow. Marrow sinusoids, *s*, and lipocytes, *f*, are surrounded by myeloid tissue. Photomicrograph, ×300.

blood stream in this manner. Most cells of myeloid tissue will be described under the topic Hemopoiesis, below.

There are other cells that do not participate in blood-cell formation. In spongy bone, especially that of young individuals, one encounters osteoblasts and osteoclasts. The lipocyte is one of the most numerous cells of red marrow.

HEMOPOIESIS

Blood formation begins at the middle of the third week of prenatal life in extraembryonic mesenchymal "blood islands." The liver becomes a site of hemopoiesis during the second month, and soon thereafter the spleen engages in this process. Hemopoiesis first occurs in the fetal bone marrow in the third month. The earlier foci are temporary and normally cease to form blood cells before birth, leaving the bone marrow and lymphatic organs as the definitive sites of hemopoiesis.

The first recognizable precursors of erythrocytes begin to form in presomite embryos. Leucocytes do not appear until the seventh or eighth week in the fetal liver and even later in lymphatic organs. Blood platelets are not encountered in human fetuses before the second half of gestation.

Hemopoiesis is the main function of adult bone marrow. The indifferent cell, from which all elements derive, is not easy to identify in stained sections. It has a large ovoid and rather lightly staining nucleus; the cytoplasm is pale, making the cell inconspicuous among the darker myeloid cells. From the indifferent cells arise not only the blood-forming elements but also macrophages, lipocytes, and the cells associated with bone.

The precursors, or "stem cells," of all blood elements are the **hemocytoblasts**. The word is appropriate because it means "blood-cell former." They are indistinguishable from most large lymphocytes, the largest measuring nearly 15 μm in diameter. One is visible in Fig. 8.3. Hemocytoblasts divide actively and, therefore, may be encountered in groups.

Origin of Agranular Leucocytes   Hemocytoblasts of bone marrow, by continuing to divide, produce medium-sized and small lymphocytes. The term **lymphoblast** is used by some writers to designate mitotic stem cells in this line. Colonies and even nodules of lymphocytes are encountered in the bone marrow of young children, but their number decreases markedly with adolescence, and it is not easy to find them in adult bone marrow.

The lymphocytes of bone marrow readily traverse sinusoidal walls and enter the blood stream. They come to lodge in such places as the thymus, spleen, lymph follicles, and lymph nodes, where they continue to proliferate to produce mature forms of lymphocytes (Chap. 13).[1]

Other agranular cells encountered in bone marrow are plasmocytes and monocytes. The former are of variable occurrence. Their number increases

[1]Some investigators believe that lymphocytes may arise from more than one type of precursor cell and that the connective-tissue indifferent cell is not their only source.

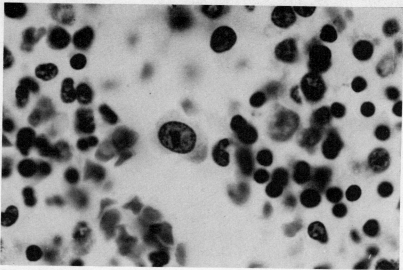

Figure 8-3 Human bone marrow section. The large cell in the center is a hemocytoblast. Photomicrograph, about ×750.

with demand for antibodies. Monocytes are no different from other free macrophages. Whether the bone marrow is the principal site of origin of monocytes is unknown, but it is possible that they are derived from lining cells of the marrow sinusoids.

Origin of Granular Leucocytes The first cells in the granulocyte line are designated **granuloblasts**. As soon as specific granules appear in their cytoplasm, it is customary to call them **myelocytes**. They are the most numerous cells of the bone marrow. The ones with neutrophilic granules outnumber those with eosinophilic or basophilic granules. Basophilic myelocytes are not seen in sections of human marrow because their granules are water-soluble and disappear during preparation of the slides. Myelocytes divide mitotically to reproduce more myelocytes of their own type. Consequently, colonies of each variety of myelocytes will be found in sections of bone marrow (Fig. 8.4). Specific granules of myelocytes first appear in the vicinity of the golgi complex. Agranular endoplasmic reticulum and free ribosomes are present but become fewer as granulocytes reach maturity.

A number of steps in the development of granular leucocytes can be seen in bone marrow. The basophilia of the cytoplasm of the early myelocyte subsides as the specific granules increase in number. The last mitotic divisions give rise to myelocytes that can scarcely be distinguished from young granular leucocytes. They have darkening U-shaped nuclei like young circulating neutrophils. Hematologists give the names "promyelocyte" and "metamyelocyte" to the early and late stages in differentiation of myelocytes. These names may be ignored for the sake of simplification, but one should keep in mind the

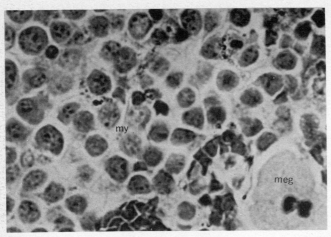

Figure 8-4 Human bone marrow section (same preparation as in Fig. 8-5), showing a colony of myelocytes, *my*, and a megakaryocyte, *meg* (lower right). Photomicrograph, ×450.

sequence of principal stages in formation of granular leucocytes: hemocytoblast → myeloblast → myelocyte → granular leucocyte. All these can be identified in thin films and sections of bone marrow.

Origin of Erythrocytes The stages in development of erythrocytes constitute another major category of bone-marrow cell. Some hemocytoblasts give rise to cells with a little hemoglobin in their basophilic cytoplasm near the large open nucleus. They are called **erythroblasts**. They undergo many mitotic divisions, gaining hemoglobin each time and losing the basophilia. The nucleus becomes more chromatic, the nucleolus disappears, components of the endoplasmic reticulum decrease in number, ribosomes become fewer and scattered, and the cell decreases in size. Hematologists call the large early erythroblasts "proerythroblasts." The late ones, which are smaller and retain a little basophilia, giving their cytoplasm a gray appearance, are designated "polychromatophil erythroblasts." Colonies of erythroblasts and the cells derived from them are encountered in sections of bone marrow (Fig. 8.5). Few isolated erythroblasts will be observed, but numerous groups of them will be seen.

Further differentiation leads to the formation of **normoblasts**. These cells are about the size of erythrocytes. The cytoplasm is filled with hemoglobin and is acidophilic. Nuclei are distinctly darker and smaller than those of their precursors. Late normoblasts have darkly stained nuclei. They have lost the ability to divide. They become erythrocytes by extrusion of the nucleus surrounded by a thin film of cytoplasm and plasmolemma. Figure 8.6 illustrates diagrammatically the sequence of formation of erythrocytes from erythroblasts.

The method of extrusion of the nucleus from normoblasts to form erythrocytes has caused speculation for many years, and the best explanation is

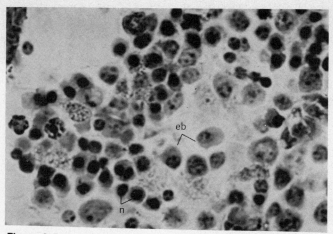

Figure 8-5 Human bone marrow section (same preparation as in Fig. 8-4) showing a colony of normoblasts, *n*, and erythroblasts, *eb*. Photomicrograph, ×450.

the following. In rabbits, the thin walls of the marrow sinusoids are known to be traversed by the blood corpuscles formed in the loose stroma outside the vascular channels of the bone marrow. The sinusoidal linings in this species possess numerous minute perforations, approximately 1 to 4 μm in diameter. The cytoplasm of normoblasts can extrude readily through these pores, but the nuclei, being denser, are retained outside. Figure 8.7 illustrates this process in the rabbit. The sinusoidal lining cells of the bone marrow are firmly attached to one another by junctional complexes. No blood cells can traverse the walls at these sites, but only do so through the pores.[2]

Some erythrocytes exhibit a cytoplasmic reticulum, with supravital staining methods, when first produced in the marrow. This may represent a remnant of the ribosomes. The corpuscles showing it are called reticulated erythrocytes or **reticulocytes**. Keep clearly in mind the distinction between reticulocyte,

[2]Other views are held on this subject. The possibility that disintegration of the nucleus by enzymatic activity as one way the erythrocyte is formed may be considered.

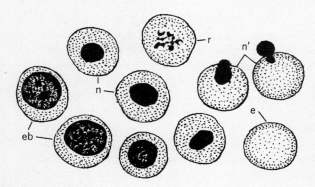

Figure 8-6 Schematic representation of formation of erythrocytes, *e*, from erythroblasts, *eb*, through condensation and extrusion of nuclear material of normoblasts, *n* and n'. One reticulated erythrocyte, *r*, is shown. About ×1,200. *(JFN)*

147

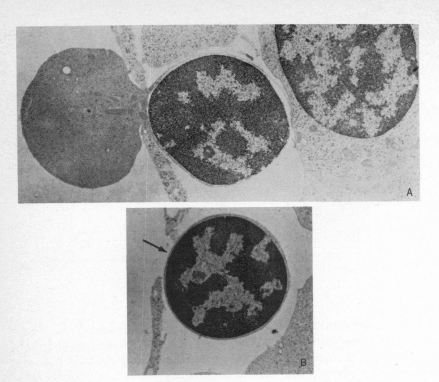

Figure 8-7 Transmural passage and enucleation of a rabbit normoblast. *A*. Nucleated cell, a normoblast, in passage through the wall of a marrow sinus, showing the cytoplasm completely within the lumen and the nucleus remaining behind. *B*. A nucleus located near a pore (*arrow*); it may have been recently lost from a passing normoblast. Electron micrograph, ×8,500. *(Contributed by W. H. Crosby and M. Tavassoli,* Science, *vol. 179, pp. 912–913, 1973. Reproduced with permission of the publishers.)*

which is a red blood corpuscle, and reticular cell, which is a connective-tissue cell of a primitive kind.

To summarize, the following stages in the development of erythrocytes are identifiable: hemocytoblast → erythroblast → normoblast → erythrocyte.

It is always a matter of surprise in studying bone marrow to find that the number of cells in the granular leucocyte line is so great in proportion to the number in the erythrocyte line. In circulating blood, there are approximately 800 erythrocytes to every granular leucocyte. Why does not a similar numerical relationship exist in the bone marrow, where both these elements are formed? The erythrocytes form and quickly get out into the circulation, where they live about 120 days—longer than most leucocytes. The precursor cells of granular leucocytes normally develop more slowly, remaining longer between mitotic divisions in the bone marrow; so there are nearly three times as many myelocytes as erythroblasts.

Origin of Blood Platelets The study of bone marrow would be easy, indeed, if all the cells could be as readily identified as the **megakaryocyte.** Aside

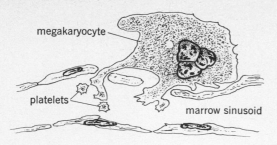

megakaryocyte

platelets

marrow sinusoid

Figure 8-8 Formation of blood platelets from pseudopodia of a megakaryocyte in the bone marrow of a kitten. The pseudopodia project into the lumen of a sinusoid through gaps in its lining. About ×600. *(Modified from J. H. Wright.) (WEL)*

from its large size, ranging up to 40 μm in diameter, and its ragged outline, the megakaryocyte is characterized by an irregularly lobulated nucleus. Young megakaryocytes with less complicated nuclei will be found. They, too, arise from hemocytoblasts.

The central cytoplasm of the megakaryocyte contains a golgi complex, lamellae of granular endoplasmic reticulum, and ribosomes in clusters—the features of protein-synthesizing cells. The peripheral cytoplasm has numerous channels of agranular endoplasmic reticulum that tend to subdivide the cytoplasm into small units. These channels serve as cleavage planes that permit pieces of the cytoplasm to break off as they are released into the sinusoids to become blood platelets.

Release of platelets is preceded by extrusion of cytoplasmic processes of the megakaryocyte through pores in the sinusoidal walls. When cleavage occurs, single platelets or clusters of them become swept away in the blood stream. Figure 8.8 illustrates this process. The function of platelets was considered in Chap. 7.

SUGGESTED READING

Bessis, M., and J. P. Thiery: Electron Microscopy of White Blood Cells and Their Stem Cells. *International Review of Cytology*, vol. 12, pp. 199–241, 1961.

Crosby, W. H., and M. Tavassoli: Fate of the Nucleus of the Marrow Erythroblast. *Science*, vol. 179, pp. 912–913, 1973.

DeBruyn, P. P. H., P. C. Breen, and T. B. Thomas: The Microcirculation of the Bone Marrow. *Anatomical Record*, vol. 168, pp. 55–68, 1970.

Steinberg, B., and B. Hufford: Development of Bone Marrow in Adult Animals. *Archives of Pathology*, vol. 43, pp. 117–126, 1947.

Stohlman, F. (ed.): *Hematopoietic Cell Proliferation*. Grune & Stratton, Inc., New York, 1970.

Weiss, L.: The Structure of Bone Marrow. Functional Interrelationships of Vascular and Hematopoietic Compartments of Experimental Hemolytic Anemia. *Journal of Morphology*, vol. 117, pp. 467–537, 1965.

———: *The Cells and Tissues of the Immune System*. Prentice-Hall, Inc., Englewood Cliffs, N. J., 1972.

Wintrobe, M. M.: Factors and Mechanisms in the Production of Red Corpuscles. *Harvey Lectures*, ser. 45, pp. 87–126, 1950.

Muscular Tissue

clear or obvi[?]
to eye or
mind.

Muscular tissue is composed of cells specialized to contract. Rapid contractility is a property of protoplasm that distinguishes animals from plants. The activity of muscles is responsible for most of the outward manifestations of animal life. Not only movements of the body but also the heartbeat, breathing, and many invisible movements of a visceral nature come about by muscle contractions. Those of the embryonic heart begin to propel blood before other muscles have developed. In walls of arteries, muscle cells help regulate blood flow. Skeletal muscles provide more than motive power. They also limit movements, brace against gravity, and maintain posture. They are always in a state of partial contraction, known as "tonus." Body heat is produced by this activity.

There are two main varieties of muscular tissue: smooth and cross-striated. The latter can be subdivided into skeletal and cardiac types. The parenchymal elements of all three types of muscle are elongated cells, designated as **muscle fibers.** They are, for the most part, arranged in layers or bundles surrounded by stromal connective tissue, but they exist singly or in small groups in some locations. The cells of all varieties of muscular tissue have a common characteristic: They exhibit myofibrils in the cytoplasm consisting of parallel arrays of microfilaments. Table 9.1 presents the principal features of the three types of muscle fiber.

Table 9.1   Principal Features of Muscle Fibers

	Smooth	Skeletal	Cardiac
Shape	Individual; long, tapering cells	Syncytial; long, straight fibers	Cells joined in long fibers
Branching	Not as a rule	Not as a rule	Nearly all fibers
Nucleus	Single, central, cigar-shaped	Multiple, peripheral, ovoid	Multiple, central, ovoid
Cell surface	Plasma membrane	Thick sarcolemma	Thin sarcolemma
Myofibrils	Unstriated, evenly distributed	Striated, often arranged in groups	Striated, usually arranged in distinct groups
Sarcoplasm	Scanty	Scanty	Considerable amount
Intercalated disc	Absent	Absent	Present
Nerve supply	Sparse; simple endings	Extensive; specialized endings	Sparse; simple endings
Blood supply	Slight	Rich	Rich, but anastomoses inadequate
Action	Involuntary	Voluntary	Involuntary, rhythmic

SMOOTH MUSCLE

Smooth-muscle fibers are the simplest of the three types. They are sometimes called "plain," because they are unadorned by cross banding. The fibers vary in length in different locations. Those of the lower vertebrates (Fig. 9.1A) are larger than those of man. In general, smooth-muscle fibers are about 6 μm wide and 15 to 500 μm long, the shortest being found in walls of small blood vessels, the longest, in the gravid uterus.

Sections parallel to the long axis show smooth-muscle fibers overlapping one another. Their nuclei, elongated and limited to one per fiber, are located in the midportion of each. In cross sections, smooth-muscle fibers appear to be of many diameters, with or without nuclei. Their appearance depends on whether they were cut through the middle or one of the tapering ends. Few intrinsic details are seen in routinely stained histologic sections of smooth muscle. Figure 9.2 shows the usual appearance.

Distinguishing smooth muscle from collagenous connective tissue in histologic sections should not be difficult. In sections stained with hematoxylin and eosin, the muscle fibers are pale gray while the collagenous fibers are light pink. Some other staining methods differentiate the two tissues more sharply.

The fine structure of smooth muscle cells has several points of interest. Cytoplasm near the nucleus contains numerous mitochondria, a golgi complex, centrioles, endoplasmic reticulum, and a few ribosomes. Glycogen granules are usually a prominent feature. More peripherally it contains parallel arrays of microfilaments, called **myofilaments** (Fig. 9.3).

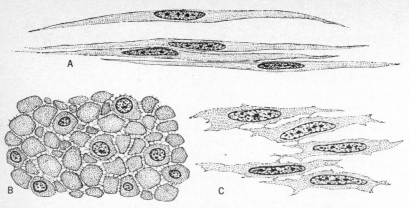

Figure 9-1 Smooth muscle: *A*, fibers isolated from a frog's bladder; *B*, cross section of fibers in the bladder of a kitten; *C*, short smooth-muscle cells isolated by macerating the aorta of a dog. ×900. *(JFN)*

The **myofibrils** of light microscopy appear to be formed by clumps of these myofilaments. Both thick and thin filaments are present in well-fixed muscle fibers, the fewer thick myofilaments often appearing to attach to **dense bodies** much as thick myofilaments attach to Z lines of striated muscle. Contractile proteins, actin and myosin, have been demonstrated chemically in smooth muscle. Contraction is believed to occur by sliding actions between filaments.

The plasmolemma of smooth-muscle cells is a unit membrane, showing vesicular indentations suggestive of pinocytosis. One cell is separated from

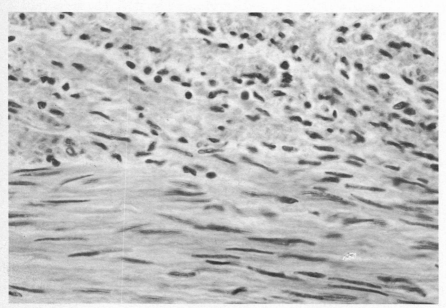

Figure 9-2 Smooth muscle of the human esophagus. Fibers are cut in cross section in the upper part of the figure and in longitudinal section in the lower part. Photomicrograph, ×600.

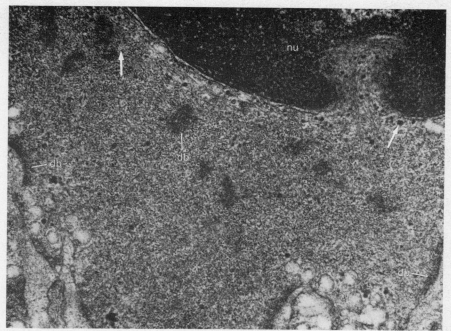

Figure 9-3 Smooth-muscle cell from intestine (toad). Cross section passing through the nucleus, *nu*. The cytoplasm is filled with thin filaments, giving it a granular appearance. Glycogen granules (*arrows*) are seen near the nuclear envelope. Dense bodies, *db*, are located centrally as well as along the plasmolemma. Electron micrograph, ×50,000. *(Contributed by J. Rosenbluth.)*

another by a little ground substance. Here and there in smooth muscle, one can see points of close contact between the cells where adjacent membranes are in close apposition in a gap junction or "nexus." Except at such places, appreciable interstitial space exists, and the ground substance separating the muscle cells contains a fine network of reticular fibers (Fig. 9.4).

Smooth muscle forms a prominent component of hollow tubular organs of gastrointestinal, respiratory, and urogenital systems. It occurs in the walls of all but the smallest blood vessels. Small groups of smooth-muscle fibers are found in the skin, notably associated with hair follicles. Special varieties of smooth muscles are located in the iris of the eye and in some glands.

Some smooth-muscle fibers can increase greatly in size as the occasion demands. During pregnancy, for example, those in the uterus become as much as eight times their original length. Denervation of smooth muscle does not lead to atrophy and disappearance of these muscle fibers.

Capillaries course in connective-tissue sheaths among groups or layers of smooth-muscle cells, but the blood supply is not so rich as in other types of muscular tissue.

The nerve supply of smooth muscle in such regions as the intestines is rather sparse. Not every muscle cell receives a nerve ending. Integration of one

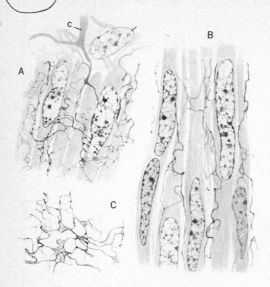

Figure 9-4 Smooth muscle in small arteries: *A* and *C*, kitten tongue; *B*, human kidney; *c*, collagenous fiber. Recticular fibers have been darkened by silver carbonate stain. ×900. *(JFN)*

cell with another appears to be effected through the gap junctions. The smooth-muscle cells of blood vessels have simple nerve endings that are more numerous than in most other organs.

The character of contraction of smooth muscle differs in various locations. That of the muscle in the walls of hollow organs, such as the intestines, is slow and sustained. In the walls of blood vessels, contraction can occur more quickly to regulate blood flow. Smooth-muscle contraction in the gravid uterus during labor can generate extraordinary force. A notable characteristic of most smooth-muscular tissue is ability to perform work for long periods with less evidence of fatigue than is exhibited by the voluntary skeletal variety.

SKELETAL MUSCLE

Skeletal muscle forms the flesh of the body, constituting over 40 percent of the total body weight and exceeding any other tissue in amount. Like other muscle, it arises from mesoderm, more specifically, from that part of each mesodermal somite known as the "myotome." Development begins in human beings at about the sixth week and ends in most muscles before birth. Further growth consists of enlargement of the fibers. Various stages of development can be seen side by side in fetal muscles. Closely packed cells of the myotomes become elongated and spindle-shaped. These cells (myoblasts) multiply mitotically and then fuse to form a multinucleated syncytial muscle fiber. The young fiber is known as a "myotube" (Fig. 9.5); its nuclei are located in the center of the fiber. Later the nuclei come to lie at the periphery beneath the cell membrane. Young myoblasts can contract as soon as myofibrils appear.

Fibers of skeletal muscle are typically long, straight, unbranching cylinders. They are among the largest cells in the body, 10 to 100 μm in thickness, and in some muscles up to many centimeters in length. Some fibers of short

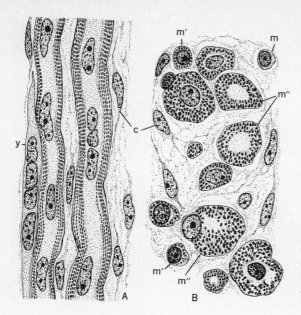

Figure 9-5 Developing skeletal-muscle fibers: *A*, longitudinal section; *B*, cross section; *c*, mesenchymal cells; *m*, *m'*, *m"*, myoblasts in several stages of development; *y*, young myoblast with four nuclei but no fibrils. ×900. *(JFN)*

muscles extend the entire length of the muscle, but most of them do not. Quickly acting muscles, such as those moving the eyes, have the thinnest fibers. The limb muscles have thick fibers. Figure 9.6 illustrates the histologic appearance of the latter.

Skeletal-muscle fibers possess many nuclei—several hundred in the largest ones. The nuclei are less elongated than those of smooth-muscle fibers. One of the features of a skeletal-muscle fiber, differentiating it from other types, is the peripheral location of its nuclei beneath the surface of the fiber in the sarcoplasm.

Skeletal-muscle fibers have a more marked longitudinally striated appearance than do smooth-muscle cells. Each fiber is composed of many myofibrils. The myofibrils are discernible with the light microscope because they measure 0.2 to 2 μm in diameter. In cross sections they are resolved as fine dots that tend to be clustered (Fig. 9.7).

A prominent feature of skeletal-muscle fibers is their cross striations. These are composites of alternating differences in fine structure of the individual myofibrils, giving the appearance of cross banding to the whole fiber. The prominent light and dark stripes are called **isotropic** and **anisotropic discs** from their appearance under polarized light. They are easily seen in ordinary histologic preparations and can be demonstrated to advantage with iron hematoxylin stain (Fig. 9.7) which darkens the anisotropic discs.

Longitudinal sections of relaxed myofibrils may show a dark line transecting the light isotropic, and a faint light zone in the dark anisotropic disc. The isotropic disc is designated I; the anisotropic, A. The dark line in the I disc is designated Z; the light zone in the A disc, H; a faint M line traverses the H zone. The portion of a myofibril between two Z lines is known as a **sarcomere**.

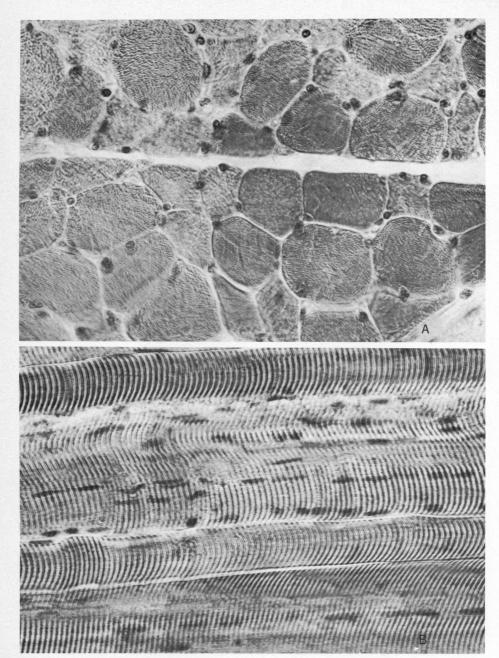

Figure 9-6 Human skeletal muscle. *A,* cross section; *B,* longitudinal section. Photomicrograph, ×600 .

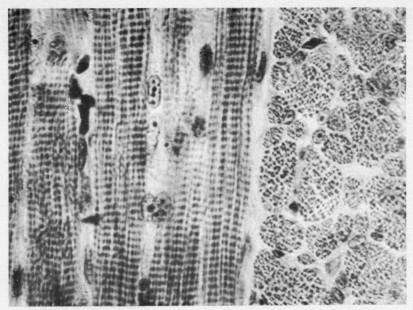

Figure 9-7 Skeletal muscle of a cat tongue; myofibrils are seen in cross section on the right and in longitudinal section on the left. Iron hemotoxylin stain. Photomicrograph, ×900.

It is the contractile unit of the myofibril. The I disc diminishes in thickness, and the H zone disappears when the muscle contracts, but the A disc remains unaffected. Details are revealed further by electron-microscopic study (Fig. 9.8).

Micrographs prepared from relaxed muscle show the myofilaments to be of two thicknesses (Figs. 9.9 and 9.10). The thicker ones, 100 to 150 Å in diameter, are confined to the A disc. Longer thin myofilaments, about 50 Å in diameter, surround each thick one in a hexagonal pattern, with minute projections of the thick filaments touching them. The thin filaments course through both I and A discs, but are interrupted in the middle of the latter during relaxation of the myofibrils, and this accounts for the H zone (Fig. 9.11*A*). Cross sections of relaxed myofibrils show only thin filament profiles in the I, both types in the A disc, and only thick filaments in the H zones (Fig. 9.11*B*).

Four of the major proteins that make up the contractile elements of muscle have been well characterized. Thick filaments are composed of several hundred macromolecules of **myosin** consisting of long and short chains. The short chains form the minute lateral projections from the filament that, in electron micrographs, appear to make contact with adjoining thin filaments. These short-chain bridges are oriented in such a way that they are not seen at the midpoint of the thick filament (Fig. 9.11*A*).

The thin filaments are composed of the other three proteins, **actin, tropomyosin**, and **troponin**. Actin molecules, the main component, are small and are arranged as long, paired, twisted strands of "beads." Slender filamentous tropomyosin molecules are aligned along the strands of actin. Globular

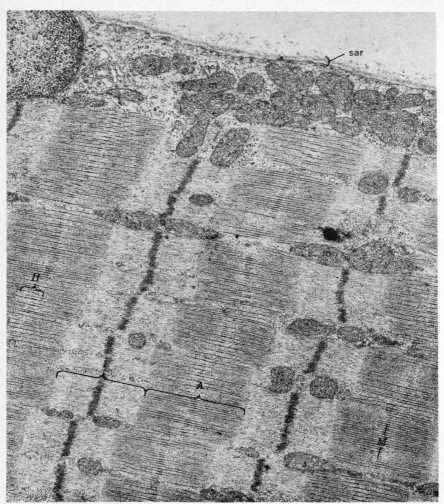

Figure 9-8   Skeletal muscle (human muscle fixed in phosphate-buffered osmium tetroxide, stained with uranyl acetate and lead citrate). Components of sarcomeres are A, I, H, and M bands and Z lines. Other abbreviations: *sar*, sarcolemma; *m*, sarcosomes, *n*, nucleus. Electron micrograph, ×20,000 *(Contributed by J. S. Resnick.)*

molecules of troponin are set periodically on the tropomyosin. Thin filaments attach to the Z lines, which are thin, transverse, protein structures. Thin filaments are absent in the middle of the sarcomere, thus accounting for the H zone. During contraction, the actin and myosin filaments slide across each other, while troponin and tropomyosin help regulate the initiation, speed, and termination of the contraction process.

Each skeletal-muscle fiber is ensheathed by the **sarcolemma.** When a fresh fiber is teased to fracture it, the myofibrils retract, and the sheath stands revealed. Electron micrographs show the sheath to be a compound structure composed of the plasmolemma of the muscle cell, and a basal lamina to which a little reticular connective tissue is adherent.

Within the muscle fiber, each myofibril is surrounded by a more or less longitudinally oriented meshwork of anastomosing tubules, cisternae, and vesicles of agranular endoplasmic reticulum to which the term **sarcoplasmic reticulum** is applied. Each sarcomere has its separate system terminating in enlarged, transversely oriented vesicles in the vicinity of junctions of A and I discs in mammals (Fig. 9.9).

Another entirely separate organelle lies between the terminal vesicles of the sarcoplasmic reticulum. It consists of a slender **transverse tubule**, forming the "T system." The transverse tubules are invaginations of the plasma membrane. The arrangement, in effect, puts the surface membrane of the muscle fiber in contact with deeply placed contractile units of the fiber. A tubule with the two associated terminal cisternae of the sarcoplasmic reticulum comprises a "triad." Figure 9.9 illustrates these structures in human skeletal muscle, where they are found at the A-I junction. In the lower vertebrates the transverse tubules lie on the Z lines (Fig. 9.12).

Highly developed, longitudinally oriented mitochondria occur beneath the sarcolemma and around the myofibrils in great numbers (Fig. 9.8), constituting the machinery for manufacturing adenosine triphosphate to satisfy the energy requirements of contraction. Glycogen granules, a storage form of glucose which provides fuel for the machinery, are numerous in the sarcoplasm (Fig. 9.12A).

Adenosine triphosphate (ATP) is hydrolized to adenosine diphosphate (ADP) and inorganic phosphate. This reaction takes place only in the presence of calcium, which is contained in the enlarged vesicles of the sarcoplasmic reticulum, especially those of the triad. Release of calcium ions occurs when membrane depolarization, incited by nerve impulses, spreads through the transverse tubules to the region of the triad. Calcium ions are instantly "pumped" back into the sarcoplasmic reticulum when the contraction stops.

These events constitute the basis for muscle contraction. When they occur, the actin filaments slide past the myosin filaments, the ends of the former colliding in the middle of the A disc and obliterating the H zone. The ends of the thick myosin filaments at the same time approach each other at the Z line in the I disc, reducing the thickness of the latter.

Contraction of a muscle fiber is triggered by an excitatory impulse generated at the motor nerve ending, passing over the plasma membrane of the fiber and, via the transverse tubules, to the interior myofibrils. Thus the signal reaches all contractile units promptly.

All skeletal muscles contract slowly at birth. Some retain this characteristic, but others become fast-contracting, so that there are two principal kinds of muscle in the adult: slow and fast. The slowly contracting muscles appear grossly to be redder in color than do the fast muscles. This difference in color results from a higher content of cytochromes, myoglobin (an oxygen-carrying protein of muscle that is similar to hemoglobin of the blood), and a denser capillary network. These constituents enable red muscles to contract for prolonged

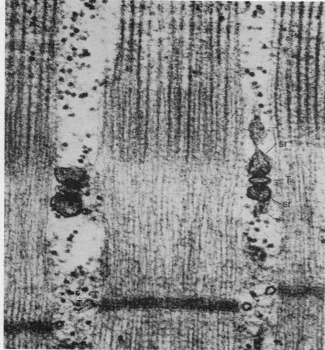

Figure 9-9 Human skeletal muscle sectioned longitudinally through parts of three myofibrils. Half of an A disc with M line through its light portion is seen above. Half of an I disc with its bisecting Z line appears below. Triad of sarcoplasmic reticulum, *sr*, on either side of a transverse tubule, *T*, is seen. Electron micrograph, ×73,000. *(Contributed by S. M. Walker.)*

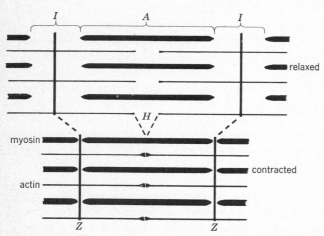

Figure 9-10 Diagram of changes occurring in a sarcomere with muscle contraction. The upper part shows myosin (*thick*) and actin (*thin*) filaments separated in the relaxed condition. The lower part shows them in the contracted state. *(CHP)*

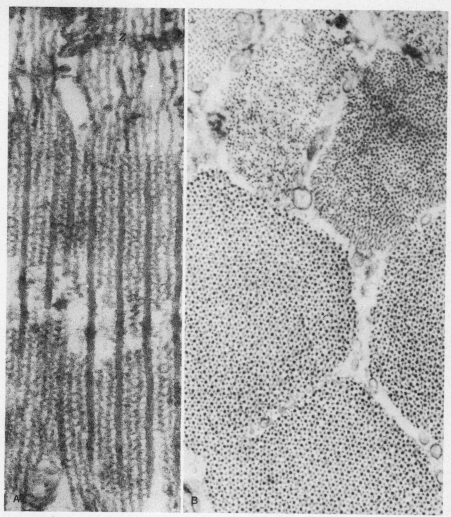

Figure 9-11   Two types of myofilaments; *A,* in longitudinal section; *B,* in transverse section. Note that the thick ones have tapering ends and that they are confined to the anisotropic disc, whereas the thin ones, attaching to the Z line, are deficient in the H. Parts of four myofibrils seen at the top of the transverse section, *B,* are cut through isotropic discs and show only the fine myofilaments. The three lower myofibrils are sectioned through anisotropic discs, showing both thick (coarse dots) and thin (fine dots) myofilaments. Electron micrographs: *A,* about ×165,000; *B,* about ×65,000. *(Contributed by H. E. Huxley.)*

periods of time (i.e., tonically) without becoming fatigued. When slow and fast muscles are examined histologically, however, it is seen that all slow fibers are red but that fast muscle fibers can be either red or white. Thus although there are two kinds of muscle, fast-white and slow-red, there are three kinds of muscle fibers, fast-white, fast-red, and slow-red (Fig. 9.13 and Table 9.2). The

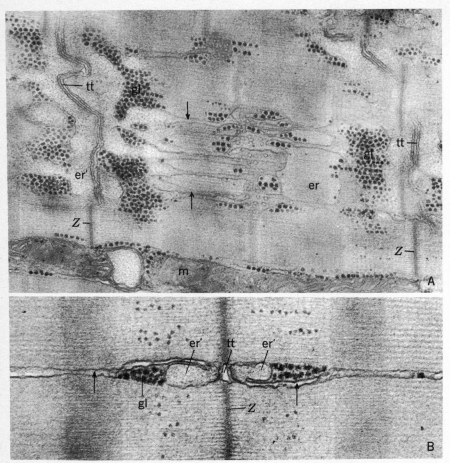

Figure 9-12 Skeletal muscle (frog) illustrating the transverse tubules (*tt*), sarcoplasmic reticulum (*er*), and glycogen (*gl*) at the junctions of sarcomeres, marked by Z lines. Note the swollen terminal cisternae of the sarcoplasmic reticulum (*er'*) containing some electron-dense particles. *A.* Tangential longitudinal section at the border of one myofibril where mitochondria, or "sarcosomes" (*m*), are visible. *B.* Longitudinal section showing components of the "triad." Confluence of terminal cisternae through narrowed intermediate portions of the sarcoplasmic reticulum are shown at the arrows. Electron micrographs: *A* ×31,800; *B*, ×60,000. *(Contributed by L. D. Peachey,* Journal of Cell Biology, *vol. 25, pp. 209–231, 1965.)*

speed of contraction (fast vs. slow) is correlated with adenosine triphosphatase (ATPase) activity, while the degree of redness reflects the ability of a fiber to contract for prolonged periods without becoming fatigued (tonic vs. phasic).

Muscles respond metabolically to neural influences as well as to demands of work. Their fibers are composed of two kinds of myosin (which accounts for the slow and fast contractions), each with a specific innervation that determines the kind of myosin in the fiber. When nerves to a slow muscle are rerouted experimentally to a fast one, the kind of myosin is reversed. Thus trophic influ-

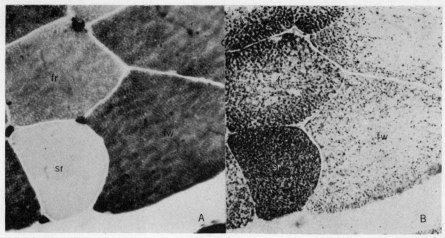

Figure 9-13 Serial sections of a cat skeletal muscle. The muscle on the left was stained to show actomyosin ATPase activity, which correlates with speed of contraction. That on the right was stained for succinic dehydrogenase activity which reveals the oxidative capacity or redness of the fibers. These preparations show that fast fibers may be red, *fr*, or white, *fw*, while slow fibers are invariably red, *sr*. Photomicrographs, ×425. *(Contributed by L. Guth.)*

ences of the nervous system can alter chemically the basic contractile protein. Although this subject is incompletely understood, it appears that neurons regulate gene expression in the muscle cell, and that the adult muscle fiber is a dynamic cell, capable of taking on a variety of phenotypic appearances under the regulation of the neurotrophic factors.

Muscles as Organs   Most skeletal-muscular tissue is found in muscles attached by tendons to parts of the skeleton. One may say that muscular tissue forms the parenchyma of muscles, and that connective tissue forms the stroma.

A good deal of areolar connective tissue invests skeletal muscles, forming the fascia or **epimysium** surrounding them and the **perimysium** that subdivides them (Fig. 9.14). Individual muscle fibers are invested, and small bundles of them are set apart, by delicate wisps of **endomysium**. The endomysium contains some reticular fibers. The connective tissue brings nerves and a rich blood-ves-

Table 9.2   Types of Muscle Fibers

Type of fiber	ATPase activity	Fatigability	Pattern of usage
Fast-White	High	Readily fatigued	Infrequent
Fast-Red	High	Fatigue resistant	Frequent
Slow-Red	Low	Fatigue resistant	Frequent

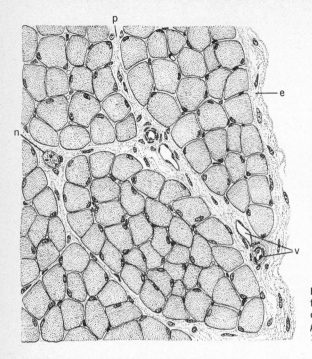

Figure 9-14 Skeletal-muscle fibers in cat gastrocnemius muscle; *e*, epimysium; *n*, small nerve; *p*, perimysium; *v*, blood vessels. ×300. *(JFN)*

sel plexus into close association with muscle fibers. There is a rich capillary bed.

Muscle fibers end freely in the connective tissue within muscles or are joined to dense connective-tissue fibers in fascia, periosteum, or tendons. At myotendinal junctions, the sarcoplasm is enclosed by the sarcolemma at the end of the muscle fiber, and the sarcolemma is firmly adherent to collagenous fibers of the tendon. Collagenous fiber bundles of the perimysial septa merge directly with the denser bundles of tendon fibers. Figure 9.15 illustrates the junction of muscle fibers with dense collagenous fibers of an aponeurosis.

Muscles are innervated by efferent (motor) and afferent (sensory) nerve fibers. Each fiber receives one motor ending at the middle of its length (Figs. 15.9 and 15.10), but this does not mean that each muscle fiber contracts individually. Each nerve fiber supplies numerous muscle fibers. When a nerve impulse comes down the fiber, the whole group of muscle fibers, constituting a **motor unit**, goes into action together. Unlike smooth muscle, that of the skeletal type is dependent upon an intact nerve supply. Not only do most skeletal muscles fail to contract after their nerves have degenerated, but the muscle fibers undergo atrophy and may disappear. Increased exercise of muscles leads to enlargement or hypertrophy of the individual fibers.

Afferent nerve fibers arise in skeletal muscles from dendrites in groups of special muscle fibers surrounded by connective-tissue sheaths. These constitute the neuromuscular spindles; they vary in size, consisting of 3 to 20 muscle fibers, which usually are shorter and thinner than the working-muscle fibers,

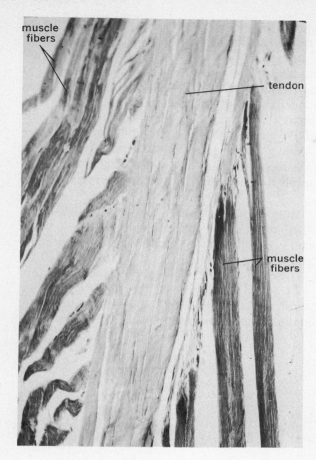

muscle
fibers

tendon

muscle
fibers

Figure 9-15 Junction of skeletal-muscle fibers with tendon.
Photomicrograph, ×150.

tend to be tapered, and may have centrally placed nuclei. The spindle fibers are
supplied by motor endings similar to those of other muscle fibers, but, in addition, dendritic branches of afferent neurons wind around them to form elaborate stretch receptors (Figs. 15.14 and 15.15). The spindle-muscle fibers do no
real pulling, but their contraction stimulates the dendrites and initiates nerve
impulses which are transmitted to the central nervous system. These impulses
are not consciously perceived, but serve reflex functions.

CARDIAC MUSCLE

Cardiac muscle composes the heart walls and is found in the large veins entering it. There is considerable structural resemblance to skeletal muscle. Although each contraction is followed by a moment of rest, the heart beats rhyth-
mically, tirelessly, and endlessly from a very early embryonic stage until death.
The nervous system exerts regulatory control over it but is not essential for the
inherent rhythmicity of the contractions and plays no part at first.

The cells of cardiac muscle are joined end to end to form the muscle fibers that branch and anastomose and falsely appear to form a syncytium. Grossly the fibers of the heart wall are arranged in layers or sheets that wind in overlapping spirals to form the myocardium. A section through the ventricular wall of the heart will cut some fibers across and others lengthwise or obliquely. Figures 9.16 and 9.17 illustrate the appearance of this type of muscle.

Longitudinal sections through cardiac muscle demonstrate the muscle fibers, separated by strands of loose connective tissue containing an extensive capillary bed that keeps this actively working muscle well supplied with blood. This connective tissue contains many reticular fibers attaching to the sarcolemma of muscle cells. The sarcolemma of cardiac muscle cells is more delicate than that of skeletal muscle.

One or two nuclei are found in each muscle cell. They resemble those of skeletal muscle but occur in the interior of the cell. Sarcoplasm is more abundant than in skeletal muscle and is equally rich in glycogen. Mitochondria are more numerous than in skeletal muscle and have a more densely packed arrangement of cristae (Fig. 9.18), commensurate with the high energy requirement of cardiac muscle.

Myofibrils resemble those of skeletal muscle, but some of them branch. They have a tendency to group in columns, especially at the periphery of the

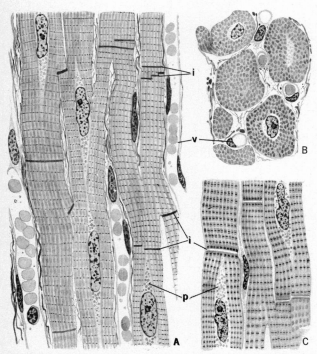

Figure 9-16 Cardiac-muscle fibers: A and B, ventricle of monkey heart; C, human heart; i, intercalated discs; p, granules of lipofuscin pigment; v, blood vessels. ×900. (JFN)

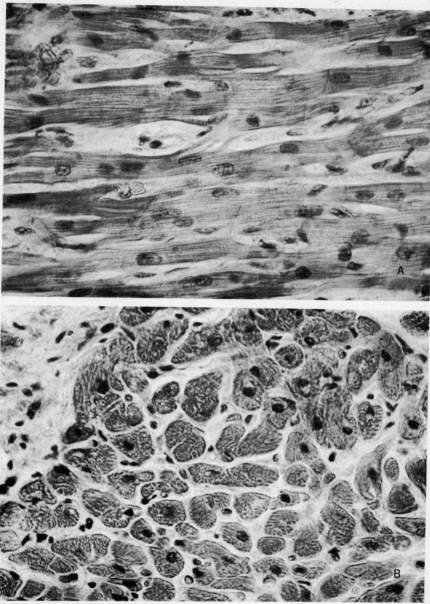

Figure 9-17 Cardiac muscle in a human heart ventricle: *A*, longitudinal section; *B*, cross section. Cross striations on the fibers are poorly stained, but central nuclei, intercalated discs, and branching fibers are seen. The epicardium is located at the upper left in *B*. Photomicrograph, ×600.

cell. Both thick and thin filaments are present, giving rise to cross banding with the same lines seen in the skeletal variety of muscle.

The sarcoplasmic reticulum forms an anastomosing system of smooth-walled vesicles and tubules that are continuous from one sarcomere to the next. The terminal dilatations, typical of skeletal muscle, are not found in cardiac muscle. However, transverse tubules—invaginations of the sarcolemma—do make contacts with membranes of the sarcoplasmic reticulum. The tubules usually are located at the Z lines of cardiac muscle, instead of at the A-1 junctions in mammalian skeletal muscle. Some of the tubules have branches extending longitudinally, thus increasing the area of membranous contact with sarcoplasmic reticulum. The space between membranes at points of contact is about 150 Å wide. The sarcolemma also makes direct contact with surface units of the sarcoplasmic reticulum.

Cardiac muscle fibers have a characteristic feature: their **intercalated discs** (Fig. 9.16). These are specializations of the plasmolemma of adjoining muscle cells, resembling desmosomes. Intercalated discs do not always extend straight across a muscle fiber, but as a rule take a stairstep course from the Z line of one myofibril to that of the next, the level shifting by the length of one sarcomere. Electron micrographs illustrate features of cardiac-muscle-cell contacts (Figs. 9.18 and 9.19).

Contractions of cardiac muscle are more prolonged and sustained than are those of skeletal muscle. Since they are automatic and occur without direct nervous action, conduction of synchronizing impulses takes place through the muscle tissue. Modified cardiac-muscle fibers[1] form a special impulse-conducting system which performs this function. They differ from the working muscle fibers in structure, being larger in diameter, swollen in appearance, and containing more sarcoplasm with relatively few myofibrils. Like other cardiac-muscle fibers, their nuclei are centrally placed, and they possess intercalated discs. Figure 9.20 illustrates their appearance. Further discussion is found in Chap. 10.

REGENERATION AND AGING

Smooth-muscle fibers are the least highly differentiated of the three types. They can regenerate to a limited extent, mainly by differentiation from indifferent cells, but partly by mitotic division of existing muscle cells. Traumatic injuries of layers of smooth muscle are healed largely by connective-tissue scar formation. Little is known about aging of smooth muscle.

Skeletal-muscle fibers can undergo some regeneration if the sarcolemma, a little of the sarcoplasm, and the nuclei are not entirely destroyed. Skeletal muscles contain an appreciable population of small uninucleated cells that have scanty cytoplasm. These cells lie alongside the muscle fibers, and for this reason are called satellite cells. During normal growth these cells divide; one

[1]These are commonly called "Purkinje fibers."

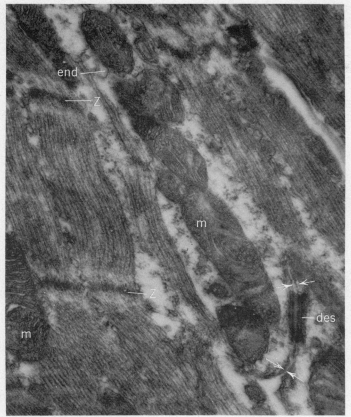

Figure 9-18 Intercalated disc of mouse cardiac muscle, *arrows* marking cell boundaries. Abbreviations: *des*, desmosomes; *end*, sarcoplasmic reticulum; *m*, mitochondria; *Z*, Z line of muscle fiber. Electron micrograph ×55,000. *(Contributed by F. S. Sjöstrand.)*

daughter cell fuses with the adjacent muscle fiber, thereby increasing the number of muscle-fiber nuclei. In this regard, the satellite cells of adult muscle resemble embryonic myoblasts. These cells may also contribute to the repair of traumatized muscle.

Maintenance requires the presence of intact motor nerves and motor nerve endings. Hypertrophy with use involves increase in muscle-fiber size rather than increase in number of fibers. The endocrine system is concerned in maintenance of healthy skeletal-muscle function. Repair of traumatic injury of skeletal muscles is effected by connective tissue. Age changes involve increase in connective tissue around muscle fibers and accumulation of pigment within the fibers.

Cardiac muscle, of all the varieties, is least able to undergo regeneration and repair, and damage to it can be most serious. Its blood supply is the richest, but in one sense it is the most precarious, because anastomoses between the ar-

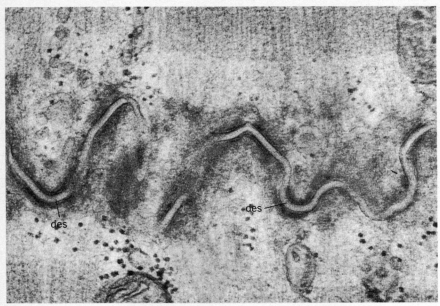

Figure 9-19 Intercalated disc, transverse portion, of cardiac-muscle fiber (cat). This represents an elaborate junctional complex between two muscle cells. Desmosomes, *des,* are prominent. Electron micrograph, about ×60,000. *(Contributed by D. W. Fawcett.)*

teries supplying it are inadequate. There is little evidence that cardiac-muscle fibers can reproduce or that they are replaced by differentiation from indifferent cells of the connective-tissue stroma. Cardiac-muscle fibers are remarkably resistant to daily wear and tear, but they show their age by accumulation of lipofuscin pigment. When the work load of the heart is maintained for long periods of time at a greater than normal level, cardiac-muscle fibers increase in diameter, but not in number.

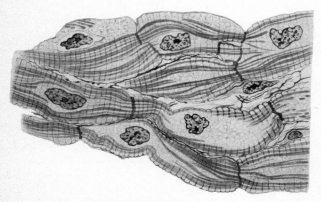

Figure 9-20 Fibers of the cardiac conduction system (monkey). Nuclei are surrounded by glycogen-filled sarcoplasm. Intercalated discs appear to constrict the fibers. ×600. *(JFN)*

SUGGESTED READING

Ashley, C. C.: Calcium and the Activation of Skeletal Muscle. *Endeavour*, vol. 30, pp. 18–25, 1971.

Bois, R. M.: The Organization of the Contractile Apparatus of Vertebrate Smooth Muscle. *Anatomical Record*, vol. 177, pp. 61–72, 1973.

Carlson, B. M.: The Regeneration of Skeletal Muscle—A Review. *American Journal of Anatomy*, vol. 137, pp. 119–149, 1973.

Dewey, M. M., and I. Barr: Intercellular Connection Between Smooth Muscle Cells: The Nexus. *Science*, vol. 137, pp. 670–672, 1962.

Guth, L.: "Trophic" Influences of Nerve on Muscle. *Physiological Reviews*, vol. 48, pp. 645–687, 1968.

Hanson, J.: Evidence from Electron Microscopic Studies on Actin Paracrystals Concerning the Origin of the Cross-striation in the Thin Filaments of Vertebrate Skeletal Muscle. *Proceedings of the Royal Society of London*, ser. B, vol. 183, pp. 39–58, 1973.

Huxley, H. E.: The Double Array of Filaments in Cross-striated Muscle. *Journal of Biophysical and Biochemical Cytology*, vol. 3, pp. 431–648, 1957.

Jean, D. H., L. Guth, and R. W. Albers: Neural Regulation of the Structure of Myosin. *Experimental Neurology*, vol. 38, pp. 458–471, 1973.

Merton, P. A.: How We Control the Contraction of Our Muscles. *Scientific American*, vol. 226, no. 5, pp. 30–37, May, 1972.

Murray, J. M., and A. Weber: The Cooperative Action of Muscle Proteins. *Scientific American*, vol. 230, no. 2, pp. 58–71, February, 1974.

Porter, K. R., and C. Franzini-Armstrong: The Sarcoplasmic Reticulum. *Scientific American*, vol. 212, no. 3, pp. 72–80, March, 1965.

Rayns, D. G., F. O. Simpson, and W. S. Bertaud: Transverse Tubule Apertures in Mammalian Myocardial Cells: Surface Array. *Science*, vol. 156, pp. 656–657, 1967.

Sjöstrand, F. S., and E. Andersson-Cedegren: Intercalated Discs of Heart Muscle, Chap. 12, pp. 421–445, in G. H. Bourne (ed.), *The Structure and Function of Muscle*, vol. 1., Academic Press, Inc., New York, 1960.

Watanabe, H., and Y. Yamamoto: Freeze-etch Study of Smooth Muscle Cells from Vas Deferens and Taenia Coli. *Journal of Anatomy*, vol. 117, pp. 553–564, 1974.

Chapter 10

Heart

The heart (cor) is an overgrown blood vessel the muscular wall of which has become differentiated for intermittent contraction. It has four chambers: two thin-walled atria, serving chiefly as reservoirs, and two thick-walled ventricles, which do most of the work. The atria receive the blood, the right atrium admitting the superior vena cava, inferior vena cava, and large heart vein, known as the "coronary sinus." Into the left atrium open the four pulmonary veins. Contraction of the muscular walls of the atria aids only slightly in passing blood on into ventricles.

The ventricles, acting as a powerful double-force pump, send the blood on its way at just the right moment and with precisely the correct force into the pulmonary artery (right) and the aorta (left). The pressure required to force blood through the systemic circulation is about three times that needed to propel it through the lungs. Correlatively, the musculature of the left ventricle is heavier than that of the right ventricle.

Fibrous Skeleton Proper functioning of the heart depends on the presence of a skeleton of dense fibrous connective tissue which prevents overdistention of orifices and provides attachments for sheets of muscle. The atria are attached to the ventricles by a fibrous plate, the atrioventricular septum. Orifices in this septum are encircled by heavy fibrous rings, to the edges of which are anchored the flaps of the right and left atrioventricular valves. Other orifices are associated with the pulmonary artery and aorta; their semilunar valves attach to fibrous cuffs which also are part of the skeleton of the heart. The dense fibrous connective tissue extends into the septum between the ventricles.

The atria and ventricles are separated by interatrial and interventricular septa. The former is thin and partly membranous and presents a shallow depression, the **fossa ovalis**, which marks the site of the aperture by which oxygenated inferior vena caval blood from the placenta entered the left atrium during fetal life.

Defective prenatal development of two overlapping septa (septum primum and septum secundum) leaves a patent foramen in the interatrial septum. This permits admixture of blood in the two atria with impaired oxygen saturation of the systemic blood. Septal defects are surgically remedial.

The interventricular septum is thick and muscular except near the atrioventricular orifices, where it receives a strong extension of the cardiac skeleton, giving it the name "septum membranaceum." Maldevelopment here produces an interventricular septal defect. Normally this septum is composed of dense fibrous connective tissue. It is inelastic, contains a few cartilagelike cells, and has a tendency to calcify or even ossify in old age. The os cordis is found here in certain large mammals.

Endocardium, Myocardium, and Epicardium   Three layers can be seen in the atrial as well as in the ventricular walls. The innermost layer is the **endocardium**, continuous with the internal coat of the vessels entering and leaving the heart. It is thicker in the atria than in the ventricles. Folds of endocardium form valves, including the flaps guarding the inferior vena cava and the coronary sinus.

The innermost component of the endocardium is endothelium on a basal lamina. Beneath this is a variable amount of fibrous connective tissue containing some elastic fibers and a few smooth-muscle cells. Blood vessels and branches of the special impulse-conducting system course in the deeper layer of the endocardium.

Structure of the cardiac wall is shown in Figs. 10.1 and 10.2. The **myocardium** is the thickest of the three coats. It is composed of cardiac muscle. The atrial myocardium is thin, and in the auricular appendages it has ridges, called pectinate muscles, extending into the lumen. Its outer layer is common to both atria.

The ventricular myocardium is more complex than that of the atria, and its arrangement can be studied best in gross specimens. There are no straight bundles of muscle fibers running from the base to the apex of the heart. Instead, the sheets of cardiac muscle are arranged spirally, deep fibers encircling each ventricle, with the thickest construction in the left. The spiral arrangement of muscle bundles makes contraction peculiarly efficient. Each heartbeat virtually wrings out the blood contained in the heart.

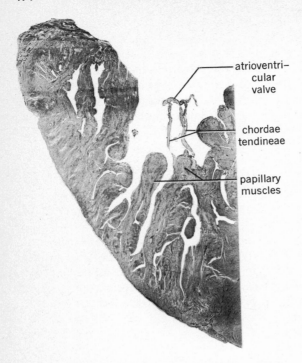

Figure 10-1 A section through the ventricular myocardium of a human infant heart. Photomicrograph, about ×3.

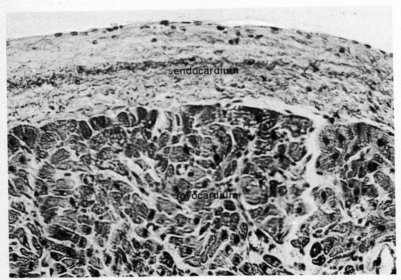

Figure 10-2 Ventricular wall of a human heart. Note the thickness of the endocardium and the endothelial cells on its surface. Photomicrograph, × 300.

The internal surfaces of the ventricles are irregular, owing to projections of the myocardium called **trabeculae carneae**. These can be seen in the low-power photomicrograph in Fig. 10.1. Extensions from these, the **papillary muscles**, give attachment to thin **chordae tendineae**, which fasten onto the free edges of the leaves of the atrioventricular valves. These cords are made of fibrous connective tissue continuous with that of the endocardium; those in the left ventricle are heavier than those in the right.

There are two papillary muscles in the left and three in the right ventricle. They control the excursion of the valve cusps during systole. When they become involved in disease, they allow too much excursion, and valvular incompetence results.

The **epicardium**, or outer coat of the heart, is the visceral pericardium. It consists of fibrous connective tissue covered with mesothelium. The main arteries, veins, and nerves of the heart, imbedded in adipose tissue, course within it.

Cardiac Valves All cardiac valves are constructed of thin leaflets of dense fibrous connective tissue covered with endothelium. The **atrioventricular valves**, tricuspid (three cusps) on the right and mitral (two cusps) on the left, are attached to the fibrous ring of the cardiac skeleton. They are inelastic but may have a few smooth-muscle fibers on the atrial side.

The **semilunar valves**, aortic and pulmonary, have elastic fibers on the ventricular side. A small fibrocartilaginous nodule is situated in the free edge of each cusp (Fig. 10.3). The microscopic structure of an aortic valve cusp is shown in Fig. 10.4.

Edges of the valve leaflets are practically avascular. The comment has been made that no living tissue could withstand the strain that is placed on the heart valves. Function of cardiac valves may be impaired when disease has affected the structure of their leaflets. Surgical repair of valves or their replacement with artificial valves is now readily accomplished.

Cardiac Vessels and Nerves The myocardium is permeated by loose fibrous connective tissue carrying blood vessels and lymphatic vessels. The capillary bed is extensive in cardiac muscle. Blood reaches it directly from the **coronary arteries**, which are the first branches given off by the aorta after it leaves the heart. This blood, fresh from the lungs, gives up more oxygen in the capillary bed of the heart than does blood in any other organ. The right coronary artery arises behind the anterior cusp of the aortic valve. The left arises behind the left posterior cusp (Fig. 10.3). The opening into the left coronary artery is slightly larger than that of the right. The branches and distribution of these vessels are described in textbooks of anatomy.

The coronary arteries anastomose freely with one another through their terminal branches, but these connective channels are small and conduct an inadequate amount of blood to nourish the myocardium after sudden occlusion of a coronary artery or one of its main branches. The part of the myocardium

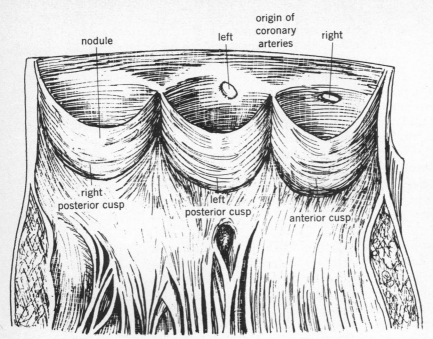

Figure 10-3 Human aortic valve. The aorta was split open lengthwise at its origin from the left ventricle of the heart. The three cusps of the valve and the openings of the coronary arteries are shown. *(CHP)*

affected by coronary occlusion then undergoes some degenerative changes that may prove fatal. Anastomotic connections between the principal branches of coronary arteries increase with age, providing improved collateral circulation. Impaired coronary blood flow often can be alleviated by surgically bypassing a region of occlusion with another blood vessel.

A number of cardiac veins accompany the arteries and join the main **coronary sinus**, returning blood to the right atrium. A rich lymphatic drainage can be demonstrated in heart muscle.

The heart is innervated by the vagus nerves and nerve fibers from the upper thoracic sympathetic ganglia. Impulses from the former retard, and those from the latter accelerate, heartbeat through their influence on the cardiac pacemaker. The cardiac nerves form a plexus in the epicardium at the base of the heart. Vagus fibers end there on nerve cells of a small parasympathetic ganglion which supplies postganglionic fibers to the heart. Nerves are distributed along the coronary vessels. Cardiac nerve fibers do not bear the same close relationship to muscle fibers as the motor nerve fibers do in skeletal muscle (Fig. 15.12).

There are sensory fibers in the cardiac plexuses; they course to the spinal cord in the sympathetic nerves (Fig. 10.5).

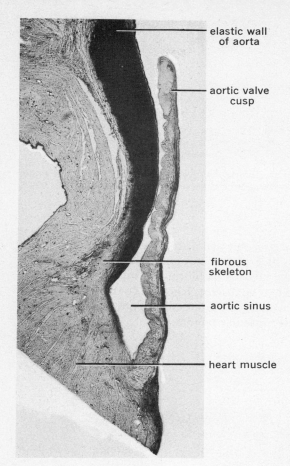

elastic wall
of aorta

aortic valve
cusp

fibrous
skeleton

aortic sinus

heart muscle

Figure 10-4 Aortic valve of a human heart. Stained for elastic fibers. Photomicrograph, × 8.

Impulse-Conducting System Regulation of contraction of the heart muscle of the four chambers is accomplished by a system of special cardiac-muscle fibers[1] composing the impulse-conducting system. The structure of these is described in Chap. 9. The conduction tissue is less easily seen in human hearts than in those of some animals, especially ungulates (Fig. 10.6).

The system may be said to start at a point between the orifices of the superior and the inferior venae cavae. There it consists of an accumulation of the special cardiac-muscle fibers, nerve fibers, and connective tissue in a mass called the **sinoatrial** or **sinus node**. From this point, impulses spread out into the atrial walls. The sinus node is called the "pacemaker"; it appears to initiate regulatory impulses for the contraction cycle of atria and ventricles.

[1]Known as "Purkinje fibers."

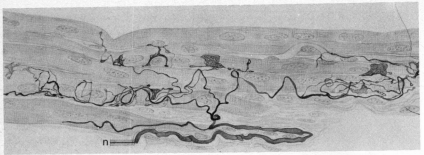

Figure 10-5 Nerve ending in the heart of a monkey. A myelinated nerve fiber, *n*, coursing in connective tissue, arises from a series of dendritic branches among cardiac muscle fibers. Silver staining; about × 300. *(JFN)*

Impulse-conducting tissue is concentrated also at an easily demonstrated **atrioventricular node** near the orifice of the coronary sinus. Thence, as the **atrioventricular bundle,**[2] this tissue crosses the fibrous atrioventricular septum to be distributed to muscle of the two ventricles. Knowledge of the distribution in the human heart has been derived largely from clinical observations of dysfunction of branches of the atrioventricular bundle.

[2] Commonly called the "bundle of His."

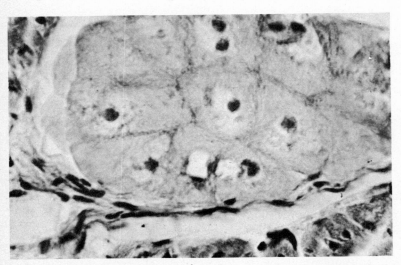

Figure 10-6 Fibers of the impulse-conducting system in a sheep heart. This cross section shows portions of a few ordinary cardiac-muscle fibers in the lower part of the picture. An artificial space and a strand of areolar tissue separate these from a bundle of the special fibers of the conduction system. Photomicrograph, × 600.

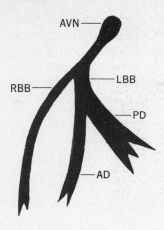

AVN

LBB

RBB

PD

AD

Figure 10-7 Schematic representation of the human atrioventricular conduction system, consisting of the atrioventricular node, *AVN,* the main atrioventricular bundle dividing into right and left bundle branches, *RBB* and *LBB.* The latter has two divisions, anterior and posterior, *AD* and *PD.* Relative thickness of branches and divisions is indicated in the schema. *(Redrawn from M. B. Rosenbaum, Modern Concepts of Cardiovascular Disease, vol. 39, 1970.)(CHP)*

Figure 10.7 illustrates schematically the branching of the conduction system in the two ventricles. The main atrioventricular bundle soon divides into right and left branches. The thinner right branch can be followed to the anterior papillary muscle of the right ventricle. The thicker left branch penetrates the septum and forms anterior and posterior divisions to supply the left ventricle. These go to the left anterior and left posterior papillary muscle, after which fibers of the conduction system deploy to other parts of the cardiac musculature.

Dysfunction of the conduction system may lead to failure of impulses to reach the ventricles, and a condition known as "heart block" ensues. The ventricles may contract at a reduced rate, or the heart may stop. Disease processes may block one or more of the three main divisions of the atrioventricular bundle. Artificial electronic pacemakers—some now powered by atomic energy—can be implanted under the skin of patients with such a problem and connected with the ventricles to restore normal rhythm and preserve life.

Great Vessels   Cardiac muscle of the myocardium extends beyond the atrial walls onto the veins that join them. A little of it may be encountered in the aorta and pulmonary arteries. Near the heart, the structure of all the great vessels is modified.

Both venae cavae have linings made up of endothelium, basal lamina, and fibrous connective tissue, as in the endocardium. They lack middle circular muscle coats, typical of most veins. Instead, they have a great deal of longitudinal smooth muscle in their outer coats. This adjusts their walls to tensions produced by the beating heart.

The pulmonary veins are relatively inelastic and possess a middle coat almost as thick as that of the branches of the pulmonary artery. Near the heart, it is formed largely by cardiac muscle. There, too, the internal coat is fibrous and thick like that within the atrium.

The aorta and pulmonary artery are elastic tubes surrounded as they leave the heart by fibrous connective tissue. The thick internal coat, continuous with the endocardium, contains elastic fibers. The muscle of the middle coat is more noticeable in infants and young individuals than it is in adults. The extensive elastic-tissue development in the middle coat is the characteristic feature of these great arteries. Further description will be found in Chap. 11.

SUGGESTED READING

Baroldi, G., and G. Scomazzoni: *Coronary Circulation in the Normal and the Pathologic Heart*. Office of the Surgeon General, Department of the Army, Washington, 1967.

Ellison, J. P.: The Adrenergic Cardiac Nerves of the Cat. *American Journal of Anatomy*, vol. 139, pp. 209–226,1974.

Hurst, J. W. (ed.): *The Heart, Arteries, and Veins*. McGraw-Hill Book Company, New York, 1974.

Page, E., and L. P. McCallister: Studies on the Intercalated Disk of Rat Left Ventricular Myocardial Cells. *Journal of Ultrastructure Research*, vol. 43, pp. 388–411,1973

Patten, B. M.: The Heart, pt. I, sec. VII, pp. 613–659, in B. J. Anson (ed.), *Morris' Human Anatomy*, 12th ed. McGraw-Hill Book Company, New York, 1966.

Rhodin, J. A. G., P. Del Missier, and L. C. Reid: The Structure of the Specialized Impulse-Conducting System of the Steer Heart. *Circulation*, vol. 24, pp. 349–367, 1969.

Rosenbaum, M. B.: The Hemiblocks: Diagnostic Criteria and Clinical Significance. *Modern Concept of Cardiovascular Disease*, vol. 39, pp. 141–146, 1970.

Talbot, L., and S. A. Berger: Fluid-Mechanical Aspects of the Human Circulation. *American Scientist*, vol. 62, pp. 671–682, 1974.

Thaemert, J. C.: Fine Structure of the Atrioventricular Node as Viewed in Serial Sections. *American Journal of Anatomy*, vol. 136, pp. 43–65, 1973.

Blood Vessels and Lymphatic Vessels

Tubes of various sizes, carrying blood from the heart through the tissues and back to the heart again, and thin-walled channels, conveying lymph, form the extensive circulatory system. They course through fibrous connective tissue to almost all parts of the body. Blood vessels are encountered in all tissues except epithelium; some parts of the body are not supplied by lymphatic vessels.

Blood vessels in the living body, except the smallest ones, are always full of blood, but many of those in fixed histologic preparations appear empty. This, of course, is an unnatural condition. Blood-vessel walls have considerable elasticity and constrict when the heart stops beating. This is especially true of the arteries. Furthermore, perfusion of fixing fluid through the vasculature of organs for histologic preparations washes most of the blood corpuscles out of the vessels. Figure 11.1 illustrates small blood vessels and lymphatic vessels that have not collapsed at the time of death and fixation of the tissues.

The largest blood vessels conduct blood under pressure. Those of intermediate size have an additional function, to regulate the flow and distribute the blood. The smallest vessels, or capillaries, allow the blood to reach tissues under little pressure. Materials carried by the blood are passed through the thin walls of the smallest vessels into the tissues.

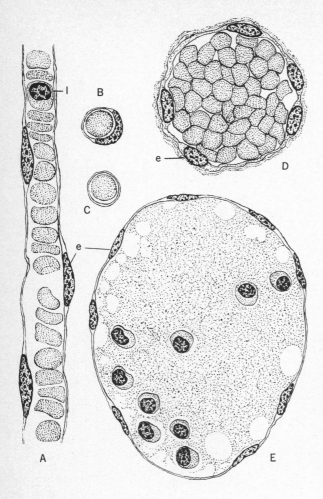

Figure 11-1 Small blood vessels and a lymphatic vessel, as they appear in histologic sections: *A,* capillary in longitudinal section; *B* and *C,* in cross section, erythrocytes and a lymphocyte, *l,* in their lumens; *D,* small venule, containing erythrocytes; *E,* lymphatic vessels with lymphocytes and coagulated lymph in its lumen. Endothelial nuclei are indicated at *e.* × 900. *(JFN)*

CAPILLARIES, PRECAPILLARIES, and SINUSOIDS

Approximately 90 percent of all blood vessels are capillaries and precapillaries. These and other small vessels are shown in Fig. 11.2. **Capillaries** are simple tubes of endothelium connecting arteries with veins. All vessels, and even the heart, begin in the embryo as capillaries, adding layers of connective tissue and muscle as they develop. Capillaries are small. Their inside diameter is approximately that of an erythrocyte, or a little wider, measuring 8 to 10 μm across, as shown in Fig. 11.1*A* to *C*. They are hard to see in ordinary histologic sections unless the cut passes through one of their nuclei or unless they are filled with blood.

The capillary wall consists of thin and elongated endothelial cells. Nuclei of these simple squamous cells are ovoid and stain rather lightly with hema-

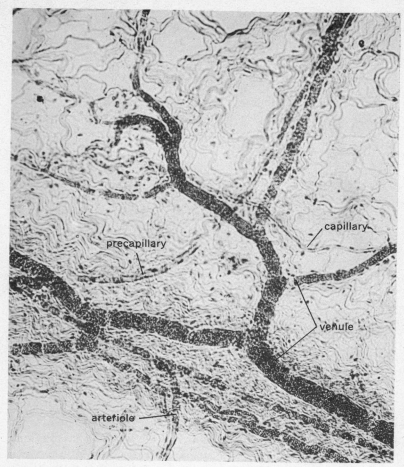

Figure 11-2 Small blood vessels in the human mesentery, spread upon a slide and stained. Photomicrograph, × 150.

toxylin. They resemble the light nuclei of fibrocytes in the surrounding connective tissue. The inner surfaces of the cells are in contact with the blood. The outer surfaces rest on a basal lamina, forming a continuous layer between the endothelium and surrounding loose fibrous connective tissue. The latter contains its usual cells—fibrocytes, macrophages, and labrocytes. Not uncommonly another type of cell, designated "pericyte," appears within the basal lamina (Fig. 11.3). Connective tissue is lacking around capillaries of the central nervous system. They are invested instead by processes of neuroglia cells.

Structure of the capillary wall differs regionally in response to requirements for passage of fluid and solutes from the blood to interstitial spaces. Thickness of the walls varies. Contacts between endothelial cells are relatively loose in many locations. Adjacent plasma membranes are separated by spaces about 200 Å wide. Gap junctions and desmosomes occur (Fig. 11.4*B*), and in

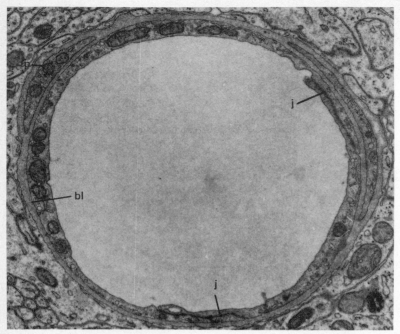

Figure 11-3 Capillary in the brain (rat). Overlapping endothelial cells exhibit tight junctions, *j*, sealing the lumen from the basal lamina, *bl*, and the brain parenchyma. Pericytes *p*, are seen in the basal lamina. Electron micrograph, × 17,000. *(Contributed by M. W. Brightman and T. S. Reese.)*

some places the endothelial cells simply overlap. Contacts between endothelial cells of capillaries in the retina and brain exhibit tight junctions, which obliterate the space between cells and ensure discontinuity between blood plasma and interstitial fluid. This is a significant feature of the blood-brain barrier (Fig. 11-4*A*).

Another type of capillary is that with fenestrated endothelium. The fenestrations are cellular "pores" bridged by thin diaphragms of electron-dense material (Fig. 11.5). The most marked fenestrations are those encountered in capillaries of the renal glomerulus (Chap. 23). There the capillary wall displays pores with diameters up to 1000 Å that lack bridging diaphragms (Fig. 23.8). A thicker basal lamina is present under the endothelium of fenestrated capillaries than is usually seen in those without fenestrations.

Most capillary endothelial cells display minute pinocytotic indentations on the lumenal border. These become vesicles beneath the cell surface, merging with elements of the agranular endoplasmic reticulum. The basal border of endothelial cells likewise often shows pinocytotic vesicles opening into interstitial spaces. Figure 11.4*B* illustrates these features in a thick-walled capillary.

Capillary permeability refers to the facility with which materials, such as oxygen, nutriments, products of cellular metabolism, and hormones, dissolved

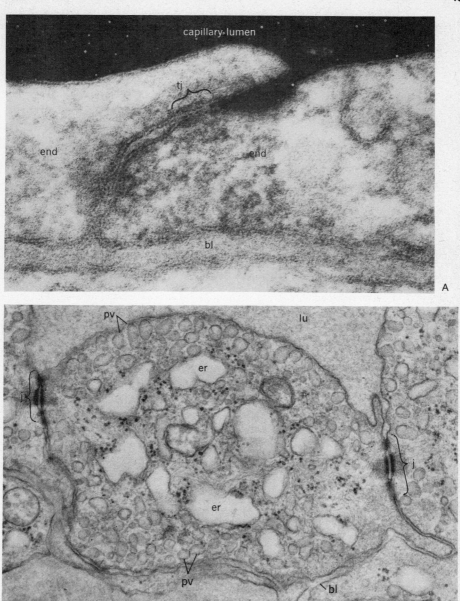

Figure 11-4 Junctions between endothelial cells of capillaries. *A.* Tight junction, *tj*, in capillary of brain (mouse). Capillary lumen contains electron-dense material (black) which failed to pass between the endothelial cells, *end*. Note basal lamina, *bl*, of capillary. Electron micrograph, ×250,000. *(Contributed by M. W. Brightman and T. S. Reese.) B.* Junctions, *j*, between endothelial cells of thick-walled capillary (fish); these consist of desmosomes. Abbreviations: *lu*, lumen; *pv*, pinocytotic vesicles; *er*, endoplasmic reticulum; *bl*, basal lamina. Electron micrograph, × 20,000. *(Contributed by D. W. Fawcett.)*

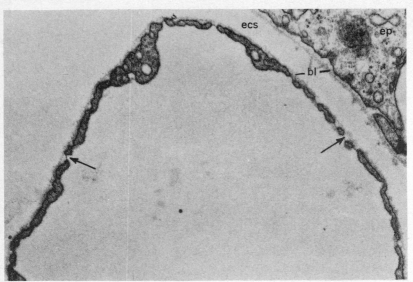

Figure 11-5 Fenestrated capillary (cross section) in the choroid plexus (mouse). Fenestrations with bridging membranes are indicated by arrows. The basal lamina, *bl*, of capillary and choroidal epithelium, *ep*, are separated by perivascular space, *ecs*. Electron micrograph, about × 17,000. *(Contributed by M. W. Brightman and T. S. Reese.)*

in blood plasma and tissue fluid, are transported across the capillary wall. Permeability not only varies with the regional differences in structural characteristics of the capillary walls, but also is influenced by humoral factors, less evident to the histologist. Variations in closeness of endothelial cell contacts and in amount of pinocytotic activity are reflected in differences in permeability. Fenestrations in capillary walls permit the most rapid rate of transudation from the blood, that in the kidney being about one hundred times that in skeletal muscle. But even the gap junctions between endothelial cells of capillaries in muscles are believed to provide adequate permeability for passage of lipid-insoluble molecules.

The network of capillaries between the smallest arteries and veins is called the **capillary bed**. Density of the capillary bed varies in different tissues. Heart muscle has a rich supply of capillaries; the muscle of the intestine has a meager capillary bed. The amount of blood passing through the capillaries of an organ increases and decreases from time to time according to degree of activity of the organ. The number of capillaries actually conducting blood at any one time is often only a fraction of the total number present, especially in organs that alternate periods of work with periods of rest. In resting muscle, most capillaries are closed, but after strenuous physical exercise, the number of open capillaries may increase as much as fiftyfold. It is well that all capillaries are not open all the time, because the volume of blood they could hold would be so great that there would be no blood left to fill the heart, and death would occur. Such a condition is known as "circulatory shock syndrome."

Opening and closing of the capillary bed is not the function of the capillaries themselves but of the smallest arteries from which they arise. No muscle cells are found in the walls of capillaries, and so capillaries have no motor nerve supply.

The next larger vessels, **precapillaries**, on the arterial side of the capillary bed, do have a few smooth-muscle cells in their walls (Figs. 11.2 and 11.8). These and arterioles are the vessels that contract and regulate the flow of blood into the true capillaries. In some places there are shunts across capillary beds, composed of precapillaries that are only slightly larger than true capillaries. When these are open, blood flow through the true capillaries stops or is slowed; when these shunts are closed by contraction of their smooth-muscle cells, blood flow through the true capillaries begins again.

The concept of the precapillary is important for understanding control of blood flow through capillaries. Precapillary spasm is responsible for one type of high blood pressure. The arterial precapillary exists in many places between the smallest arterioles and true capillaries, even though its length may be slight. Anatomists recognize it as an artery because its wall contains a few scattered smooth-muscle cells. Some physiologists classify it as a capillary because it is scarcely larger than the true capillaries and its wall is permeable. It is difficult to recognize this vessel in the living animal unless one is able to stimulate its smooth-muscle cells.

A venous postcapillary has been described by some authors, just to make the series complete. It is nothing more than a big capillary about to join a venule.

The vascular connections between arteries and veins in the liver, spleen, bone marrow, and some endocrine glands are wide channels, often 30 μm or more in diameter. The wall structure of these **sinusoids** rarely resembles that of capillaries. The lining may be roughened by projecting phagocytic cells. The endothelial lining of some sinusoids is incomplete and has many gaps. Basal laminae are lacking, and the blood plasma comes into direct contact with interstitial spaces around the parenchymal cells. Sinusoids course in a tortuous fashion through beds of reticular rather than loose fibrous connective tissue. Blood flow is often sluggish through the sinusoids and may cease for some time and begin again. More is said about them in later chapters.

ARTERIES

All arteries large enough to be seen without magnification have walls consisting of three coats. The internal coat, or **tunica intima**, is the endothelial lining with basal lamina and some connective tissue beneath it. The middle coat, or **tunica media**, is formed by smooth muscle and connective tissue, principally elastic fibers, arranged in circular fashion. The external coat, or **tunica adventitia** (tunica externa), is fibrous connective tissue with other structures in it, arranged longitudinally. The three coats may be separated by elastic membranes, internal and external.

Muscular Arteries These are sometimes called "distributing arteries."

Table 11.1 Comparison of Adult Blood Vessels

	Elastic artery	Muscular artery	Arteriole
Diameter	More than 1 cm	Less than 1 cm	0.5 mm or less
Tunica intima	Thick; fibrous connective tissue; muscle cells	Thin; some fibrous connective tissue	Very thin; little or no fibrous connective tissue
Internal elastic membrane	Double; often indistinguishable from media	Heavy	Incomplete in smallest
Tunica media	Thick; fenestrated elastic membranes and muscle	Thickest tunic; up to 40 muscle layers	Most characteristic layer
External elastic membrane	Indistinguishable	Well defined	Absent
Tunica adventitia	Thin; few or occasional muscle cells	Thinner than media; longitudinal muscle in some	One-fourth as thick as media
Vasa vasorum	Present	Present	Absent
Blood pressure (mmHg)	100 +	90 to 50	50 to 30
Blood velocity (mm/sec)	300	→	→

They can regulate blood flow to different regions by contraction and relaxation of the smooth muscle in their walls. They vary in size from vessels as big as the brachial or femoral arteries to those so small that they bear no specific name. Although all adhere to the general plan just outlined, there is considerable variation.

One of the characteristics of muscular arteries is the ability to grow in size when the occasion demands. When circulation to a region is impaired by occlusion of the main arteries supplying it, smaller collateral arteries take over and increase in size to carry the necessary volume of blood. Another important characteristic is the ability to contract spastically when injured, which may thus prevent fatal hemorrhage.

The smallest arteries, **arterioles**, are members of the muscular-artery class. The tunica intima consists of endothelium, basal lamina, and an internal elastic membrane that may be incomplete in the smallest arterioles. In cross sections, the elastic membrane appears as a corrugated, highly refractive line throwing the endothelium into folds which bulge into the lumen (Figs. 11.6 and 11.7). The tunica media is a distinct muscular coat. The adventitia is about one-third or one-fourth as thick as the muscular coat and merges with surrounding con-

Capillary	Venule	Vein	Venae cavae
8 to 10 μm	10 μm to 1 mm	2 mm and more	More than 1 cm
Endothelium; basal lamina	Very thin; little fibrous connective tissue	Thick in largest; valves in many	Thick
Absent	Absent	Not prominent	Present
Absent	Present in those 50 μm or larger in diameter	Present, but relatively thin tunic	Very thin; little muscle; absent in some places
Absent	Absent	Usually absent	Absent
Absent	Relatively thick	Thick; muscle in largest	Principal tunic; prominent longitudinal muscle
Absent	Absent	Present	Numerous
30 to 15	15 to 10	10 to 4	4 to 0
5	→	→	60

nective tissue. It is ill-defined in the smallest arterioles, in which the muscular coat consists of only two or three layers of short muscle fibers. Although a few elastic fibers appear in the wall of the arteriole, no external elastic membrane can be seen. The smallest arterioles merge with precapillaries and capillaries. The upper size limit is arbitrarily defined as 0.5 mm. Examples of arterioles are seen in Fig. 11.8 and in other illustrations in this book.

The structures of large and medium-sized muscular arteries are shown in Figs. 11.9 and 11.10. The tunica intima is formed by endothelium, basal lamina, and a subendothelial layer of fibrous connective tissue. The internal elastic membrane is a well-developed fenestrated membrane. A few special arteries contain longitudinal smooth-muscle fibers in the tunica intima.

The muscle fibers of the tunica media are spirally arranged and may form 20 to 40 layers, more in the arteries of the lower extremity than in those of the upper. Elastic fibers are interspersed among muscle fibers, and a few collagenous and reticular fibers are demonstrable. The muscle fibers predominate in the smaller muscular arteries, but the elastic fibers crowd in among them in the larger vessels, such as the external iliac arteries, so that no sharp line of demarcation exists between typically muscular and typically elastic arteries.

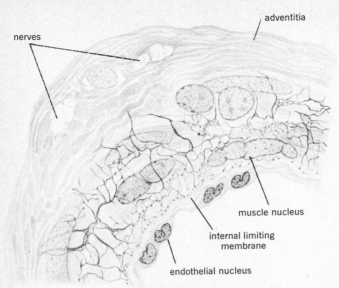

Figure 11-6 Arteriole with a muscular coat consisting of two or three layers of smooth-muscle fibers. Note the origin of reticular fibrils from collagenous fibers of the adventitia. Silver carbonate stain. × 900. *(JFN)*

The tunica adventitia consists of fibrous connective tissue with a longitudinal orientation. Where smooth muscle occurs in it, fibers are arranged longitudinally.

Muscular arteries, especially the larger ones, require a blood supply of their own. Consequently, **vasa vasorum** are encountered in the adventitia. These are arterioles that distribute blood to capillary beds in the arterial wall. They are small and less numerous in arteries than in veins.

Lymphatic vessels are not seen in the tunica media of the arteries, but occur in the adventitia where they are not subjected to much pressure.

Muscular arteries are supplied by nerve fibers, both motor fibers from the autonomic ganglia and sensory fibers from cranial and spinal nerves. Vasoconstriction, effected reflexly through the central nervous system, diminishes distribution of blood to the capillary bed. Vasodilatation, on the other hand, results in increased blood flow into the capillaries. It, too, is controlled reflexly. Vasoconstriction and vasodilatation play important parts in regulation of blood pressure (see the discussion of precapillaries above).

The muscular arteries vary not only in size but also in amount and distribution of elastic, collagenous, and muscle fibers in the walls. The cerebral arteries are thin and resemble veins. They have little elastic tissue except in the internal membrane and show only a meager adventitia. Branches of the pulmonary arteries also are thin-walled vessels with little elastic tissue.

On the other hand, the coronary artery walls are thick and have much elastic tissue, even an extra fenestrated elastic membrane in the tunica media. A heavy tunica intima is commonly present, and longitudinal smooth muscle is

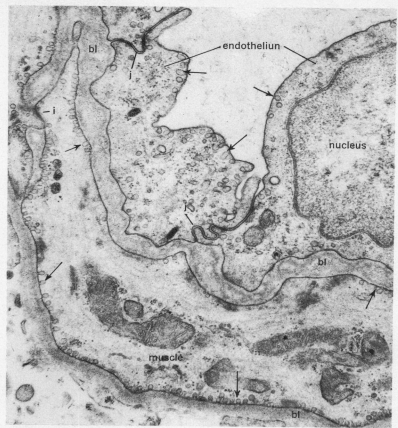

Figure 11-7 Part of an arteriole in the liver showing two junctions, *j*, between endothelial cells (one nucleus is visible); basal laminae, *bl*, appear between endothelium and smooth-muscle cells; and a gap junction, *i*, between two muscle cells is seen. Note particularly the many pinocytotic vesicles (*arrows*). Electron micrograph, × 36,000. *(Contributed by J. A. Freeman.)*

sometimes found in the intima. A heavy outer longitudinal or spiral layer of muscle may be present, as seen in Fig. 11.11. Even at birth, coronary arteries of males are said to have thicker intima than those of females.

At puberty the arteries of the penis undergo development of the intima and media, with longitudinal muscle appearing in the thickened intima. Similarly, bands of longitudinal muscle occur in the intima of the uterine spiral arteries. The renal arteries exhibit an unusual amount of elastic tissue for vessels of their size. Arteries that are tortuous, such as the splenic, and the large branches of elastic arteries, are apt to have longitudinal smooth muscle in the tunica adventitia.

Elastic Arteries These are the large vessels conducting blood from the heart to the muscular distributing arteries. They are located deep in the body,

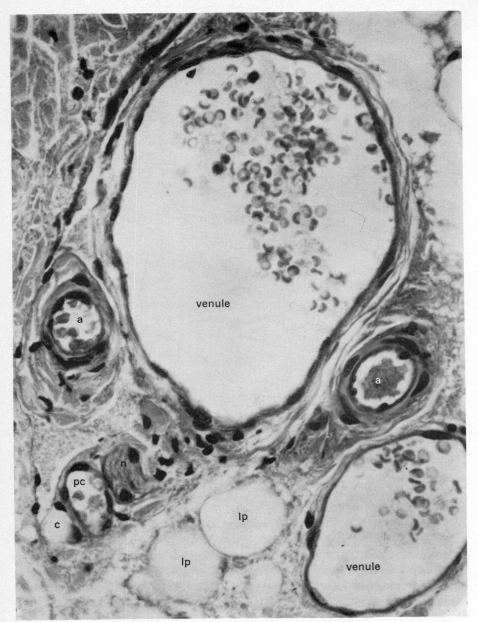

Figure 11-8 Arterioles, *a*, and venules in subcutaneous tissue; lipocytes, *lp,* capillary *c,* precapillary, *pc,* and small nerve, *n,* also are shown. Photomicrograph, × 600.

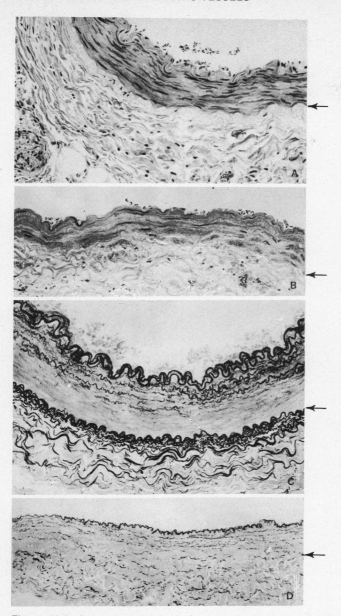

Figure 11-9 Intercostal artery (*A, C*) and vein (*B, D*): *A* and *B,* hematoxylin stain; *C* and *D,* stained for elastic fibers. Arrows mark the boundaries between muscularis, above, and adventitia, below. Photomicrographs, × 130.

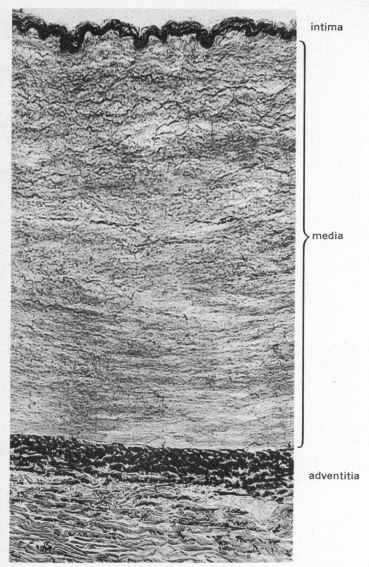

intima

media

adventitia

Figure 11-10 Human femoral artery; elastic-fiber stain. Compare with the femoral vein in Fig. 11-14. Photomicrograph, × 130.

and thus enjoy some degree of protection from superficial wounds. Their walls are fibrous and cannot constrict to obstruct and obliterate the lumen when severed. Besides the aorta and pulmonary arteries, other elastic arteries are the innominate, common carotid, subclavian, and common iliac. All resemble the aorta, but the smaller members of the group possess more smooth muscle and fewer elastic membranes. In branching to form smaller vessels, the structure changes grandually to that of the muscular type.

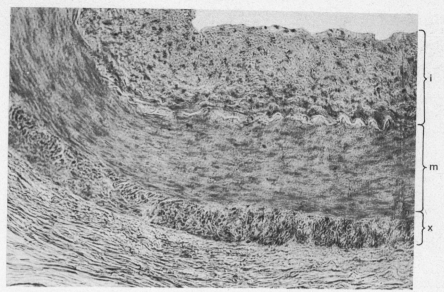

Figure 11-11   Human coronary artery, showing thick intima, *i*, and extra longitudinal smooth muscle at *x*, outside the media, *m*. Photomicrograph, × 130.

The only great conducting artery that is nonelastic is the highly muscular ductus arteriosus connecting the pulmonary artery and aorta of the fetus. It is disposed of after birth when it contracts and becomes permanently obliterated. Occasionally the ductus arteriosus remains patent, permitting blood from the aorta to enter the pulmonary system because of the lower pressure prevailing in the latter. This condition lends itself to surgical repair.

The tunica intima of elastic arteries is thick and contains a considerable amount of connective tissue and occasionally a few longitudinal smooth-muscle cells. It is bordered by the internal elastic membrane, which merges with the tunica media and is often double.

The tunica media contains smooth muscle, mostly circular but some longitudinal. However, the muscle is inconspicuous because its cells are crowded apart by many fenestrated membranes and elastic networks. There may be as many as 65 of these membranes in the arch of the aorta. Sections stained with orcein and other special elastic-fiber stains reveal them (Fig. 11.12), but they are clearly visible in ordinary preparations because of their size and high refractive index. Compare Fig. 11.13*A* and *B*. Networks of reticular fibers occur among other elements of the tunica media.

The tunica adventitia of the elastic arteries is relatively thin but tough, limiting the amount of dilatation of the tunica media. It is made up of collagenous fibers arranged in long, loose spirals. Among these are small blood vessels, the vasa vasorum. The adventitia merges with surrounding loose fibrous connective tissue.

The walls of elastic arteries are much thinner in relation to size of lumen than are those of muscular arteries. By virtue of their great elasticity, they act

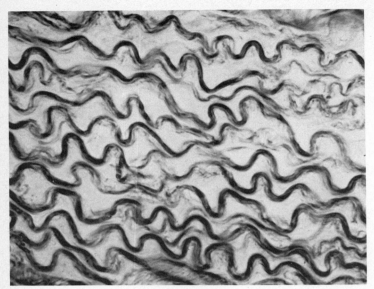

Figure 11-12 Fenestrated elastic membranes in the aorta (female lion cub), stained for elastic fibers. Photomicrograph, × 450.

as shock absorbers or compression chambers, smoothing out the flow of blood by dilating passively with each systole and resuming their original diameter during diastole of the heart. Were it not for their elastic construction, blood would move intermittently, instead of continuously, through the small vascular channels. As a matter of fact, in extreme degrees of sclerosis of elastic arteries, the pulse can be observed in capillaries, although it is never visible there normally.

Changes in Structure with Age   The structure of some large blood vessels changes with age. Obliteration of the ductus arteriosus at birth is an example of aging. The aorta is a muscular vessel at birth. The elastic membranes of its tunica media increase in prominence with passage of time and are not completely differentiated until about the twenty-fifth year. Likewise, the muscular arteries exhibit changes during the same period. The muscular coat becomes thicker; the vessels acquire more connective tissue in the adventitia and some in the intima beneath the basal lamina of the endothelium. These are physiologic changes.

It is said that "man is as old as his arteries," but the vascular changes that occur with time are more often pathologic than physiologic. Some people reach advanced age without marked alterations in their blood vessels. Others are less fortunate. Their large arteries, especially the aorta but also the coronary, common carotid, and internal and middle cerebral arteries, are prone to acquire lipid deposits in the intima that increase its thickness as time goes on and narrow the vessel lumen. This disease condition, known as "atherosclerosis," is

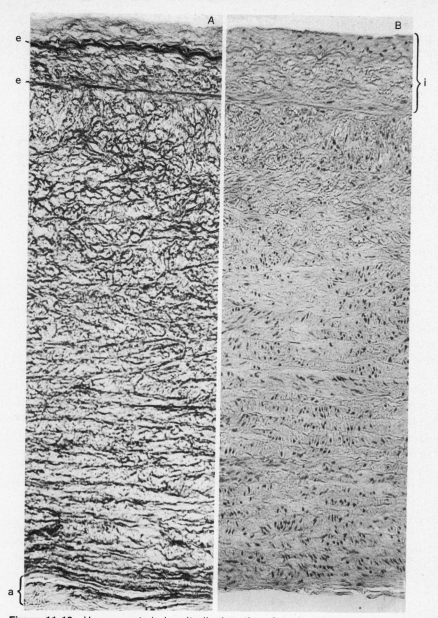

Figure 11-13 Human aorta in longitudinal section. *A*, stained for elastic fibers; *B*, the same preparation with hematoxylin stain. The intimal layer *i*, contains two prominent elastic membranes, *e*; a small part of the adventitia, *a*, is shown in *A*; the rest of the wall is media. Photomicrographs, × 130.

one of the major causes of death in North America. Surgical replacement of weakened and bulging segments of diseased vessels with tubes of synthetic material has become a procedure that is usually successful and results in reestablishing normal blood flow.

VEINS

Veins are the comparatively thin-walled tubes conducting blood from the capillary bed back to the heart. Blood flows more slowly and is under less pressure than in the arteries, and the lumen of veins is greater. Veins do not adhere closely to the general blood-vessel plan. Some depart markedly from it. Most veins are formed principally by fibrous connective tissue with no strong fenestrated elastic membranes. Furthermore, there is little circular smooth muscle. Special mechanisms in veins aid the return of blood to the heart.These are the valves and longitudinal bands of smooth muscle, most prominent where the force of gravity is to be overcome.

Little veins are called **venules** (Fig. 11.2). The smallest resemble large capillaries, but their walls have some fibrous connective tissue forming a thin layer outside the endothelium. Their function is similar to that of capillaries. Venules 40 to 50 μm in diameter have a few isolated smooth-muscle cells wrapped circularly about them. A complete muscular tunic is absent in venules smaller than 0.2 mm in diameter. Little veins of this size have relatively thick adventitial coats.

Medium-sized veins usually course with muscular arteries. They vary structurally in different locations. The tunica intima is thin in the smaller members of this group (Fig. 11.9), and although elastic fibers can be demonstrated, a true internal elastic membrane is lacking as a rule. It is difficult to see a division into tunica intima and tunica media in most veins. The femoral vein is shown in Fig. 11.14 as an example of a medium-sized vein.

Valves are formed by folds of the tunica intima. They occur in most veins that are 2 mm or more in diameter and conduct blood against the force of gravity. They are absent in some of the visceral veins and in those of the brain, spinal cord, and meninges. Valves are illustrated in Fig. 24.13.

The tunica media of veins is thin in contrast with that of accompanying arteries (Figs. 11.9 and 11.14). It may be absent altogether. It consists of circularly arranged smooth-muscle fibers with some fibrous connective tissue, but the number of elastic fibers is small. Veins of the lower extremities, pulmonary veins, and the veins of the gravid uterus exhibit a well-developed layer of smooth muscle in the tunica media. Veins of the cranium, retina, and bones and those of the deep layers of the maternal placenta have no muscle. The tunica media is missing in the superior vena cava as well as in much of the inferior vena cava (Fig. 11.15).

The adventitia is the thickest coat of the veins. It is formed largely by fibrous connective tissue but contains longitudinal smooth-muscle fibers in many locations. Elastic fibers occur, too, although no external elastic mem-

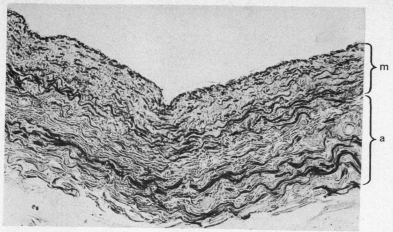

Figure 11-14 Human femoral vein stained for elastic fibers. It is difficult to differentiate the adventitia, *a*, from the media, *m*. Photomicrograph × 130.

brane is present. The venae cavae and other large veins have much longitudinal smooth muscle in the adventitia, rather evenly distributed. Prominent longitudinal bundles of muscle are found in the outer coat of the portal and renal veins and especially in the suprarenal veins; in cross sections these give a lopsided appearance to the vessel wall.

Nerve fibers accompany veins, supplying their smooth muscles and probably controlling tonicity of the muscles in compensation for blood pressure and volume changes.

Walls of veins are supplied with blood by small arterioles constituting their vasa vasorum. These vessels are larger than those of corresponding arteries, and their branches penetrate deeper into the wall of the veins, some reaching the tunica intima. Lymphatic vessels are present in all layers of the large veins.

ARTERIOVENOUS ANASTOMOSES

Capillaries connect arteries and veins in most tissues of the body, but they are not the only channels by which blood circulates. In many locations, arterioles anastomose directly with venules and provide short-circuiting mechanisms aiding in regulating peripheral blood flow and decreasing peripheral resistance.

Most **arteriovenous anastomoses** are located in the skin of exposed parts of the body and in the walls of the intestinal tract. In the latter place they are thought to reduce blood flow through the mucous membrane when digestion is not in progress. In the skin, they are prevalent in the nose, lips, finger tips, and toes, but especially in the nail beds. The cavernous spaces of erectile tissue are a type of arteriovenous anastomosis.

The **coccygeal body**, located ventral to the tip of the coccyx, is a highly developed arteriovenous anastomosis (Fig. 11.16). This consists of a group of vessels arranged in a mass of dense fibrous connective tissue. The walls of anastomosing vessels are thick and muscular and make possible a complete

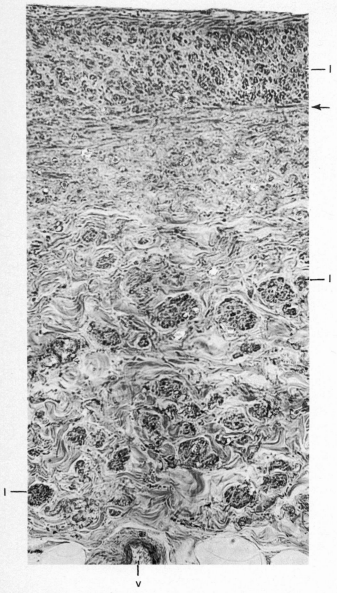

Figure 11-15 Inferior vena cava from human abdomen. The wall is mainly connective tissue with a few circular smooth-muscle fibers (*arrow*) and many longitudinal muscle bundles, *l*. A blood vessel, *v*, supplies the wall. Photomicrograph, ×150.

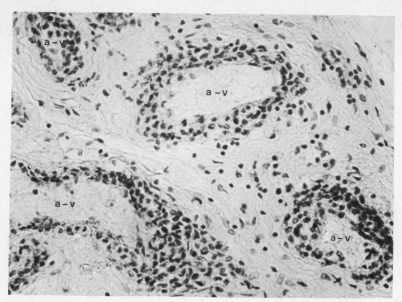

Figure 11-16 Arteriovenous anastomoses (*a-v*) in the human coccygeal body. Smooth-muscle nuclei of very short muscle fibers are numerous, giving the vessel walls an endocrine appearance. Photomicrograph, ×300.

occlusion when not needed. The smooth-muscle cells are short and somewhat hypertrophied. They are abundantly supplied with motor nerve fibers, and some sensory fibers occur among them.

CAROTID AND AORTIC BODIES

The **carotid body** is a small glomus located in the wall of the internal carotid artery at its origin from the common carotid artery. Similar structures, known as **aortic bodies**, are found on the arch of the aorta. These are not arteriovenous anastomoses, but are elaborate chemoreceptors. Each consists of a series of irregular cords of epithelioid cells closely associated with wide capillaries. The capillaries of the carotid body receive blood from a small branch of the carotid artery. A sensory nerve supply comes from the glossopharyngeal nerve to the carotid body, and from the vagus nerves to the aortic bodies (Fig. 11.17).

Chemoreceptors of the carotid and aortic bodies respond to changes in oxygen tension in the arterial blood traversing them. The nerve impulses from them initiate cardiovascular and, especially, respiratory responses.

The carotid body should not be confused with the **carotid sinus**, which is a dilatation in the wall of the internal carotid artery near its origin. There is a rich network of nerve endings in the outer part of the thinned tunica media of the artery at this place, and this constitutes a baroreceptor. Changes in blood pressure stimulate the end organ and result in vasomotor responses which are part

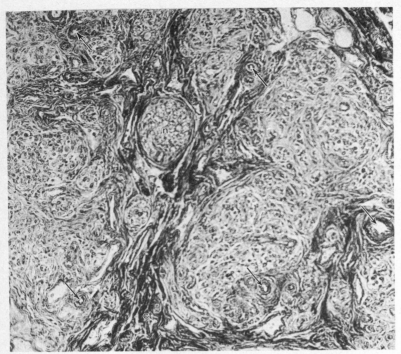

Figure 11-17   Human carotid body. Note the many small blood vessels (*arrows*), a nerve, *n*, and connective-tissue stroma, *ct*. Photomicrograph, × 150.

of the mechanism for regulation of blood pressure; overstimulation of the carotid-sinus endings, under certain abnormal conditions, will produce fainting attacks—the "tight-collar syndrome."

LYMPHATIC VESSELS

Lymphatic vessels make up a one-way collateral system of channels through which fluid and some of the formed elements of blood are transported from the tissues to the vascular system. Some of the fluid leaving the blood stream and entering interstitial spaces returns directly into blood capillaries, but a considerable amount of fluid—approximately 1 ml/kg/hr—after being collected by lymphatic capillaries, rejoins the blood by way of the thoracic and right lymph ducts. These empty into the subclavian veins at the base of the neck.

All lymphatic vessels course through layers of fibrous connective tissue and are especially numerous in the skin and subcutaneous tissues. They are confined to the capsule and septa of organs with highly cellular parenchyma, such as the liver. No lymphatic vessels are found in the brain and eyeball, where spaces contain special tissue fluids of the second order.

Lymphatic capillaries resembel blood capillaries, although they are wider and appear collapsed in histologic sections. They branch and anastomose to form plexuses. The lymphatic capillaries consist simply of thin endothelium with no basal lamina and no pericytes. Their cells adjoin one another without specialized junctional complexes, often overlapping. Pinocytotic vesicles are not often encountered. Transport by diffusion through the intercellular spaces seems to be the rule. The permeability of lymphatic capillaries in the skin can be enhanced by warming and by mild trauma.

Collecting lymphatic vessels receive lymph from the lymphatic capillaries and conduct it through lymph nodes to lymphatic vessels of larger size, and ultimately to the main lymph ducts. Small collecting lymphatic vessels are thin walled, resembling venules. Comparisons can be made in Fig. 11.1*D* and *E* and in Fig. 11.18. Three coats can be recognized in those greater than 0.2 mm in diameter, but the middle and outer layers are incomplete. The tunica intima is formed by endothelium and a little loose fibrous connective tissue. The tunica media has no more than an occasional spirally arranged smooth muscle cell. The tunica adventitia is principally collagenous with a few elastic fibers. Boundaries between coats are indistinct. Numerous valves give collecting lymphatic vessels a beaded appearance. Figure 11.19 shows the structure of a large lymphatic vessel.

The largest collecting lymphatic vessel is the **thoracic duct**. As seen in Fig. 11.20, its wall resembles that of a vein. Compare it with the vein in Fig. 11.14. It and other large lymphatic vessels are supplied with blood vessels and motor nerves innervating their scanty smooth muscle. Prominent valves guard the

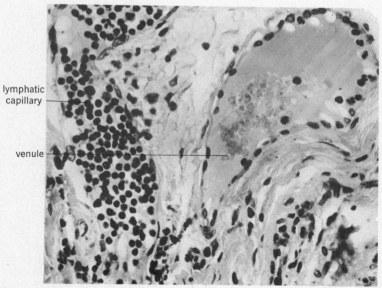

lymphatic capillary

venule

Figure 11-18 Lymphatic capillary full of lymphocytes, and venule containing a little blood; from the stroma of a human tonsil. Photomicrograph, × 300.

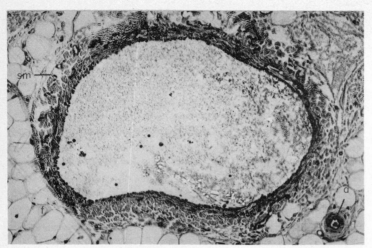

Figure 11-19   A large lymphatic vessel (monkey thoracic duct) surrounded by adipose tissue, *f*. The adventitia contains a few bundles of smooth muscle cells, *sm*. The lumen is filled with coagulated lymph. Note an arteriole, *a*, in the lower right corner of the figure. Photomicrograph × 130.

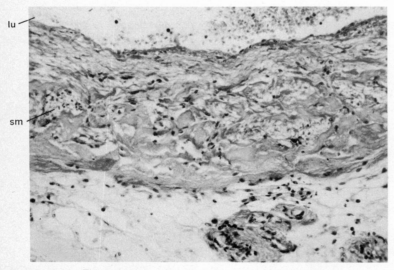

Figure 11-20   Thoracic duct of a 20-year-old woman. This section was taken close to the junction of the duct with the subclavian vein. Blood corpuscles entered the lumen, *lu*, after death. There is no true media, but there is a little smooth muscle. The adventitia has longitudinal bundles of smooth muscle, *sm*. Note the difference in thickness of the wall in monkey and human specimens (compare with Fig. 11-19). Photomicrograph, × 130.

openings of thoracic and right lymph ducts into the subclavian veins, effectively preventing blood from flowing into them.

The fluid conveyed by peripheral lymphatic capillaries and small collecting lymphatic vessels is clear, but it contains lymphocytes after it has traversed lymph nodes that occur along the course of the collecting vessels. Fluid from the liver, drained by the hepatic lymphatic vessels, has a high content of protein. Lymphatic capillaries in the villi of the small intestine are known as "lacteals." During digestion of fatty meals, they and the mesenteric lymphatic vessels contain a white lymph, called "chyle." Entering the blood, the lipid particles are known as chylomicrons.

Lymph is not propelled by the force of the heartbeat, but is moved by contraction of skeletal muscle in the vicinity of the small lymphatic vessels and by tissue-fluid pressure generated by filtration of fluid from the blood capillaries. Transport of lymph from the periphery along the system of lymphatic vessels is surprisingly rapid; dye injected into a dog's hind foot, for example, has been found in the thoracic duct in a matter of seconds. Under natural conditions transport is probably slower.

The rich cutaneous lymphatic plexuses provide a useful portal of entry to the body for certain type of therapeutic agents. Immunity-stimulating antigens, for example, find ready entrance into the lymphatic system from patches applied to scarified areas of skin.

SUGGESTED READING

Abraham, A.: *Microscopic Innervation of the Heart and Blood Vessels in Vertebrates Including Man.* Pergamon Press, Oxford, 1969.

Abramson, D. J.: *Blood Vessels and Lymphatics*; Academic Press, Inc., New York, 1962.

Bennett, H. S., J. H. Luft, and J. C. Hampton: Morphological Classifications of Vertebrate Blood Capillaries. *American Journal of Physiology*, vol. 196, pp. 381–390, 1959.

Boggon, R. P., and A. J. Palfrey: The Microscopic Anatomy of Human Lymphatic Trunks. *Journal of Anatomy*, vol. 114, pp. 389–405, 1973.

Brightman, M. W., and T. S. Reese: Junctions between Intimately Apposed Cell Membranes in the Vertebrate Brain. *Journal of Cell Biology*, vol. 40, pp. 648–677, 1969.

Clark, E. R., and E. L. Clark: Caliber Changes in Minute Blood Vessels Observed in the Living Mammal. *American Journal of Anatomy*, vol. 73, pp. 215–250, 1943.

Rhodin, J. A. G.: Ultrastructure of Mammalian Venous Capillaries, Venules, and Small Collecting Veins. *Journal of Ultrastructure Research*, vol. 25, pp. 452–500, 1968.

Zweifach, B. W.: The Microcirculation of the Blood. *Scientific American*, vol. 200, no. 1, pp. 54–60, January, 1959.

Chapter 12

Lymphatic Tissue and Organs

Lymphatic tissue is a secondary tissue, related, like blood and bone marrow, to connective tissue. It is diffusely arranged beneath certain epithelia, but elsewhere is more compacted into lymphatic organs. The parenchyma of the latter consists of lymphocytes, plasmocytes, their stem cells, and phagocytes enmeshed in a stroma of reticular cells and fibers. Lymphatic organs are encapsulated by fibrous connective tissue. Lymphatic tissue and organs, with the exception of the thymus, are encountered in places where antigens from infective organisms are prone to enter the body and along routes they travel, once having entered. All lymphatic tissue except that of the thymus exists in underdeveloped form before birth and remains so in animals born and reared in germ-free environments. Maturation requires a varying length of time, at least several months. For a comparison of the principal lymphatic organs, see Table 12.1.

SUBEPITHELIAL LYMPHATIC TISSUE

The loose tissue beneath epithelia of the alimentary, upper respiratory, and, to a lesser extent, urogenital tracts contains indifferent and reticular cells. Some of the latter are phagocytic and belong to the reticuloendothelial system. The stem cells of lymphocytes and plasmocytes spring from others. Not all lymphocytes arise locally. Some of them, notably large lymphocytes, come from other places

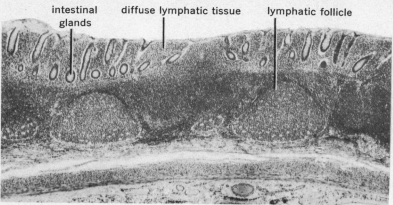

Figure 12-1 Diffuse lymphatic tissue and lymphatic follicles in a longitudinal section of the human appendix. Photomicrograph, × 40.

by way of the blood. Subepithelial lymphatic tissue consists of a loose arrangement of reticular fibers and reticular cells enmeshing the lymphocytes. This gives it the name **diffuse lymphatic tissue**. It can be recognized by the darkly staining nuclei of its small lymphocytes.

Diffuse lymphatic tissue forms a continuous layer beneath the epithelium of the adult intestine (Fig. 12.1), but it is not well developed at birth. Here and there more densely packed lymphocytes form small nonencapsulated ovoid masses in it, called **lymphatic follicles.**[1] Solitary follicles are prevalent, but occasionally they are grouped as aggregate follicles, especially in the pharynx, lower small intestine,[2] and appendix. Lymphatic follicles form structural units in lymphatic organs. They are represented at birth by simple accumulations of lymphocytes, but no plasmocytes are present at that time. Full development depends on functional requirements, lymphatic follicles undergoing cyclic changes throughout life.

As large immature lymphocytes proliferate in diffuse lymphatic tissue, they crowd the more mature, darkly staining, small lymphocytes aside. Small lymphocytes formed by cells in this **germinal center** of a lymphatic follicle accumulate around it in darkly staining rings or crescents, as seen in Fig. 12.1. The cells of these rings are more compactly arranged. Active proliferation is indicated by the presence of mitotic figures in the centers. A germinal center is lighter than the surrounding lymphatic tissue because its cells, including plasmocytes, have more cytoplasm than mature lymphocytes, and their nuclei are less chromatic.

Involution of a lymphatic follicle may be associated with cessation of mitotic activity in the germinal center, which stains lightly when its stem cells disappear, leaving only reticular cells and usually a few macrophages.

[1]Lymphatic follicles were formerly called "lymphatic nodules."
[2]Aggregate follicles of the lower small intestine are often called "Peyer's patches." They are an important source of cells secreting immunoglobulin A.

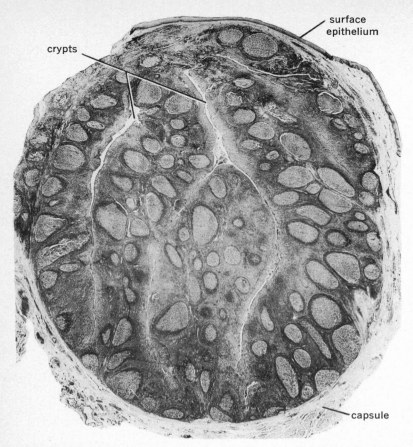

Figure 12-2 Human palatine tonsil. The mucous membrane has been torn away on the left. Photomicrograph, × 8.

Tissue fluid filters through the diffuse lymphatic tissue and follicles of mucous membranes and enters lymphatic capillaries that course away from the lymphatic tissue. Efferent lymphatic capillaries are prominent in regions containing large aggregates of follicles.

A feature of the diffuse lymphatic tissue beneath epithelium is migration of its lymphocytes into the epithelium and on through the epithelium into the lumen of the organ. This migration may be so extensive that the epithelium appears eroded, as it does in the crypts of the tonsils (Fig. 12.3).

Tonsils   The aggregates of lymphatic follicles of the pharynx form large masses, called tonsils. In the lateral pharyngeal wall they form the **palatine tonsils** (Fig. 12.2). Similar accumulations of lymphatic follicles are found in the posterior wall of the nasal pharynx, around the opening of the auditory tubes, and at the root of the tongue. These are the **pharyngeal**, **tubal**, and **lingual tonsils**.[3]

[3]The masses of aggregate follicles guarding the pharynx compose "Waldeyer's ring."

The palatine tonsils are compound aggregates of lymphatic follicles, about 20 mm long and 15 mm wide, encapsulated in dense fibrous connective tissue continuous with that of the pharyngeal submucosa. The tonsilar surface is covered with stratified squamous epithelium, invaginated into the subjacent lymphatic tissue to form pits of varying depths. These invaginations are the tonsilar crypts, each of which may branch into a number of subdivisions. Figure 12.3 shows a crypt in the human palatine tonsil.

Little fibrous connective tissue is seen in the lamina propria of the tonsils

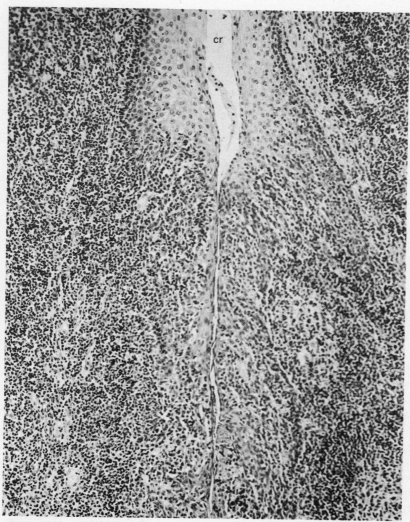

Figure 12-3 Crypt of the palatine tonsil. In the upper one-third of the crypt, *cr,* the stratified squamous epithelium is intact and its basal cells can be seen; the dark nuclei in the epithelium belong to invading lymphoctyes. The crypt epithelium is almost obliterated by lymphocytes in its lower two-thirds. Photomicrograph, × 150.

because of the abundance of lymphocytes. Lymphatic follicles with germinal centers abound beneath the tonsilar epithelium. Invasion of the epithelium by lymphocytes and escape of lymphocytes into the crypts are prominent features of the tonsils. Desquamated epithelial cells, lymphocytes, bacteria, and detritus will be seen in the crypts of even the healthiest tonsils. Tonsils lack afferent lymphatic vessels, but they have efferent vessels that convey great numbers of lymphocytes to the blood stream (Fig. 11.18).

Tonsils are by no means useless organs. Their function is production of lymphocytes and of antibodies in response to antigens of the oral and nasal cavities.

The pharyngeal tonsil is similar in structure and function to the palatine tonsil. It is located on the posterior wall of the nasal pharynx and is covered with pseudostratified epithelium. Enlargement of the pharyngeal tonsil forms the "adenoids," especially prominent during childhood. All the tonsils undergo involution with age.

LYMPH NODES

Lymph nodes are encapsulated masses of lymphatic tissue measuring 1 to 30 mm in diameter, found along the course of lymphatic vessels. They are easily seen in the mesenteries, axilla, and groin and occur in many other places as well. Their structure varies with their size and location. Typically they are little organs with a stroma of fibrous connective tissue and reticular tissue and a parenchyma of lymphocytes and plasmocytes. Arterioles enter the lymph node at an indentation called the hilum and course along with venules, through trabeculae of fibrous connective tissue, which are septal projections of the capsule.

The capsule and trabeculae of the lymph node consist of fibrous connective tissue containing, occasionally in the largest organs, a few smooth-muscle cells. Small nodes have slight trabeculae. Large nodes have heavier connective tissue subdividing the lymphatic tissue into compartments. Trabeculae, shown diagrammatically in Fig. 12.4, form the major skeleton of the lymph node.

The finer stroma is formed by reticular cells and fibers, as in other lymphatic tissue. Reticular fibers become continuous with collagenous fibers under the capsule and along the trabeculae, where the reticular stroma is particularly well defined.

Lymphatic tissue of the lymph node usually is divisible into an outer, more compact **cortex** and an inner, looser **medulla**. The medulla reaches the surface of the node only at the hilum. The cortex contains a variable number of lymphatic follicles which, several months postnatally, develop germinal centers (Fig. 12.5). Diffuse lymphatic tissue passes from the cortex toward the hilum to form medullary cords. The cells in these include many plasmocytes. Surrounding the larger cortical masses and separating these and the smaller medullary cords from the capsule and trabeculae are the **lymphatic sinuses**.

The sinuses are fluid-filled spaces containing relatively few lymphocytes.

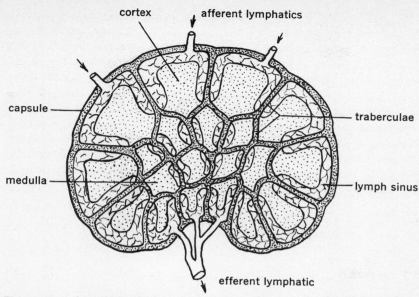

Figure 12-4   Diagram to illustrate structural plan of a lymph node. *(MWS)*

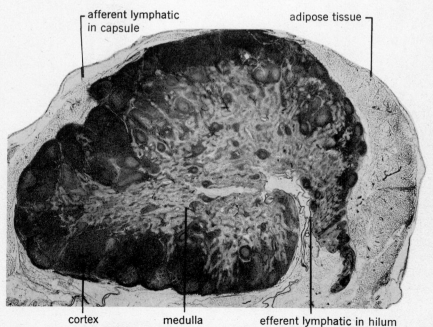

Figure 12-5 Human mesenteric lymph node sectioned through the hilum. Photomicrograph, ×10.

In them the reticular stroma is usually clearly seen. They are extensively baffled channels through which lymph circulates slowly. In addition to the reticular cells and fixed macrophages that form the sinus walls, there are free macrophages extending into the lumen. Lymph sinuses are seen in Fig. 12.6.

The lymph nodes are the only lymphatic organs into which lymph flows from other regions. Lymph enters the peripheral cortical sinuses from afferent lymphatic vessels that perforate the capsule. Endothelium of these vessels merges with the reticular lining network of the lymphatic sinuses. Valves controlling direction of lymph flow occur in the afferent vessels near their entrance into the nodes. Lymph filters through the cortical and medullary lymphatic sinuses, where the macrophages phagocytize foreign material that may be in it.

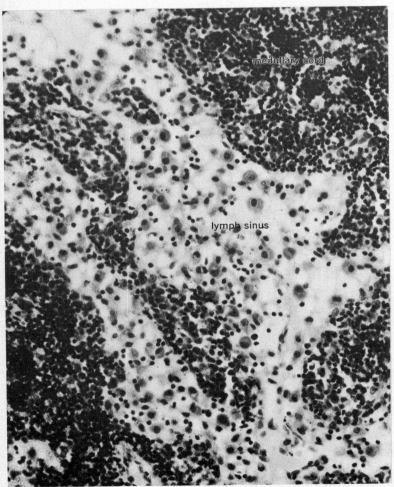

Figure 12-6 Medullary cords and a lymphatic sinus of a human lymph node. Photomicrograph, × 300.

Lymph leaves the lymph node at the hilum by way of efferent lymphatic vessels. These, too, possess valves, permitting lymph to flow only away from the node. If the lymph entering the node has not previously passed through a node, it is almost noncellular; but it leaves with many lymphocytes acquired in the sinuses. Afferent and efferent lymphatics are shown in Figs. 12.4 and 12.5.

Lymph nodes are among the principal sites of lymphocyte production. The roles of lymphocytes and plasmocytes in the immunity system are considered in the next chapter.

Hemal Nodes   Hemal nodes, resembling small lymph nodes but containing blood in their sinuses, occur in some species. They probably are not present in human beings. However, hemorrhagic lymph nodes are sometimes found and diagnosed as hemal nodes. These should not be difficult to differentiate from tiny accessory spleens which are encountered once in awhile.

SPLEEN

The spleen (lien) is the largest lymphatic organ, differing from lymph nodes by virtue of the fact that it has blood sinusoids rather than lymph sinuses. Production of granulocytes, erythrocytes, and blood platelets occurs in the spleen of a few species of animal and is a prominent feature of the human fetal spleen, but this function is normally lost before birth.

The spleen has a heavy capsule covered by mesothelium and firmly attached by trabeculae that pass into its substance and tend to subdivide it into a series of compartments or lobules. The capsule and trabeculae are composed of dense fibrous connective tissue containing unusually large numbers of elastic fibers and some smooth-muscle cells scattered throughout, individually and in small groups. Arteries, veins, and nerves enter the spleen at a slitlike hilum and course for some distance in the system of branching trabeculae. Their finer branches leave the trabeculae and enter the parenchyma. Lymphatic vessels are found only in the connective-tissue framework of the organ.

The splenic lobules are filled with **red pulp**; this is a modified lymphatic tissue of the diffuse type arranged in poorly defined cords. The red pulp consists of the usual elements of lymphatic tissue, that is, reticular cells and fibers, macrophages, lymphocytes, and plasmocytes. In addition, one finds all types of cells of circulating blood. Monocytes are numerous. The blood gives it its color. The term **splenic cord**, used to designate strands of red pulp, is a little misleading. The red pulp really constitutes the bulk of the splenic parenchyma through which run innumerable sinusoids.

The small arteries leave the trabeculae and traverse the splenic lobules. Around some of them are thick sheaths of compact lymphatic tissue forming the **white pulp**. The terms red and white pulp refer to appearance in the fresh condition. In histologic sections, the white pulp appears as isolated circular masses, called **splenic follicles**,[4] stained dark with basic dyes. Germinal centers

---

[4]Formerly known as "Malpighian corpuscles."

are found in some splenic follicles, especially during the early years of life. The white pulp undergoes cyclic changes, as does compact lymphatic tissue in other places. That seen in Fig. 12.7 represents a relatively inactive state. The structure of a follicle is illustrated in Figs. 12.8 and 12.9. The function of splenic follicles is like that of lymphatic follicles elsewhere in the body: production and storage of lymphocytes. There are no afferent lymphatic vessels, but the splenic white pulp is drained by efferent lymphatic vessels that accompany trabecular arteries and veins.

A good way to study the structure of the spleen is to follow its blood vessels and their branches. Subdivisions of the **splenic artery** enter the hilum and undergo further branching; these branches are distributed throughout the trabecular system as small muscular trabecular arteries. Their adventitial coat blends with the dense fibrous connective tissue of the trabeculae. They are accompanied by trabecular veins that drain blood from the spleen.

When the arteries leave the trabeculae, the fibrous adventitia is replaced by reticular connective tissue, and this becomes packed with lymphocytes to form the white pulp. These little vessels, eccentrically placed in the splenic follicles, are called **central arterioles**. They are not accompanied by veins. Occasionally two central arterioles are seen in one follicle near a point of branching (Fig. 12.8).

Branching continues for some distance, and smaller arterioles ultimately

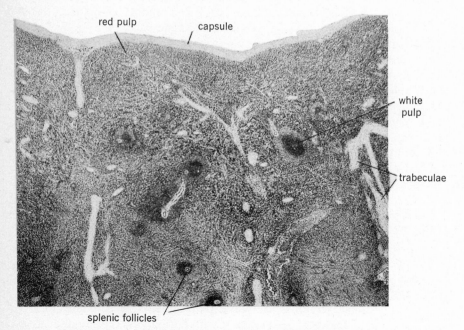

Figure 12-7 Human spleen. Note the heavy capsule and trabeculae (light bands), the splenic follicles (dark spots), and red pulp (main gray bulk). Photomicrograph, ×25.

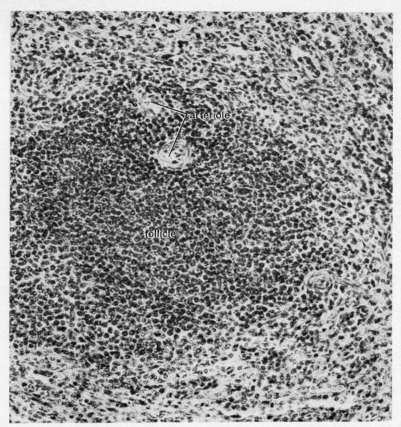

Figure 12-8 Splenic follicle, showing an eccentrically placed central arteriole, above which is a smaller branch. Photomicrograph × 300.

pass among cords of red pulp, having lost the adventitia with its white-pulp lymphocytes. The diameter of the artery diminishes from about 200 μm, as it leaves the trabeculae, to 40 μm, as it leaves the white pulp. During the first and longest part of their course through the red pulp, branching sprays of arterioles with single layers of smooth muscle but no adventitia are formed. These are the **pulp arterioles.** When the muscle disappears with further branching, a peculiar thickened wall appears as a consequence of addition of concentrically arranged reticular connective-tissue cells adjacent to the lining cells. These vessels are usually called **sheathed "arteries,"** although their structure is not at all that of true arteries. They are more prominent in some other species than in man, in whom arterial capillaries are the finest ramifications of the arterial tree. The arterial capillaries connect with the splenic sinusoids. Other arterioles and capillaries provide shunts between the arterioles and venules to bypass the sinusoids. The course of blood is shown in Fig. 12.10.

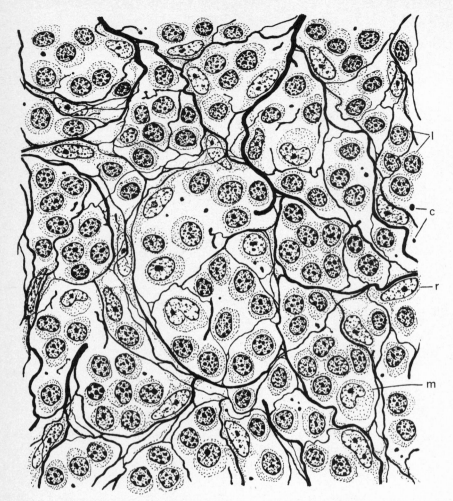

Figure 12-9 Reticulum of a splenic follicle: *c*, reticular fibers in cross section; *l*, lymphocytes; *m*, monocyte; *r*, reticular cell. Silver carbonate stain. ×600. *(JFN)*

Splenic sinusoids are wide, tortuous channels with walls formed by elongated cells that bulge into the lumen. These cells resemble the staves of a barrel. Circularly arranged reticular fibers form the hoops. The lining cells are not like endothelial cells of capillaries or venules. They are more elongated and are not joined firmly to one another by junctional complexes. The lining cells, called "littoral cells," are phagocytic and are classified with elements of the reticuloendothelial system; they are fixed macrophages (Fig. 12.11).

The lining cells abut each other while blood pressure in the sinusoid is low, but readily separate as it is raised. Thus openings between the "staves of the barrel" appear, allowing blood to pass freely out of the sinusoids into the tissue

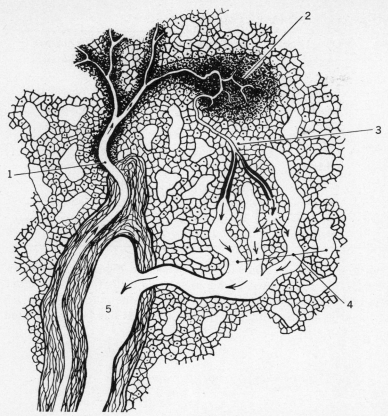

Figure 12-10 Diagram illustrating the course of blood through the spleen. Note that both open and closed channels through the red pulp are shown. 1. Branch of splenic artery leaving a trabecula to enter the white pulp. 2. White pulp. 3. Arteriole entering red pulp. 4. Sinusoids. 5. Trabecular vein. *(Modified from A.H. Ham,* Histology, *6th ed, J.B. Lippincott Company, Philadelphia, 1969.)(CHP)*

spaces of the red pulp cords. The circulation of blood through the splenic red pulp has preferential channels, and the flow can go both ways: out of the sinusoids into the pulp cords and back again into the sinusoids. The splenic sinusoids occupy a considerable amount of space in the red pulp, as is shown in Figs. 12.11 and 12.12. They connect with small venules in the pulp which, in turn, drain blood into larger venules in the trabeculae. Sphincters have been described at the junction of sinusoids and vessels.

The splenic red pulp acts as a blood filter (Fig. 12.13). Blood leaking into the pulp cords becomes static; that entering the sinusoids flows sluggishly or may become static when sphincters on the arteriolar shunts and at the venous ends of the sinusoids close. Littoral cells and other macrophages of the sinusoids and pulp cords phagocytize blood corpuscles whose lives are spent and other particulate matter in the blood. The number of macrophages avail-

Table 12.1   Comparison of Principal Lymphatic Organs

	Lymph node	Tonsil	Spleen	Thymus
Capsule	Present	Present	Marked	Present
Trabeculae in parenchyma	Present	Absent	Marked	Absent
Separate lobes	Absent	Absent	Absent	Present
Hilum	Present	Absent	Present	Absent
Cortex and medulla	Present	Absent	Absent	Present
Germinal centers	Present	Present	Present	Absent
Lymph sinuses	Present	Absent	Absent	Absent
Blood sinusoids	Absent	Absent	Present	Absent
Lymphatic vessels	Afferent and efferent	Efferent only	Only in stroma	Efferent only

able for this purpose is great. When erythrocytes are digested by macrophages, products of the breakdown of hemoglobin are distributed to other places—notably, bile salts to the liver and iron to the bone marrow.

Storage of blood is another function of the spleen. It has been estimated

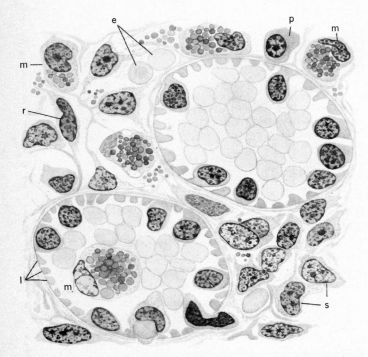

Figure 12-11   Splenic sinusoids and red pulp: *e*, erythrocytes in pulp; *l*, thin cytoplasmic portions of cells lining a splenic sinusoid; *m* and *s*, macrophages in the pulp and in a sinusoid, *p*, plasmocyte; *r*, reticular cell. × 600. *(JFN)*

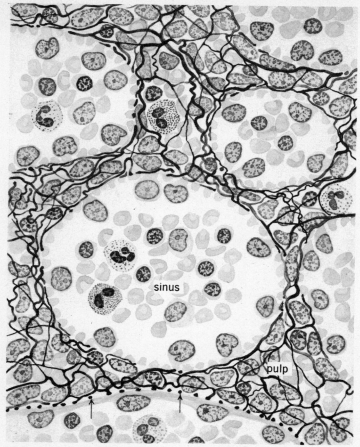

Figure 12-12 Splenic sinusoids (*sinus*) and red pulp, showing reticular fibers. The sinusoids contain blood corpuscles. The sinusoid at the bottom is sectioned longitudinally and shows its encircling reticular fibers cut across (*arrows*). Silver carbonate stain. About × 600. *(JFN)*

that nearly one-sixth of the total blood volume of the cat can be stored in the distended spleen. It is much less in human beings. Intermittent closure of shunts permits engorgement of the splenic sinusoids and subsequent concentration of the formed elements of the blood as some of the plasma filters through the thin walls. Large volumes of erythrocytes can be concentrated in this way. As the sphincters of the sinusoids open again and as arterioles and smooth muscle of the capsule and trabeculae contract, the concentrated blood of the sinusoids moves out into the splenic veins.

The role of the spleen in antibody production is of major importance. The organ responds to antigens in the blood just as lymph nodes respond to antigens in lymph. Plasmocytes quickly form when the call for antibodies comes. Although the spleen has these important functions, it is not a vital organ. Its removal is followed by transfer of its functions to the bone marrow.

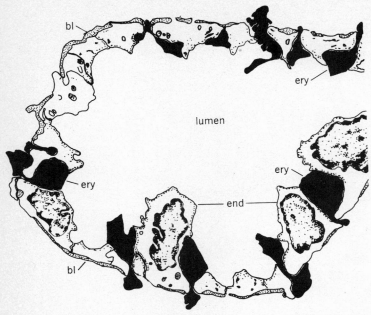

Figure 12-13 Splenic sinusoid with loosely joined endothelial cells, *end*. Erythrocytes (black), *ery*, are squeezing out into the pulp spaces between endothelial cell junctions and across the basal lamina, *bl*. This illustration is a tracing of portions of an electron micrograph. The erythrocytes that fill the lumen have been eliminated from the tracing. *(Contributed by L. T. Chen and L. Weiss.)*

SUGGESTED READING

Brooks, R. E., and B. V. Siegel: Normal Human Lymph Node Cells: An Electron Microscopic Study. *Blood*, vol. 27, pp. 687–705, 1966.

Chen, L. T., and L. Weiss: Electron Microscopy of the Red Pulp of Human Spleen. *American Journal of Anatomy*, vol. 134, pp. 425–458, 1972.

Clark, S. L., Jr.: The Reticulum of Lymph Nodes in Mice Studied with the Electron Microscope. *American Journal of Anatomy*, vol. 110, pp. 217–257, 1962.

Edwards, V. D., and G. T. Simon: Ultrastructural Aspects of Red Cell Destruction in the Normal Rat Spleen. *Journal of Ultrastructure Research*, vol. 33, pp. 187–201, 1970.

Knisely, M. H.: Spleen Studies. *Anatomical Record*, vol. 65, pp. 23–50, 1936.

Weiss, L.: The Structure of the Intermediate Vascular Pathways in the Spleen of Rabbits. *American Journal of Anatomy*, vol. 113, pp. 51–92, 1963.

Wenk, E. J., D. Orlic, E. J. Reith, and J. A. G. Rhodin: The Ultrastructure of Mouse Lymph Node Venules and the Passage of Lymphocytes Across Their Walls. *Journal of Ultrastructure Research*, vol. 47, pp. 214–241, 1974.

Chapter 13

Thymus and the Immune System

The thymus is a lymphoepithelial organ with a key role in immunity. The immune system is composed of it and a number of other organs, chief of which are the bone marrow and the various lymphatic organs described in the preceding chapters. Precursors of all components of this system are found in bone marrow, some giving rise there to the myeloid stem cells from which granulocytes, erythrocytes, and megakaryocytes are derived, and others becoming lymphoid stem cells. The latter are of two types: those leaving the marrow for other sites in lymphatic tissue, where they are destined to produce humoral-antibody-secreting cells, and those migrating to the thymus, where they become the lymphocytes responsible for cell-mediated immunity.

THYMUS

The thymus is located in the upper thorax behind the sternum. It consists of two main lobes lightly encapsulated by connective tissue. Its parenchyma is subdivided into many lobules by septa conveying blood vessels and the accompanying nerve fibers. The thymus lacks the fine stroma of reticular tissue that is encountered in other lymphatic organs. Thymic lobules are composed of darkly staining cortex and lightly staining medulla, sharply delineated from each other,

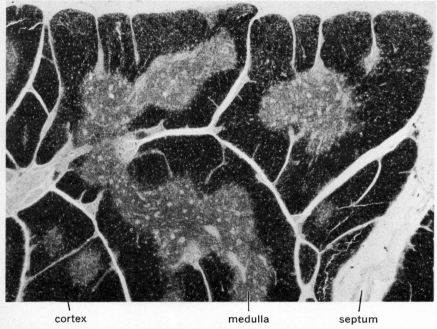

cortex   medulla   septum

Figure 13-1 Thymus of a child. Photomicrograph, × 25.

as seen in Fig. 13.1, a photomicrograph taken at low magnification. One does not need the microscope to recognize a stained section of thymus.

The thymus arises embryologically from outgrowths of the third branchial pouches. These primordia are the source of the epithelial cells that form its intrinsic framework.

The **thymic cortex** is a compact arrangement of small lymphocytes among which few other cells can be recognized in the usual preparation. The epithelial cells are more easily observed in the medullary regions than in the cortex. Occasionally they form compact masses, as seen in Fig. 13.2. They are separated by lymphocytes in the cortex but do retain contacts with one another, so that they appear to form a meshwork, called a "cytoreticulum." Epithelial cell junctions are formed by desmosomes, and tonofibrils are present in the cytoplasm. Electron micrographs show cytoplasmic granules that may be secretory.

One of the most characteristic features of the medulla of this organ is the **thymic corpuscle.**[1] This is a rounded mass of flattened epithelioid cells concentrically arranged, as seen in Fig. 13.3. Thymic corpuscles vary in diameter from 30 to 100 μm. Since they stain pink by eosin, they may be confused with venules filled with erythrocytes.

[1]Often called "Hassall's corpuscle."

The **thymic medulla** contains many clusters of lymphocytes, less compactly arranged than in the cortex. They infiltrate among the epithelial cells somewhat as lymphocytes do in the tonsils. Macrophages are present in considerable numbers in the thymic parenchyma. After puberty, adipose tissue is associated with the thymic connective tissue (Fig. 13.4).

The usual description of the thymus applies to the organ during infancy and childhood (Fig. 13.1). Its appearance changes with age. Relatively largest in the fetus, it reaches maximum actual size during adolescence. It weighs about 12 g at birth, triples in weight by the fifteenth year, returns to birth weight

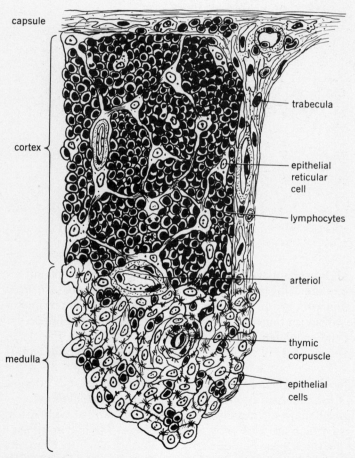

Figure 13-2 Portion of a thymic lobule in which the medulla consists mainly of epithelial cells. The medulla is filled with lymphocytes among which are epithelial cells of stellate shape, the so-called "epithelial reticular" cells. *(Drawing modified from L. Weiss,* The Cells and Tissues of the Immune System, *Prentice-Hall, Inc., Englewood Cliffs, N. J., 1972.) (CHP)*

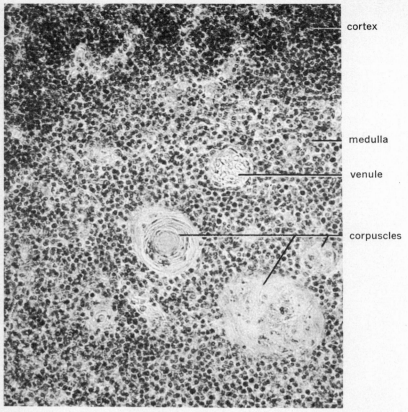

cortex

medulla

venule

corpuscles

Figure 13-3 Thymic corpuscles in the medulla of the thymus of a 14-year-old girl. Photomicrograph, × 300.

by age 45 or 50. Involution begins with a gradual thinning of the cortex and replacement by adipose tissue. This is normally a slow process. The gross form of the organ is often maintained by the replacing adipose tissue, as is illustrated in Fig. 13.4. Sometimes fibrous connective tissue takes the place of adipose tissue, as is the case of the specimen from an old individual shown in Fig. 13.5. Thymic involution in early life may occur accidentally as the result of debilitating disease.

There are no afferent lymphatic vessels entering the thymus, but efferent ones can be found in the subdivisions of the fibrous stroma. Arterial blood vessels enter through interlobular septa and branch into thick-walled capillaries, the endothelial cells of which are united by tight junctions. Thymic epithelial-cell processes invest the thick basal lamina of the capillaries. All these elements together appear to form a blood-thymus barrier somewhat like the blood-brain barrier.

The thymus has both lymphocytogenic and endocrine functions. Lympho-

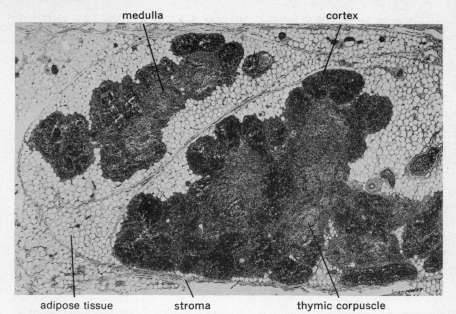

Figure 13-4 Thymus of a 39-year-old man, showing partial involution and replacement of outer portions of lobules by adipose tissue. Compare with Fig. 13-1. Photomicrograph, × 25.

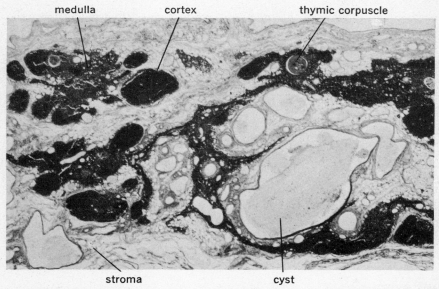

Figure 13-5 Old human thymus showing marked involution. Cortex and medulla are still visible. Adipose tissue has been largely replaced by fibrous connective tissue. Several epithelium-lined cysts are present. Photomicrograph, × 25.

cytes can first be identified in the fetal thymus at the end of the third month of gestation. Precursors of lymphocytes apparently do not arise in situ but are derived from stem cells that migrate to the thymus from hemopoietic organs—at first from the fetal liver, while that organ is producing blood cells, and later from the bone marrow.

Lymphocytes are produced in the young thymus at a more rapid rate than in other lymphatic organs. However, most of them die and are disposed of by macrophages before they can make their way into the circulation. Those that are released live for years, circulating and recirculating throughout the body. These **thymus-derived lymphocytes** become lodged in other lymphatic organs. Removal of the young thymus results in loss of lymphocytes in lymph nodes, spleen, and other lymphatic tissue, and the number of lymphocytes in the blood is greatly reduced.

The thymus is deficient or absent at birth in an occasional infant who, therefore, lacks the means of acquiring cell-mediated immunity. Transplantation of fetal thymic tissue has successfully rectified this deficiency in some instances. More recently administration of thymic hormone has been successfully employed.

The thymus-derived lymphocyte is usually called a "T cell." Lymphocytes of bone-marrow origin are known as "B cells." One cannot tell them apart in routinely prepared histologic preparations or blood films. However, the thymus-derived lymphocytes bear a distinctive marker (theta antigen) on their surface; this makes it possible to distinguish them from other cells by special techniques of immunology.

The second function of the thymus is production of **thymosin**, a hormone that stimulates lymphocyte production in lymphatic tissue generally. Thymic epithelial cells have characteristics of cells in some other endocrine organs— notably their cytoplasmic granules. These cells are believed to be the source of thymosin. Its production, like that of other endocrine secretions, appears to be regulated by a hypophyseal hormone.

Antibody production does not occur to any extent in the thymus, even though an occasional plasmocyte can be identified (mainly in connective-tissue septa). Germinal centers, which are sites of antibody production in other lymphatic organs, are not found in the normal human thymus.

Activities of the thymus decrease as the organ undergoes involution. It is presumed that adequate numbers of thymus-derived lymphocytes have populated the other lymphatic organs by the time of marked thymic involution. Thymosin levels in the blood decrease as the organ undergoes involution. It has been suggested that this change may be related to the process of physiologic aging.

IMMUNE SYSTEM

This is essentially a dual system, one component of which is concerned with cell-mediated immunity by thymus-derived lymphocytes. The other component has to do with the production of antibodies. The latter are immunoglobulin macromolecules commonly circulating in the blood. Progenitors of cells of the immune system are among elements of reticular tissue in the bone marrow. They can give rise to myeloid stem cells (for granulocytes, erythrocytes, and megakaryocytes) or to lymphoid stem cells.

Cells that can phagocytize foreign material are part of the immune system. The functions of granular leucocytes, monocytes, and macrophages in defending against invading microorganisms were discussed in previous chapters. Other cells, no less important, are lymphocytes that function in cell-mediated immunity and plasmocytes that secrete antibodies in defense against antigens.

A foreign antigen can be any molecule that differs from those of the body's own and can damage tissues upon entering the body. When it is recognized as "not self," the body's defenses can be brought into play to inactivate it. A major function of the immune system is that of guarding against foreign antigens.

Surfaces of the body's own cells normally contain small protein molecules known as "histocompatibility antigens" (e.g., β_2-microglobulin). These ordinarily do not provoke immune responses, but under certain circumstances they can elicit a reaction, for example, transplant rejection. The histocompatibility antigens that exist in places sequestered from elements of the immune system can function as autoantigens when the barrier between the sequestered cells and the blood stream becomes damaged.

Antigens on the surface of cells provide binding sites for antibodies. Those in the plasma membrane of erythrocytes identify the cells as members of one of the blood groups.

There are untold numbers of foreign antigens with different molecular specificities, each of which requires a separate antagonist to render it harmless. Lymphocytes of the immune system carry the genetic information required for production of antibodies for any and all.

Antibodies are protein macromolecules of immunoglobulin secreted by cells derived from lymphocytes and by plasmocytes. These immunoglobulins circulate in the plasma as humoral antibodies, and are bound to surface receptors of certain lymphocytes. Several general classes of immunoglobulins have been recognized, of which only three will be considered here.

Immunoglobulin M is a large macromolecule (molecular weight 950,000) that binds with antigens during an initial immune response. It is the first antibody formed by the newborn infant. An electron micrograph of this molecule is seen in Fig. 13.6. **Immunoglobulin G,** a smaller macromolecule, is the main weapon of defense in the delayed immune response; it becomes available after cells of the immune system have been triggered to go into "mass production."

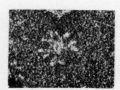

Figure 13-6 A molecule of human immunoglobulin M (19S). Electron micrograph, × 300,000. *(Contributed by Sven-Erik Svehag.)*

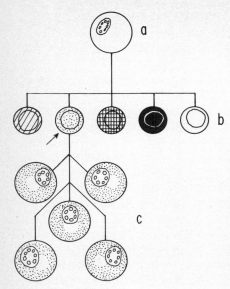

Figure 13-7 Diagram illustrating clonal selection. Stem cells of reticular tissue in bone marrow or lymphatic organs, *a*, multiply and differentiate into numerous immunologically committed small lymphocytes, *b*. The different shading indicates that, although the lymphocytes look alike, they have antibody receptors of different specificities on the surface. When stimulated by an antigen (*arrow*), the lymphocytes become able to divide and form clones, *c*, of daughter cells capable of secreting the particular antibody. *(CHP)*

Immunoglobulin A is secreted by plasmocytes in the subepithelial connective tissue of the alimentary tract, passing into the lumen to react with antigens there.[2]

The plasma of adult human beings contains humoral antibodies able to bind immediately with a number of antigens. This occurs during the initial immune response. However, antibodies do not preexist in sufficient quantity or diversity in the plasma to bind with each and every antigen that may appear. They must be provided upon demand, and this appears to be accomplished by means of **clonal selection**, a process illustrated by the diagram in Fig. 13.7.

Specific cells, already committed to produce the appropriate antibody, are stimulated by invading antigens. Each cell secretes an antibody of a specific character. Stimulation of cell division and immunoglobulin synthesis follows the interaction between antigen and cell. The antibodies produced by each of the proliferated cells in the clone are identical with those that met the invading antigen.

The body is able to respond to far more antigens than it will ever be exposed to. The genetic information is available for synthesis of a great many immunoglobulin molecules with specific binding sites, not all of which can be detected in the blood. Vast numbers of its small lymphocytes are **immunocompetent**,[3] and can be transformed into antibody-secreting cells that produce one specific antibody per cell. Most immunocompetent lymphocytes circulate while waiting for an invading antigen that may never appear.

When a small lymphocyte meets a specific antigen and "recognizes" it, the

[2]These three immunoglobulins are commonly designated "IgM," "IgG," and "IgA."
[3]Immunologically competent cells are those that have become able to "recognize" an antigen and be influenced by it; that is, they can respond to an inductive stimulus in their environment.

lymphocyte enlarges, and its cytoplasm increases in amount and becomes more basophilic because of great numbers of ribosomes in it. This cell has been called a "pyroninophilic cell" because it stains readily with the dye pyronin. Its cytoplasm contains few elements of the endoplasmic reticulum at this stage, but it soon acquires granular endoplasmic reticulum and thereby becomes a plasmocyte, or it stimulates some other cell (plasmoblast) to become a plasmocyte.

The immune system contains cells that can bind with antibodies and cells that secrete antibodies. Figure 13.8*A* is a fluorescence photomicrograph of a group of immunoglobulin-secreting cells, and Fig. 13.8*B* shows a lymphocyte

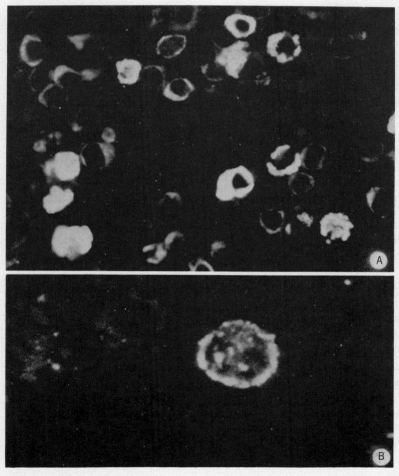

Figure 13-8 *A*. Fluorescence photomicrograph of a section through the medulla of a lymph node. Numerous immunoglobulin-secreting cells appear as light objects against a dark background. *B*. Fluorescence photomicrograph of a small lymphocyte, on the surface of which antibodies are bound and revealed as light particles against a black background. *(Contributed by R. A. Good, Harvey Lectures, 1973. Reproduced with permission of Academic Press, Inc., New York.)*

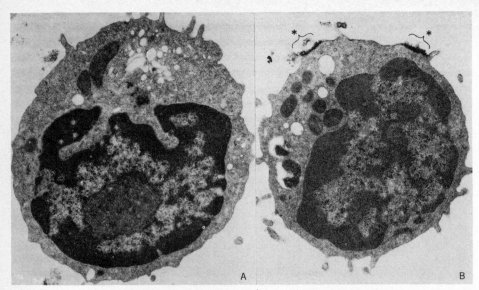

Figure 13-9 Two lymphocytes of a mouse. That in *A* does not bind an antigen-antibody complex. That in *B* binds the complex, as shown by the electron-dense plaques that are bracketed and indicated by asterisks (*). Electron micrographs, × 16,000. *(Contributed by L. T. Chen and L. Weiss.)*

with fluorescing antibodies on its surface. The binding sites to which antigen-antibody complexes adhere are demonstrated on mouse-lymph-node lymphocytes but not on mouse-thymus lymphocytes in Fig. 13.9.

Isotope-tagged markers have been used to identify the two types of small lymphocyte. Those derived from bone marrow cells (B lymphocytes) accumulate in diffuse lymphatic tissue and in follicles of lymph nodes, spleen, and aggregates of follicles in the lower small intestine. Deep cortical regions of lymph nodes and periarteriolar white pulp of the spleen, on the other hand, are sites of accumulation of thymus-derived small lymphocytes (Fig. 13.10).

Antibody production begins after birth when antigens engage the appropriate cells—first those beneath the epithelium of mucous membranes. The newborn infant's blood contains humoral antibodies that were made by its mother and passed through the placenta. These provide passive immunity until the newborn's own immune system can take over.

The other component of the dual system, namely, cell-mediated immunity, is best demonstrated by the phenomenon of allograft rejection. Success in tissue transplantation and organ transplantation depends on finding the means to prevent thymus-derived lymphocytes from interfering with acceptance of the foreign tissue by the recipient.

Transplantation can be carried out successfully when the donor and recipient are the same person (autograft) or are closely related persons who have genes derived from the same ovum and sperm, as in the case of identical twins

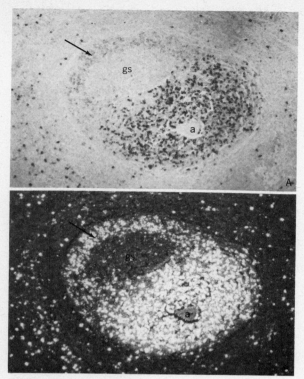

Figure 13-10 Radioautographs of white pulp of the spleen (rat) 48 hours after an intravenous injection of 10^9 normal thoracic-duct lymphocytes that had been labeled in vitro with uridene-3H. Heavily-labeled small lymphocytes (thymus-derived) have localized around the arteriole, *a*. Lightly-labeled (marrow-derived) small lymphocytes have accumulated (*arrow*) around the germinal center, *gs*. A. Bright-field view. B. Dark-field view of same; approximately × 90. *(Contributed by J. L. Gowans,* The Journal of Experimental Medicine, *vol. 135, pp. 200–219, 1972. Reproduced with permission of the publishers.)*

(isograft). When donor and recipient are unrelated members of the same species, the procedures (allograft) can be done successfully only by suppressing the immune response, thus preventing the recipient's immune system from recognizing the donor's tissue antigens (autoantigens) as foreign and causing rejection. Blood transfusion, for example, is a type of tissue transplantation, techniques for which have been well established (Chap. 7).

Dysfunction of the immune system sometimes occurs. An autoimmune phenomenon that appears when the body turns its defenses against itself can lead to tragic consequences, now often avoidable because of increasing understanding of the complexities of the immune system. A case in point is the recent conquest of the dread Rh hemolytic disease of the human fetus and newborn infant, which occurs when erythrocytes from an Rh-positive fetus cross the placental barrier and induce an immune response in an Rh-negative mother. Anti-Rh antibodies secreted by her then may traverse the placenta to the fetuses of subsequent pregnancies and destroy their erythrocytes. An effective Rh vaccine (the 7S fraction of gamma globulin) is now available for administration to women before they become sensitized to the Rh factor.

Immunodeficiency diseases are yielding to replacement therapy. Marrow cells can be aspirated from the bones of a compatible donor and implanted in an immunodeficient recipient. This technique, still in early stages of development, offers hope to many patients whose blood diseases now doom them to early death.

SUGGESTED READING

Edelman, G. M.: Antibody Structure and Molecular Immunology. *Science*, vol. 180, pp. 830–840, 1973.

Goldstein, A. L., J. A. Hooper, R. S. Schulof, G. H. Cohen, G. B. Thurman, M. C. Mc-Daniel, A. White, and M. Dardenne: Thymosin and the Immunopathology of Aging. *Federation Proceedings*, vol. 33, pp. 2053–2056, 1974.

Good, R. A.: Immunodeficiency in Developmental Perspective. *Harvey Lectures, Ser.* 67 (1971–1972), pp. 1–107, 1973.

Jerme, N. K.: The Immune System. *Scientific American*, vol. 229, no. 1, pp. 52–60, July, 1973.

Lucky, T. D. (ed.): *Thymic Hormones.* University Park Press, Baltimore, 1973.

Marx, J. L.: Immunology: Role of β_2-Microglobulin. *Science*, vol. 185, pp. 428–429, 1974.

Mayer, M. M.: The Complement System. *Scientific American*, vol. 229, no. 5, pp. 54–66, November, 1973.

Miller, J. F. A. P.: The Thymus and the Development of Immunologic Responsiveness. *Science*, vol. 144, pp. 1544–1551, 1964.

Norsal, G. F. V.: How Cells Make Antibodies. *Scientific American*, vol. 211, no. 6, pp. 106–115, December, 1964.

Porter, R. R.: Structural Studies of Immunoglobulins. *Science*, vol. 180, pp. 713–716, 1973.

Trainin, N.: Thymic Hormones and the Immune Response. *Physiological Reviews*, vol. 54, pp. 272–315, 1974.

Weiss, L.: *The Cells and Tissues of the Immune System.* Prentice-Hall, Inc., Englewood Cliffs, N.J., 1972.

Williamson, A. R.: Clones of Antibody-forming Cells: Natural and Experimental Selection. *Endeavour,* vol. 31, pp. 118–122, 1972.

Zimmerman, D. R.: *Rh. The Intimate History of a Disease and Its Conquest.* The Macmillan Company, New York, 1973.

Nervous Tissue

Nervous tissue is the last fundamental tissue to be considered. It is composed of cells of three main types, associated with elements of other tissues to form the "nervous system." Nervous tissue forms the parenchyma of the nervous system, the stroma of which is connective tissue and its blood vessels. The nervous system consists of the brain and spinal cord (central nervous system) and the nerves, ganglia, and nerve endings (peripheral nervous system). Peripherally the components of nervous tissue extend into the skin, muscles, and nearly all other organs. Although nervous tissue is encountered almost everywhere, it makes up only about 3 percent of the body weight.

Neurons are the most prominent and largest cells of nervous tissue. Their total number is estimated to be about 12 billion. Smaller and several times more numerous, the **neuroglia cells** are associated with them in the central nervous system. Another type of nervous-tissue cell occurs in ganglia and nerves of the peripheral nervous system. This is the **neurolemma cell**.[1] Neurons, neuroglia, and neurolemma have a common embryonic origin from the ectoderm of the neural plate.

[1]Commonly called "Schwann cell."

NEURONS

Neurons typically consist of an elongated fiber, or **axon**, along the course of which—in most cases, near one end—a swelling, the **cell body,** is located. Axons vary in length. Some run less than a millimeter, but the longest ones course for more than a meter and are 10,000 times as long as the diameter of the cell body. Many are two hundred times as long. Although each seems incredibly small when viewed in cross section, calculations indicate that the whole axon may contain one hundred times as much protoplasm as the cell body. These points are illustrated in Fig. 14.1.

The cell body is the trophic center of the neuron, containing the machinery for metabolic activities including protein synthesis. Other parts of the neuron are more directly concerned with its primary functions, i.e., reception of stimuli, generation and transmission of the nerve impulse, and induction of a response, either in another neuron or in an effector organ, such as a muscle fiber or gland cell. Relatively short branches, **dendrites**, receive stimuli at the proximal end of the neuron either from receptor organs or from terminal endings of other neurons. This results in generation of the nerve impulse at the point where the axon begins. The axon then conducts the impulse to the distal end of the neuron, where its terminal branches, **telodendria,** make contacts with an effector or with another neuron in the latter's dendritic zone.

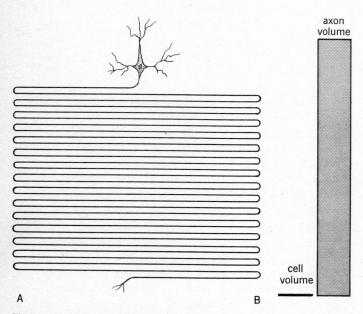

Figure 14-1 Schematic diagram illustrating quantitative relationships between the nerve-cell body and its main process. *A*, the axon, gathered into folds, is two hundred times as long as the diameter of the cell body from which it arises. *B*, the axon contains one hundred times as much protoplasm as the cell body. *(WEL)*

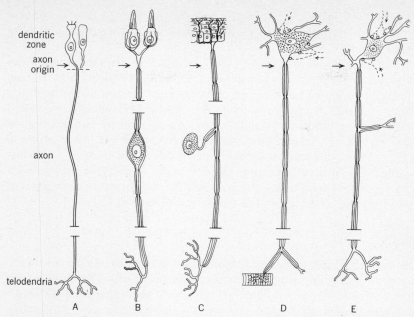

dendritic
zone

axon
origin

axon

telodendria

A   B   C   D   E

Figure 14-2 Diagram of a variety of neurons showing points in common. The cell body is in the dendritic zone of the olfactory, *A,* motor neuron, *D,* and interneuron, *E;* in the axon of the auditory neuron, *B;* and separated from the axon of the cutaneous sensory neuron, *C.* *(Redrawn from D. Bodian.) (CHP)*

The cell body is commonly found in the dendritic zone, as in peripheral olfactory neurons and in most neurons of the central nervous system. It is in the axon itself in neurons of the vestibulocochlear nerve. In the spinal ganglia it is located away from the axon and attached to it by a stalk (Fig. 14.2).

Neurons exhibit greater variation in shape and size than other cells. The diameter of the smallest nerve-cell body is only about 4 μm, while that of the largest is 135 μm or more. As a rule, the axons of large neurons are longer and thicker than those of small neurons. Various shapes and sizes will be seen in illustrations accompanying this and the succeeding two chapters.

Neurons are long-lived cells. Specialized to the extreme, they have lost the power to divide. There is no evidence that cell division occurs in human neurons after birth. As though to compensate for inability to provide replacements, it would seem that there is an enormous excess of neurons in some parts of the nervous system. Perhaps the loss of an occasional neuron with the passage of time may not be noticed. However, most of them survive for life. They are quite resistant to the ravages of time and a succession of minor insults by noxious agents, but they are sensitive to traumatic injury of their processes. Furthermore, their metabolism requires a continuous oxygen supply, without which they quickly die.

Most axons arise and terminate within the brain and spinal cord. Others enter the central nervous system from the periphery. Only the axons of motor neurons arise in the central nervous system (or in sympathetic ganglia) and pass into the nerves.

Because its axon commonly extends for considerable distances away from the cell body, it is never possible to observe a neuron in its entirety in histologic sections. The cell bodies of neurons are often grouped in clusters in the brain, called "nuclei," as well as clusters outside the central nervous system, called "ganglia." The axons tend to run parallel to one another in bundles, called "fiber tracts" in the central nervous system and "nerves" in the peripheral nervous system. It is convenient to study cell bodies and axons of neurons separately, speaking of them as **nerve cells** and **nerve fibers**. One must not let this artificial separation lead to misconceptions. Nerve fibers are main parts of neurons, and they die when separated from the cell bodies.

NERVE CELLS

Nerve cells vary so widely in size and shape that selection of any one as a typical example for description of intrinsic structure is arbitrary. The smallest are smaller than lymphocytes; the largest are visible to the naked eye. Globoid, piriform, spindle-shaped, pyramidal, and stellate nerve cells are encountered in the nervous system. Cells with many processes, i.e., multipolar, particularly the stellate variety, outnumber other types. Those measuring 40 μm or more in diameter most clearly portray details of cell structure (Fig. 14.3).

A plasmolemma encloses the nerve-cell protoplasm, or **neuroplasm**, which contains a variety of organelles. Mitochondria are numerous, and a golgi complex can be readily observed in electron micrographs; the latter consists of clusters of flattened cisternae distributed around the nucleus rather than concentrated at one pole (Fig. 2.17A). Although nerve cells do not undergo mitosis, centrioles may be seen occasionally. Lysosomes are present, and so are lipofuscin-pigment bodies, the latter being prominent in nerve cells of old individuals (Fig. 2.11). Melanin pigment is encountered in certain regions of the nervous system. Granular endoplasmic reticulum, free ribosomes, microfilaments, and microtubules are prominent organelles in the neuroplasm. Fine structure is illustrated in Fig. 14.4.

The three most characteristic structures seen in nerve cells under the light microscope are the nucleus, neurofibrils, and chromophil substance. The cytoplasm of a nerve cell is designated its **perikaryon** (the nucleus being the "karyon").

The **nucleus** usually is located centrally. Its diameter varies to some extent with the size of the nerve cell. It stands out prominently in histologic sections, mainly because of its vesicular appearance (Fig. 14.3A). There are few clumps of chromatin in it, the chromosomes being dispersed, but it has a distinct nucleolus that stains metachromatically. Most nerve cells contain a single nucleus, but binucleate and even multinucleate cells are encountered occasionally in certain regions (Fig. 2.26).

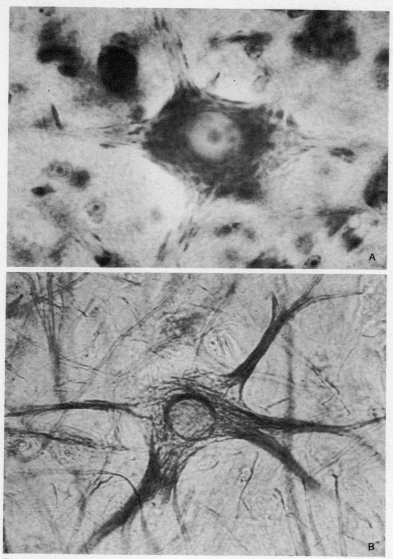

Figure 14-3 Multipolar motor neurons of the spinal cord: *A*, guinea pig; *B*, newborn kitten. Chromophil substance stained in *A;* neurofibrils stained in *B*. Photmicrographs, × 900.

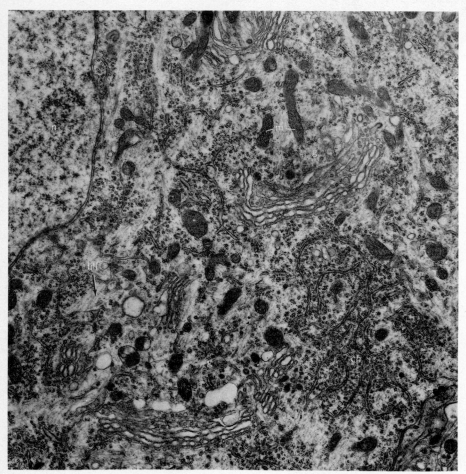

Figure 14-4 Part of a nerve cell in the ventral horn of the spinal cord (young mouse). An extensive golgi complex, *g,* occupies the perikaryon adjacent to the nucleus, *n.* Clusters of ribosomes (polysomes) associated with endoplasmic reticulum constitute the chromophil substance, *ch;* mitochondria, *m,* and neurofilaments, *fil,* are present. Electron micrograph, about × 18,000. *(Contributed by D. S. Maxwell.)*

Neurofibrils are observed in the cytoplasm of all neurons specifically stained by silver methods (Fig. 14.3*B*). These structures cannot be identified as such in electron micrographs of well-fixed preparations. Probably they represent clumped microfilaments that were agglutinated by the fixing reagent prior to staining. **Neurofilaments** are arranged in parallel arrays in the cytoplasm of the cell body as well as in all processes of the neuron (Fig. 14.13). **Neurotubules** course parallel to neurofilaments, and can be seen to advantage in the axon (Fig. 14.21).

The **chromophil substance** of the neuroplasm is ordinarily encountered as small flakelike masses[2] (Fig. 14.3*A*). Its patterns are relatively constant within groups of nerve cells of similar function but vary from one group to another. Chromophil substance is composed of granular endoplasmic reticulum and is intensely basophilic. Electron micrographs reveal numerous ribosomes, not only on the surface of the cisternae of endoplasmic reticulum, but also as free polysomes (especially in developing nerve cells). The extensive ribosomal component, the numerous mitochondria, and the dispersed state of chromosomes all signify that the neuron is an active cell.

Chromophil substance responds to sudden imposition of changes in metabolic requirements, as when the axon is severed from the cell body, by undergoing a marked change. Trauma, asphyxia, and toxic agents cause dispersion and alteration of the pattern of the chromophil substance. The nerve cells are said to undergo **chromatolysis** when flakes of it disappear. The process begins in a few hours, proceeds to death of the cell, or reaches its peak in 4 to 6 days and subsides as recovery takes place. Figure 14.5 shows chromatolysis.

Nerve cell bodies located in the dendritic zone of multipolar neurons of the brain and spinal cord have chromophil substance extending into parts of all the major processes except the axon. Where the axon springs directly from the cell body, there is a cone-shaped region, the **axon hillock**, lacking chromophil substance (Fig. 14.6). Similarly, a hillock may be found at the origin of the process of large unipolar cells in spinal ganglia (Fig. 14.7). Multipolar nerve cells, from whose dendritic processes axons spring, usually exhibit no axon hillocks.

Neuroplasm of the axon is the medium of communication between the protein-synthesizing machinery of the cell body and the distant parts of the neuron. Two main types of movement have been recognized. Outgrowth of processes of the neuroplasm, for example during embryonic development, involves **axoplasmic flow.** This is slow, occurring at a rate of only a few millimeters or less per day. Within the processes of neurons, on the other hand, there is a different type of flow for rapid **axoplasmic transport** of material synthesized in the nerve cell. This occurs at rates up to 410 mm per day. Moreover, there is a reverse transport mechanism that accounts for movement of substances from the distal end of the axon toward the perikaryon.

Slow axoplasmic transport of macromolecules maintains the structural constitution of the neuron. Glycoprotein and protein materials essential to production of new unit membranes, mitochondria, and presynaptic vesicles are transported rapidly. It is probable that different mechanisms are involved in the two types of transport. There is a system of agranular endoplasmic reticulum composed of long continuous tubules running from the perikaryon through the axon to its terminations. Figure 14.8 is a thick-section, high-voltage electron micrograph showing part of this system. The tubules of agranular endoplasmic reticulum appear to provide the mechanism by which rapid axoplasmic transport is accomplished.

[2]These are usually referred to as "Nissl bodies."

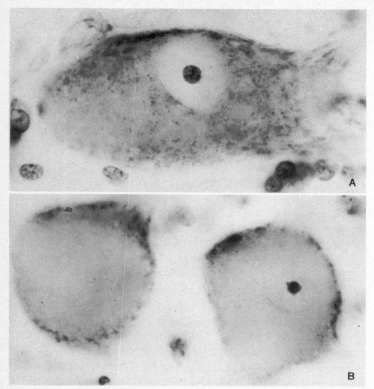

Figure 14-5 Chromatolysis: *A*, in a motor nerve cell of the spinal cord of a cat, 6 days after concussion; *B*, two cells of the red nucleus of the brainstem of a guinea pig, 4 days after their axons were severed. Thionine stain. Photomicrograph, × 900.

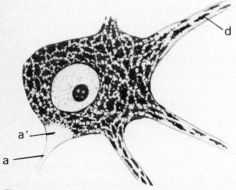

Figure 14-6 Large, multipolar nerve cell from the spinal cord. Note clear nucleus containing dark nucleolus. Cytoplasm is filled with flakes of chromophil substance extending into dendrites (d) but absent in the axon (a) and axon hillock (a'). Approximately × 900. *(JFN)*

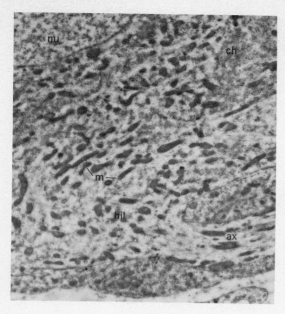

Figure 14-7 Axon hillock, *hil,* and axon, *ax,* of a spinal-ganglion cell (rat). The nucleus, *nu,* is visible at the top of the picture. The perikaryon is filled with dark rod-shaped mitochondria, *m;* a clump of chromophil substance, *ch,* is seen. Electron micrograph, × 8,000. *(Contributed by J. Rosenbluth and S. L. Palay.)*

Precursors of neurons are called **neuroblasts**. These cells are able to migrate, their locomotion being accomplished in the manner of other free cells. With the formation of their dendrites, the neuroblasts become anchored in definitive places in the nervous system, but their axons continue to grow slowly in length. The processes of cell locomotion and cell elongation are fundamentally different. Locomotion is characterized by ruffling activity of the plasmolemma, whereas elongation is associated with **growth cones** exhibiting microspike formation at the tips (Fig. 14.9). A nervous-tissue protein that appears to be involved in the process of elongation has been identified. It is similar to, though not identical with, actomyosin of muscle, having the ability to convert chemical energy to mechanical energy.

Neurons, having been derived from an epithelial primordium, the embryonic ectoderm, possess secretory properties to a greater or lesser extent. The most notable examples of **secretory neurons** are found in the hypothalamus of the brain in close proximity to the hypophysis. Secretory products are elaborated in hypothalamic nerve cells and pass through their axons to the neurohypophysis, or are transported to capillaries that carry them to the adenohypophysis (Chap. 24).

A full complement of neurons is reached by the human infant before birth. Individual neurons, however, do not stop growing. Protein synthesis continues, and so does axoplasmic flow. The cell processes increase in length and thickness. Degenerative and regenerative activities are thought to involve

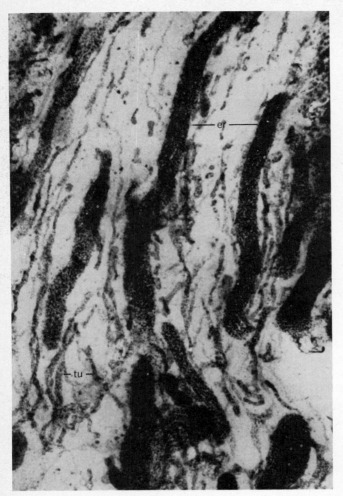

Figure 14-8 Agranular endoplasmic reticulum, *er,* appearing as long, tubular structures in the initial segment of an axon. Neurotubules, *tu,* are seen among them. The electron micrograph was made with a 1-million-volt instrument employing a section 1 µm thick. Approximately ×60,000. *(Contributed by A. Droz, from unpublished findings of A. Rambonsy.)*

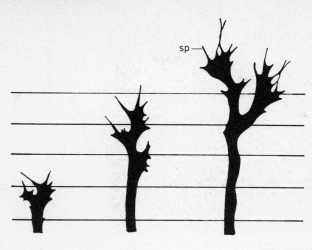

Figure 14-9 Three stages in elongation of a growing nerve fiber in tissue culture, showing microspike formation, *sp. (Modified from P. Weiss.)*

neurons well beyond the time of birth. To what extent the microspike activity at tips of telodendria continues as an ongoing function of adult neurons is not known. However, it is known that the potential for sprouting is not lost at maturity.

SYNAPSES

It is possible, with appropriate methods and by means of the light microscope, to see the minute endings of some telodendria upon parts of adjacent neurons in their dendritic zones. Electron micrographs, however, have done much to develop our concepts of structural contacts between neurons, called **synapses**.

Several types of synapse are recognized. The contacts may be between axonal telodendria and the surface of the cell body (axosomatic), surface of a dendrite (axondendritic), or surface of another axon (axoaxonic). Other characteristics of synapses are illustrated in Fig. 14.10. A form of synapse commonly encountered in the spinal cord involves multiple **end-bulbs** (Fig. 14.11)—minute swellings of the axonal terminations.

The fine structure of the synapse is illustrated in Fig. 14.12. The plasmolemma of the axon terminal and that of the cell with which it makes a synapse are darker and thicker at the points of contact than elsewhere. The dark portions are called **presynaptic** and **postsynaptic membranes,** respectively, depending upon their position. The telodendritic swelling on the presynaptic side contains many microvesicles and more than the usual number of mitochondria. On the postsynaptic side, the cytoplasm is deficient in these **synaptic vesicles,** although numerous microfilaments may be seen there. A space about 200 Å wide intervenes between the synaptic membranes. This contains some electron-dense material.

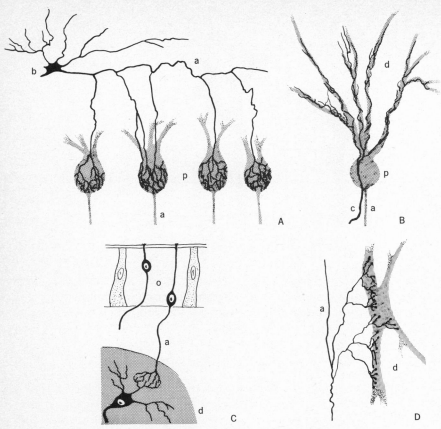

Figure 14-10 Four types of synapse: *A*, between endings of the axon, *a*, of a cerebellar basket cell, *b*, and the cell bodies of four purkinje, *p*, neurons; *B*, between a climbing fiber, *c*, and the dendritic tree of a purkinje neuron; *C*, between the axon terminals of an olfactory sensory neuron, *o*, and dendrites, *d*, of a nerve cell of the olfactory bulb; *D*, between end-bulbs of axon collaterals and the body of a nerve cell in the spinal cord. *(WEL)*

The synapse provides a mechanism by which electrical activity of a neuron can initiate electrical activity in another neuron or in a muscle or epithelial cell of some effector organ. Transmission across this synaptic cleft is chemical. A transmitter substance, usually acetylcholine or norepinephrine, is released by exocytosis from the presynaptic element, traverses the cleft, and on the postsynaptic element finds receptor sites that respond by initiating electrical activity in that neuron or end-organ cell. The presynaptic vesicles contain the chemical transmitter that was manufactured in the perikaryon and that reached the ending via the rapid axoplasmic transport system.

Two varieties of synaptic vesicle have been described on the basis of the appearance of their contents in electron micrographs. Clear vesicles are as-

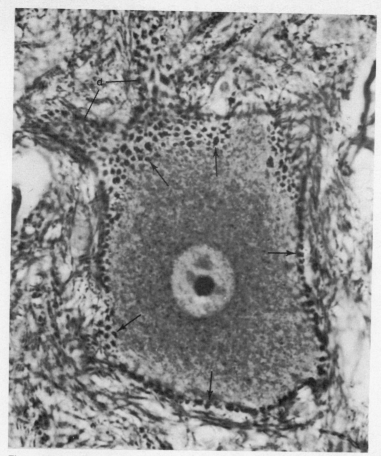

Figure 14-11 Synapses formed by end-bulbs (*arrows*) on the surface of the cell body and dendrites, *d*, of a multipolar neuron in the medulla oblongata of a cat. The specimen was stained by a silver method. Photomicrograph, × 900. *(Contributed by G. L. Rasmussen.)*

sociated with acetylcholine (cholinergic), while vesicles with electron-dense contents are related to norepinephrine (adrenergic). Furthermore, round vesicles are believed to be present in excitatory synapses, while oval vesicles are located in inhibitory synapses.

NERVE FIBERS

The term "nerve fiber" is reserved for long axons with their sheaths. Each nerve fiber has a core, its axis cylinder, consisting of a drawn-out portion of the neuroplasm of the neuron. The neuroplasm of the **axis cylinder** is known as "axoplasm." It is bounded by a plasmolemma sometimes called the "axolemma,"

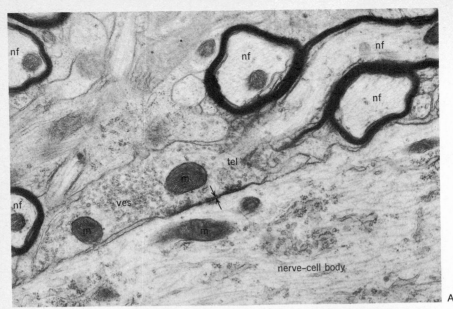

A

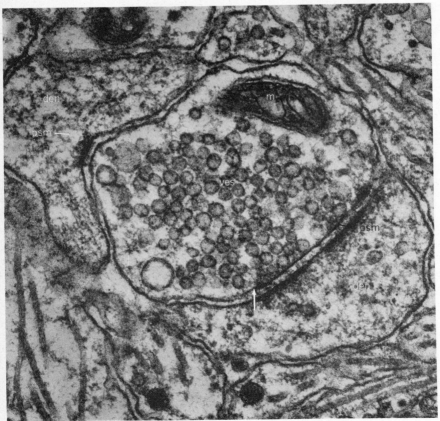

B

though no different from other plasma membranes. The axoplasm contains long tubules of agranular endoplasmic reticulum, and many parallel arrays of neurofilaments and neurotubules, but no chromophil substance and few mitochondria. The fine structure of axis cylinders is shown in Figs. 14.13 and 14.21.

Many nerve fibers are sheathed axis cylinders. Throughout the entire nervous system, myelin sheaths are prevalent. **Myelin** has a high lipid content giving the living or freshly killed myelinated nerve fiber its white, glistening appearance. The white matter of the brain and spinal cord contains great numbers of nerve fibers with myelin sheaths. The largest myelinated fibers are 11 to 20 μm in diameter; the smallest measure 2 to 4 μm.

The myelin sheath is acquired by the axis cylinder during development. Myelination is incomplete at birth and continues for many years, but at a decreasing rate. Myelin becomes an integral part of the nerve fiber, adding considerably to its total bulk. Not all nerve fibers acquire myelin sheaths. Many unmyelinated nerve fibers are found in both peripheral and central nervous systems. Table 14.1 presents a comparison of nerve fibers.

Certain structural features of myelin sheaths can be observed in peripheral nerve fibers stained by appropriate methods. The lipids of myelin are dissolved by solvents used in most procedures. Those used in silver techniques leave only spaces where myelin was once located (Fig. 14.14). Sheath stains, especially solutions of osmic acid, darken myelin, as shown in Fig. 14.15. When not dissolved in fixing fluid and dehydrating agents, the sheath remains intact, and after staining with hematoxylin and eosin has the appearance seen in Fig. 14.16. Viewed in longitudinal planes with the light microscope, the myelin sheath appears to have diagonal clefts passing from the outer surface inward to the axis cylinder (Fig. 14.17A). These, the **myelin incisures**,[3] are seen best in fibers stained with osmic acid. The myelin incisures have been identified with the electron microscope in well-fixed tissue. After staining by hematoxylin and other dyes, a network of some refractive substance may appear in place of the myelin. This is called "neurokeratin" and probably is the precipitated protein component of myelin. It is shown in the teased preparation of Fig. 14.17B.

[3]Myelin incisures are often called "incisures of Lantermann" or "Schmidt-Lantermann lines."

Figure 14-12 A. Synapse in the ventral horn of the cervical spinal cord of a rat. Myelin sheaths of three nerve fibers, *nf*, are seen on the right (others on the left); the middle one is sectioned longitudinally; a telodendron, *tel*, slips out of this myelin sheath and expands into a terminal ending on the surface of a motor nerve cell. The terminal contains numerous synaptic vesicles, *ves*, and two mitochondria, *m*. Synaptic membranes, shown at *arrows*, are thickenings of the plasmolemma of the terminal and the nerve cell. Electron micrograph, ×19,000. *(Contributed by S. L. Palay.)* B. Synapse in central nervous system of a toad. Terminal ending of axonal telodendron is filled with synaptic vesicles, *ves*, and contains a mitochondrion, *m*. Dendrites, *den*, show postsynaptic membrane thickenings, *psm*, and lack vesicles. Note electron-dense material in the synaptic interspaces. Electron micrograph ×100,000. *(Contributed by J. Rosenbluth.)*

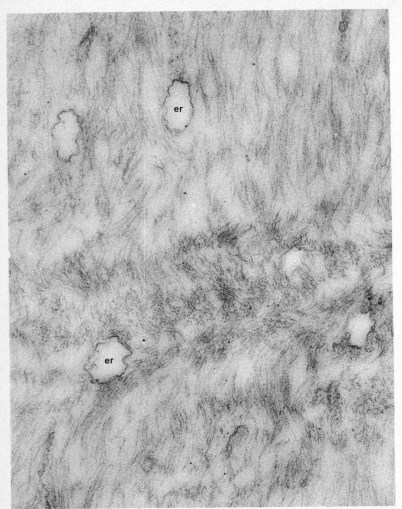

Figure 14-13 Axoplasm of a nerve fiber from a goldfish, showing undulating parallel arrays of neurofilaments. A few components of the agranular endoplasmic reticulum, *er,* are present. Electron micrograph, × 50,000. *(Contributed by S. L. Palay and S. M. McGee-Russell.)*

Table 14.1 Comparison of Nerve Fibers

	Unmyelinated		Myelinated	
	Peripheral nerves	Central nervous system	Peripheral nerves	Central nervous system
Cells of origin	Small	Small	Medium and large	Medium and large
Fiber diameter	Very small	Very small	Small, medium, and large	Small, medium and large
Fiber length	Long	Many short fibers	Long	Predominantly long
Neurolemma cells	Present; several fibers in one cellular strand	Absent	Present; one cell per segment	Absent
Functions	Afferent: pain Efferent: postganglionic autonomic	Various functions	Afferent: all sensory modalities Efferent: large, somatic motor; small fibers, preganglionic autonomic	Various functions

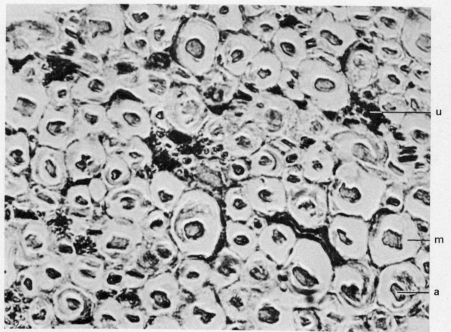

Figure 14-14   Nerve fibers of a peripheral nerve sectioned transversely and stained with silver: *a*, axis cylinder; *m*, myelin sheath; *u*, group of unmyelinated fibers. Photomicrograph, × 900.

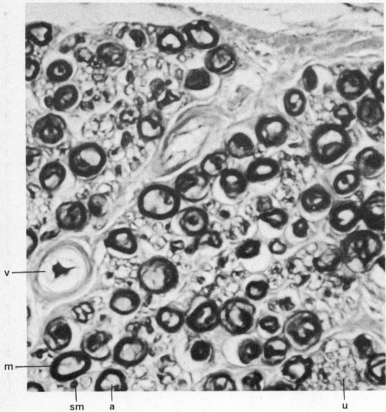

Figure 14-15 Nerve fibers of a peripheral nerve sectioned transversely and stained for myelin sheaths with osmic acid: *a,* unstained axis cylinder; *m,* myelin sheath; *sm,* small myelinated; *u,* unmyelinated fibers; *v,* blood vessel in perineurial septum. Photomicrograph, × 900.

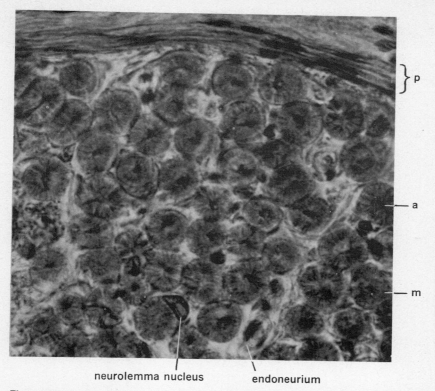

neurolemma nucleus   endoneurium

Figure 14-16 Nerve fibers of a peripheral nerve sectioned transversely and stained with hematoxylin and eosin: *a*, axis cylinder; *m*, myelin sheath; *p*, perineurium. Photomicrograph, × 900.

All nerve fibers of peripheral nerves are closely associated with **neurolemma** cells that form a delicate sheath[4] over the myelin, as shown in Fig. 14.17*C*. The nuclei of neurolemma cells can be seen in preparations of tissues stained by ordinary methods. Each neurolemma cell is related to a variable linear extent of a peripheral myelinated nerve fiber. Each has a thin coating of ground substance comparable with the basal lamina of epithelial cells. At the point where two cells meet, they constrict and pinch the myelin sheath to form a **node**,[5] as in Figs. 14.17 and 14.18. Thin basal laminae extend across nodes. Excrescences of the myelin sheath are often seen at the node. The peripheral myelinated nerve fibers resemble sausage chains with long, thin links, the internodal segments, 80 to 600 μm in length. The thicker the fiber, the longer the internodal segments and the faster the nerve impulse is conducted. The thin unmyelinated, peripheral nerve fibers course through strands of neurolemma

[4]Often referred to as the "sheath of Schwann."
[5]Commonly designated the "node of Ranvier."

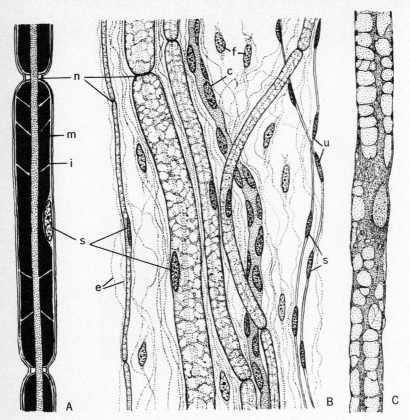

Figure 14-17 Nerve fibers of peripheral nerves, teased preparation stained, *A,* with osmic acid; *B,* with hematoxylin after alcohol fixation to show neurokeratin; *C,* by a special method to show a neurolemma cell. Abbreviations: *c,* capillary; *e,* endoneurium; *f,* fibrocytes; *i,* incisure; *m,* myelin; *n,* nodes; *s,* neurolemma nuclei; *u,* unmyelinated fibers. *A* is a diagram; drawings *B* and *C,* about × 900. *(JFN)*

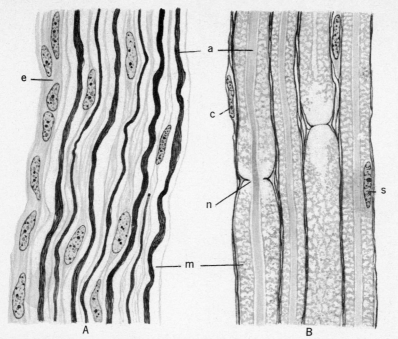

Figure 14-18 Nerve fibers of peripheral nerves in longitudinal sections, *A*, stained by silver; *B*, stained by connective-tissue stain. Abbreviations: *a*, axis cylinders, black in *A* and gray in *B*; *c*, fibrocyte nucleus; *e*, endoneurium; *m*, myelin; *n*, node in myelin sheath; *s*, neurolemma nucleus. × 900. *(JFN)*

cells. Branching of peripheral myelinated nerve fibers takes place only at nodes. Nerve fibers of the central nervous system lack neurolemma cells, but branching occurs, and nodelike formations have been observed.

Studies with the electron microscope provide quite a different conception of myelin and its formation than is possible with the light microscope. Myelin is a lamellated structure composed of neurolemma-cell membranes. The neurolemma cells have marked affinity for axis cylinders, apply themselves closely, and engulf them, as it were (Figs. 14.19 and 14.20). At the same time, their cytoplasm flows around the axis cylinder. The resulting invagination of the plasmolemma forms a spiral, at first one, then a few layers, and later many layers thick. Thus the myelin sheath is actually part of the neurolemma unit membrane with its lipid and protein layers. Myelin in the central nervous sys-

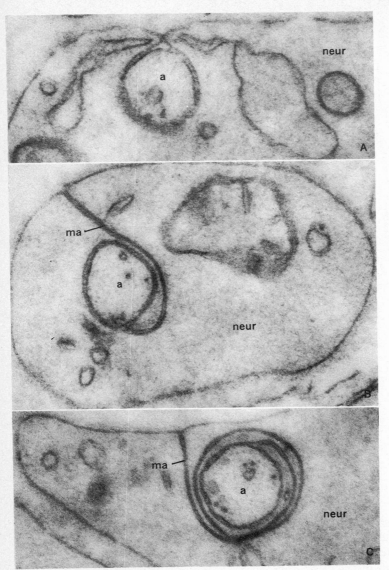

Figure 14-19 Development of myelin as seen in electron micrographs: *A,* a neurolemma cell, *neur,* has surrounded an axis cylinder of a nerve fiber, *a; B* and *C,* a "mesaxon," *ma,* has been formed, and coiling by the doubled plasma membranes of the neurolemma cell has begun to provide the first lamellae of the myelin sheath. Electron micrographs, × 54,000. *(Contributed by J. D. Robertson.)*

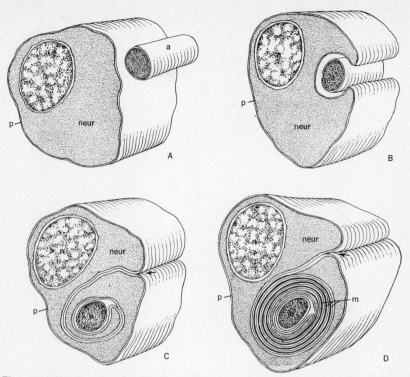

Figure 14-20 Schematic diagrams illustrating the relationship between an axis cylinder, *a*, of a developing peripheral nerve fiber and part of a neurolemma cell, *neur;* the nucleus, of the neurolemma cell, *n*, is shown; the plasma membrane, *p*, is double and exaggerated in thickness. The axis cylinder lies next to the cell in *A;* beginning invagination is shown in *B*, and at arrows in *C* and *D;* the spiraling, or "jelly-roll," formation appears in *C.* Myelin lamellae, *m*, consisting of the plasmolemma of the neurolemma cell, are seen in *D.* Compare with Fig. 14-19. *(Redrawn from B. O. Filho, based on data by J. D. Robertson.) (WEL)*

tem, likewise lamellated (Fig. 14.21), is laid down by neuroglia cells. Unmyelinated nerve fibers in the peripheral nerves are clothed in cytoplasm of neurolemma cells, several often being embedded in one strand of cells, as shown in Fig. 14.22.

The sheath of the nerve fiber is known to have a relationship to speed of conduction. With increasing fiber diameter, the speed of propagation of the nerve impulse is increased. The impulse appears to travel along the surface of a nerve fiber, and its speed over the large myelinated fibers is as great as 150 meters per second, or about 337 miles per hour.

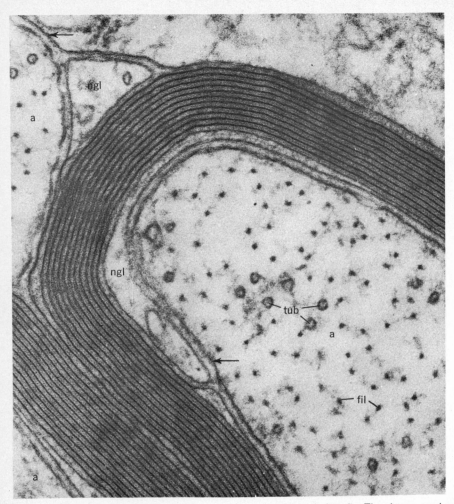

Figure 14-21 Myelinated nerve fiber of the spinal cord (toad). The inner and outer "mesaxons" (*arrows*), and 13 concentric lamellae surrounding the axis cylinder, *a,* represent the plasmolemma of a neuroglia cell, small portions of whose cytoplasm, *ngl,* are visible. Portions of adjacent nerve fibers are present (left). The axis cylinders contain neurofilaments, *fil,* and neurotubules, *tub.* Electron micrograph, × 112,500. *(Contributed by J. Rosenbluth.)*

SUGGESTED READING

Bodian, D.: The Generalized Vertebrate Neuron. *Science,* vol. 137, pp. 323–326, 1962.

Bray, D.: The Fibrillar Proteins of Nerve Cells. *Endeavour,* vol. 33, pp. 131–136, 1974.

Caley, D. W., and A. B. Butler: Formation of Central and Peripheral Myelin Sheaths in the Rat. *American Journal of Anatomy,* vol. 140, pp. 339–347, 1974.

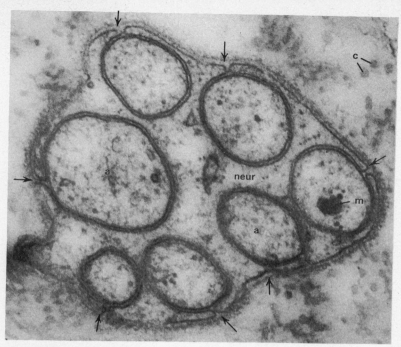

Figure 14-22 A group of unmyelinated nerve fibers in the adventitia of an artery (bat). This electron micrograph shows seven axis cylinders, *a* (one containing a mitochondrion, *m*), enclosed by invaginations of the plasmolemma of a neurolemma cell, *neur.* The points of invagination are marked by arrows. Collagen fibrils, *c,* surround the neurolemma cell. Micrograph, about × 50,000. *(Contributed by D. W. Fawcett.)*

Driscoll, B. F., A. J. Kramer, and M. W. Kies: Myelin Basic Protein: Location of Multiple Independent Antigenic Regions. *Science,* vol. 184, pp. 73–75, 1974.

Eccles, J.: The Synapse. *Scientific American,* vol. 212, no 1, pp. 56–66, January, 1965.

Harrison, R. G.: The Outgrowths of the Nerve Fiber as a Mode of Protoplasmic Movement. *Journal of Experimental Zoology,* vol. 9, pp. 787–846, 1910.

Lim, R., and K. Mitsunobu: Brain Cells in Culture: Morphological Transformation by a Protein. *Science,* vol. 185, pp. 63–66, 1974.

Palay, S. L., and G. E. Palade: The Fine Structure of Neurons. *Journal of Biophysical and Biochemical Cytology,* vol. 1, pp. 69–88, 1955.

Peters, A., S. L. Palay, and H. deF. Webster: *The Fine Structure of the Nervous System. The Cells and Their Processes.* Hoeber Medical Division, Harper & Row, Publishers, Incorporated, New York, 1970.

Uzman, B. G., and S. Nogueira-Gref: Electron Microscope Studies of the Formation of Nodes of Ranvier in Mouse Sciatic Nerve. *Journal of Biophysical and Biochemical Cytology,* vol. 3, pp. 589–598, 1957.

Williams, P. L., and S. M. Hall: In Vivo Observations on Mature Myelinated Nerve Fibers of the Mouse. *Journal of Anatomy,* vol. 107, pp. 31–38, 1970.

Chapter 15

Peripheral Nervous System

Division of the nervous system into peripheral and central portions is arbitrary and is mainly for convenience of description. The peripheral nervous system is not a separate entity. Most of its neurons either arise in the central nervous system and pass to the periphery or arise in the periphery and enter the brain and spinal cord. Some are entirely peripheral. The peripheral nervous system is the sum of all nerves, ganglia, and specialized end organs. The autonomic nervous system is a subdivision of it. Figure 15.1 shows the human peripheral nervous system nearly in toto. The relationship of peripheral to central nervous system is illustrated diagrammatically in Fig. 15.2.

NERVES

Nerves are bundles of nerve fibers coursing together in fibrous connective tissue supplied with blood vessels and lymphatic vessels. They contain unmyelinated as well as myelinated fibers. Nerves usually consist of several bundles, called "fascicles." The fibrous connective tissue surrounding the whole nerve and holding the fascicles together constitutes the **epineurium.** A denser form of fibrous connective tissue, the **perineurium,** encases each fascicle, often sending septa into the larger fascicles, partially subdividing them.

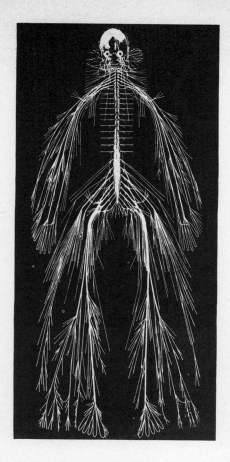

Figure 15-1 The human peripheral nervous system. A photograph of a dissection of a female subject by R. B. Weaver, of Hahneman Medical College, Philadelphia, made in 1888. Originally complete, the autonomic components and the distal parts of intercostal nerves were removed to prevent obscuring the rest of the nerves. *(Courtesy of R. C. Truex and Hahneman Medical College.)*

Both epineurium and perineurium are illustrated in Fig. 15.3. Within each fascicle, the individual nerve fibers are separated from one another by wisps of loose fibrous connective tissue containing reticular fibers. This loose component is the **endoneurium;** it can be seen in Fig. 15.4. Blood vessels and lymphatics, supplying nerves, pass into the fascicles in the perineurial septa and form branches with longitudinal orientation.

Nerves vary in their fiber composition, and the **cranial** and **spinal nerves** consist of fibers of many different diameters. Some of the small peripheral nerves are made up wholly of unmyelinated fibers, while others are entirely myelinated. Some nerves conduct motor impulses to muscles, while others carry sensory messages from the skin to the central nervous system. To a limited extent, the diameter of nerve fibers can be correlated with function.

The 31 pairs of spinal nerves are attached to the spinal cord by dorsal and ventral **nerve roots,** which unite to form the spinal nerve (Fig. 15.5). Dorsal roots are composed of fibers conducting sensory impulses only, while ventral roots are purely motor in function. Nerve fibers of the roots of all typical cranial and spinal nerves lose their association with neurolemma cells as they enter the brain or the spinal cord and become associated with neuroglia cells.

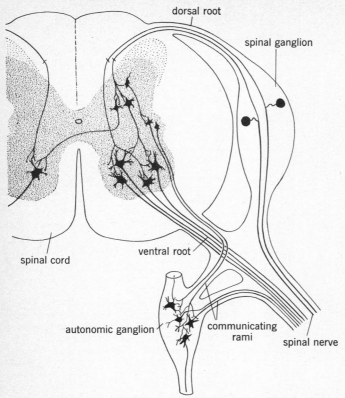

Figure 15-2 Diagram to show the relation of the spinal cord to spinal ganglion, nerve roots, and autonomic ganglion. *(WEL)*

GANGLIA

Nerve cell bodies grouped in the path of a nerve form a local swelling known as a **ganglion**. Most of the cranial and all spinal nerves have ganglia near their connections with the central nervous system. Those in the cranium have specific names, while those on the spinal nerve roots are simply called **spinal ganglia** (Fig. 15.5). Besides nerve cell bodies and their fibers, the ganglia contain neurolemma cells, fibrous connective tissue, blood vessels, and lymphatic vessels.

Each ganglion is surrounded by dense fibrous connective tissue, forming its epineurium and perineurium. Septa of connective tissue convey blood vessels and lymphatic vessels into the ganglion. The nerve cells tend to be arranged about the periphery as well as in clusters more deeply placed among fascicles of nerve fibers.

The ganglion cells in most cranial and spinal ganglia, having a single process, are unipolar (Fig. 15.6), but in the vestibular and cochlear ganglia they are bipolar. Ganglion cells usually are globoid and vary from about 20 to 100 μm in

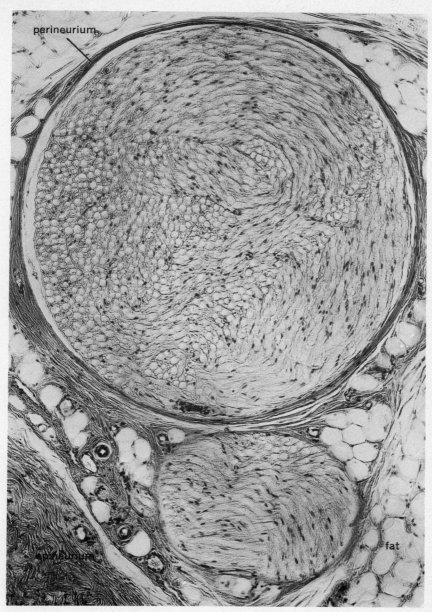

Figure 15-3 Two fascicles of the human femoral nerve, stained with hematoxylin. Note the dense fibrous-connective-tissue sheaths of perineurium around them. Photomicrograph, × 150.

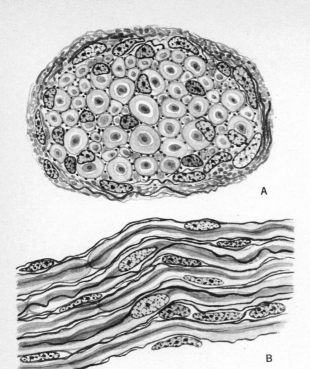

A

B

Figure 15-4 Nerve fascicles from tongue (kitten). Silver carbonate stain. Note the reticular fibers of the endoneurium among the nerve fibers. These appear as fine black dots in *A* and as wavy lines in *B*. × 900. *(JFN)*

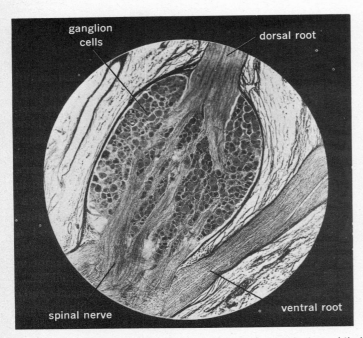

ganglion cells

dorsal root

spinal nerve

ventral root

Figure 15-5 Spinal ganglion, dorsal and ventral nerve roots, and their union to form a spinal nerve. *(Photomicrograph by George A. Piersol.)*

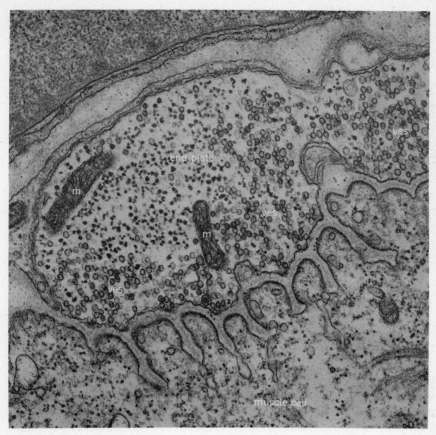

Figure 15-10 Motor end plate in *Triturus irridescens.* Synaptic vesicles, *ves*, and mitochondria, *m*, occupy the end plate. The muscle surface is extensively folded and separated from the end plate by ground substance. Electron micrograph, × 32,000. *(Contributed by T. L. Lentz, Journal of Cell Biology, vol. 55, pp. 93–103, 1972.)*

groups. Those stimulated by changes in the internal environment are **interoceptive.** Those telling of degrees of tension, pressure, and orientation are **proprioceptive.** Changes in the external environment are registered by the **extroceptive** end organs. Rarely does one become conscious of the messages received by the interoceptive, visceral end organs. Proprioceptive end organs are concerned with automatic functions, although the impulses from some deep pressure endings do reach a level of consciousness and cause awareness—the position of the limbs, for example. Everyone is acutely aware of the messages initiated by the exteroceptive end organs, which include the visual, auditory, touch, pain, and temperature receptors.

Interoceptive organs are formed by rather simple dendritic arborizations in the walls of some of the hollow organs and blood vessels. Many of the free endings in deeper parts of the body belong to this group. Examples of interoceptive

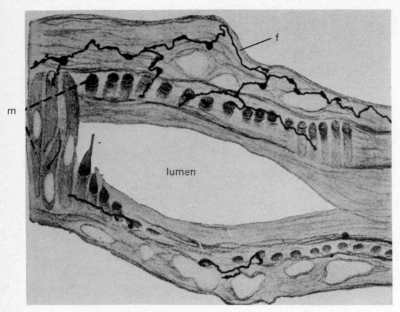

Figure 15-11   Efferent nerve endings, *f*, on smooth-muscle cells *m*, of an arteriole. About
×600.

endings are the chemoreceptors in the carotid body and the baroreceptors in
the adventitia of the carotid sinus and in other large blood vessels. Figure 15.13
illustrates an end organ of the latter type. Taste and smell may be considered
special varieties of interoceptive sensation; taste receptors are described under
Oral Cavity in Chap. 19, and receptors for smell are described under Nasal
Cavity and Nasopharynx in Chap. 22.

Proprioceptive end organs occur in muscles, tendons, joints, and deep connective-tissue layers. Three examples are the muscle spindle, tendon spindle,

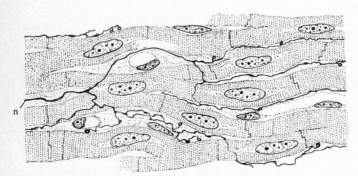

Figure 15-12   Efferent nerve endings on cardiac muscle; *n*, nerve fiber. Silver stain. About
×600. *(JFN)*

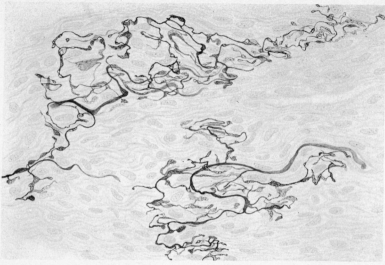

Figure 15-13 Interoceptive end organ in the subendothelial layer of the superior vena cava (cat). Silver stain. × 300. *(JFN)*

and lamellated corpuscle. The special end organs of the vestibular nerve belong in this category. They are described in Chap. 17.

Muscle spindles are complicated receptors in skeletal muscles composed of little groups of muscle fibers of smaller diameter than the working-muscle fibers, encapsulated in a thin layer of fibrous connective tissue (Fig. 15.14). The muscle spindles are about 2 to 4 mm long. Each is supplied by one or more (commonly two or three) myelinated nerve fibers, which arise, before piercing the capsule, from a number of fine dendrites exhibiting little varicosities that

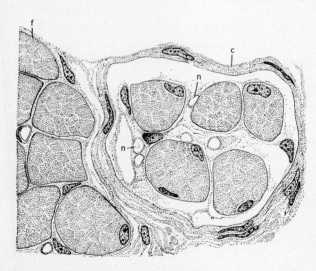

Figure 15-14 Muscle spindle in cross section of cat gastroc-nemius muscle: *c*, capsule of the muscle spindle; *f*, working muscle fibers; *n*, nerve fiber. About × 900. *(JFN)*

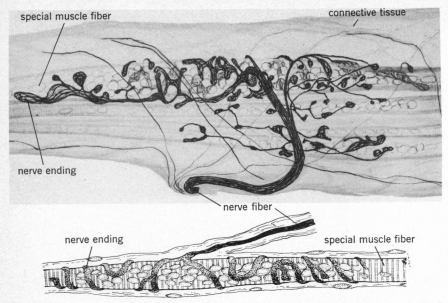

Figure 15-15 Sensory end organ in skeletal muscle. Part of one muscle spindle from a human fetus of 6 months; the afferent nerve fiber branches, and the branches entwine around the special muscle fibers of the spindle. The thin fibers probably are autonomic fibers to smooth muscle of blood vessels, not illustrated. Below this, a schematic drawing shows mode of origin of one afferent neuron. *(Upper drawing made by the late Prof. Francisco Tello and contributed by A. P. Rodriguez-Pérez.)*

are applied to the muscle fibers of the spindle. Some of the dendrites are arranged as ribbons wound about the muscle fibers (Fig. 15.15). Small motor end plates are found on the spindle-muscle fibers; they represent telodendria of a myelinated motor nerve fiber. When the working muscle contracts, its spindle-muscle fibers contract. Their contraction stimulates the sensory dendrites wrapped about them.

Tendon spindles occur near the junction of muscles and tendons as well as in other dense fibrous connective tissue (fascia). They, too, are lightly encapsulated end organs containing dendrites of myelinated nerve fibers. Some are much like muscle spindles. Others have dendrites forming palisades among the tendon fibers. Tendon spindles are shorter than muscle spindles, measuring a little more than 1 mm in length. Stretching the tendon or pulling on the fascial investments by muscles stimulates these end organs.

Other types of end organs occur in muscles, tendons, and fascia. Among these, the most striking is the **lamellated corpuscle**[2] found in connective tissue beneath the skin, around the viscera, in the peritoneum, and in many other places. The corpuscles are large. Some of them measure 3 or 4 mm in length and are visible to the naked eye. Lamellated corpuscles consist of many concentrically arranged layers of connective-tissue fibers and cells with ground

[2]These are often called "Pacinian corpuscles."

substance between the layers (Fig. 15.16). This onionlike bulb has a core called the "inner bulb," which is penetrated by a dendritic process of a large myelinated nerve fiber. The axon acquires its myelin sheath just outside the bulb, and occasionally a small branch accompanies the main fiber into the inner bulb. The corpuscles are stimulated by pressure.

Many kinds of exteroceptive end organs record changes in the external environment. Visual and auditory functions involve special receptors, and are considered with the histology of the eye and ear in Chap. 17. Other end organs mediate pain, touch, and temperature. Both encapsulated and **free nerve endings** are concerned with these senses. The latter are the most widely distributed of all the dendritic endings, occurring even in the walls of blood vessels and in the viscera, where pain may be perceived on occasion. In the epidermis, the free endings are confined to the germinative stratum. Figure 15.17*A* illustrates their appearance in this location. Free endings are not specific for the modality of pain, which can be induced by stimulating sensory endings of various kinds, depending on the strength of stimulus and threshold of the centers reached by the impulses generated. Some superficial regions, such as the cornea of the eye, are supplied only by free endings and are exquisitely sensitive to pain-inducing stimuli, but other sensations can be elicited by adequate stimulation. Most free nerve endings represent dendritic terminals of small myelinated and unmyelinated afferent nerve fibers.

There are several other types of nonencapsulated afferent endings that represent modifications of the free endings of the skin. The two most commonly encountered are present among epithelial cells of the epidermis and in the outer root sheath of hair follicles (Fig. 15.17*B* and *C*). Both of these are primarily tac-

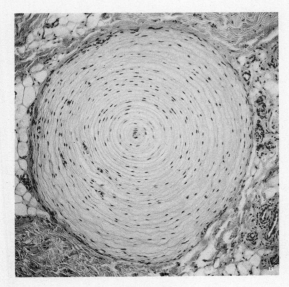

Figure 15-16 Lamellated corpuscle in the human labia majora. Photomicrograph.

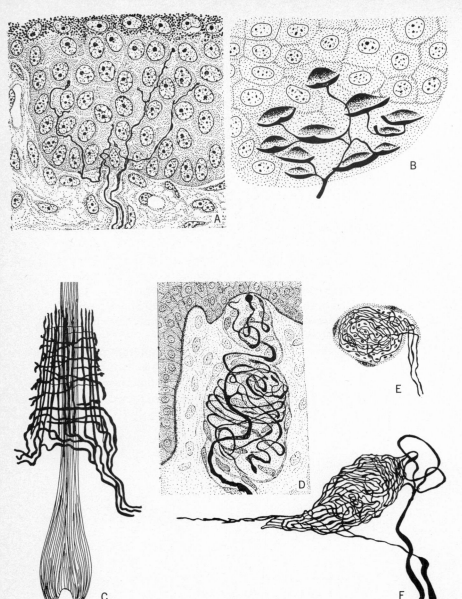

Figure 15-17 Exteroceptive end organ (semidiagrammatic): *A*, free endings in the stratum germinativum of epidermis; *B*, tactile discs; *C*, dendrites about hair; *D*, tactile corpuscles; *E*, "end-bulb of Krause"; *F*, "corpuscle of Ruffini." *A* and *D (JFN); B, C, E,* and *F (CHP).*

tile. The **tactile discs**[3] are minute plaques at the ends of dendritic arborizations. **Palisade endings** about hairs are activated by movements of the hairs and constitute receptors for light touch.

The most highly specialized touch end organs are the **tactile corpuscles,**[4] 50 to 100 μm long. They are found in the papillae of the dermis of the skin, especially the skin on the volar surface of the fingers and toes (Fig. 15.17D). A tactile corpuscle of this type is formed by a number of layers of special-connective-tissue cells lying transverse to the long axis of the corpuscle. These cells are encapsulated by a small amount of fibrous connective tissue. Dendrites, ramifying among the cells of the corpuscle, converge to form an axon which leaves the corpuscle to become a myelinated nerve fiber.

Pressure touch is mediated by lamellated corpuscles located in the deep layers of the skin. These corpuscles have the same structure as the lamellated corpuscles of proprioceptive function.

End organs specifically stimulated by warm and cold objects have not been identified with certainty.[5]

DEGENERATION, REGENERATION, AND AGING

When a peripheral nerve is severed, the nerve fibers in that portion distal to the site of the cut degenerate, and the nerve cells whose axons are cut undergo chromatolysis. This may be so severe that the whole neuron dies, but often it is followed by complete recovery of the pattern of chromophil substance in a few weeks. The neurons do not wait for this process to be complete before they make an effort to regenerate. The proximal ends of the cut fibers fray out, and little sprouts grow out of the axis cylinder just back of the cut (Fig. 15.18).

The progress of degeneration distal to the cut is shown in Figs. 15.19 and 15.20. The axis cylinders disintegrate in the first few days. The myelin breaks up into short ovoid segments during the first 3 or 4 days and becomes further subdivided during the next week. Its chemical composition changes with production of neutral fats. Macrophages invade the nerve and engulf the particles of degenerating axis cylinder and myelin. The neurolemma cells do not degenerate, but proliferate to form nucleated strands that replace the nerve fibers. In the course of 4 to 6 weeks the degenerative process is nearly complete.

Regeneration begins before the degenerative process in the distal stump is well under way. The new sprouts from cut fibers of the proximal stump penetrate the distal portion of the nerve and gradually make their way within proliferating neurolemma strands, ultimately replacing the degenerated distal portion of the nerve (Fig. 15.21). Should the two cut ends of the nerve be separated by

[3]The "tactile endings of Merkel."
[4]The "corpuscles of Meissner."
[5]The "end-bulb of Krause" (Fig. 15.17E) and the "corpuscle of Ruffini" (Fig. 15.17F) have been suggested for cold and warmth, respectively.

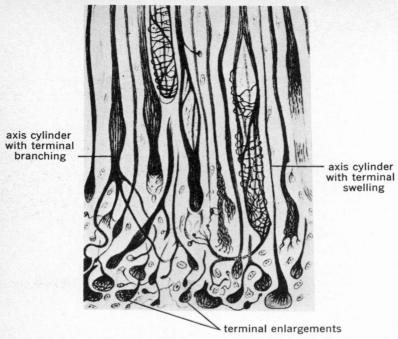

axis cylinder
with terminal
branching

axis cylinder
with terminal
swelling

terminal enlargements

Figure 15-18   Regeneration beginning in the central stump of a nerve cut 2½ days previously. *(Drawing by S. Ramón y Cajal.)*

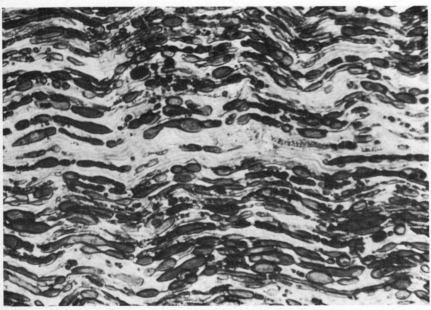

Figure 15-19   Degeneration in a peripheral nerve distal to a cut made 3 to 5 days previously. *(Photomicrograph contributed by A. Elwyn.)*

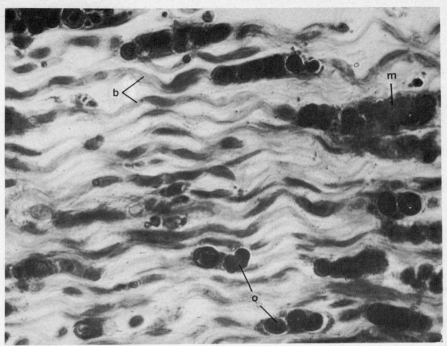

Figure 15-20 Degeneration in a peripheral nerve distal to a cut made 12 to 15 days previously. High-power view shows several nucleated neurolemma strands, *b*, with macrophages, *m*, and myelin-sheath remnants, *o*. *(Photomicrograph contributed by A. Elwyn.)*

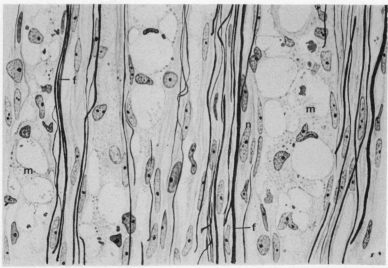

Figure 15-21 Regeneration of nerve fibers, *f*, in the distal stump of a peripheral nerve, approximately 30 days after severance and union. Remnants of degenerating myelin, *m*, and proliferating neurolemma cells are shown. *(JFN)*

an appreciable space, a fibrous scar is formed between them, preventing successful regeneration. The new nerve fibers grow out the distal portion of the nerve at the rate of 1 or 2 mm a day when they find conditions favorable.

The peripheral end organs degenerate along with the nerve fibers of the distal portion of the nerve. When new growths of neurons reach the site of these degenerated structures, new end organs are constituted.

Myelination of nerve fibers is incomplete at birth. The size of the fiber increases as the body grows. The number of fibers that can be counted in ventral spinal nerve roots of the cat is no less in aged animals than in young adults. Whether this holds true for human beings is unknown. Although connective-tissue components of ganglia and nerves may undergo the same alterations encountered elsewhere, the ganglion cells show little effect of age except an accumulation of lipofuscin pigment.

SUGGESTED READING

Cauna, N., and G. Mannan: The Structure of Human Digital Pacinian Corpuscles (corpuscula lamellose) and Its Functional Significance. *Journal of Anatomy,* vol. 92, pp. 1–20, 1958.

Cockett, S. A., and J. A. Kiernan: Acceleration of Peripheral Nervous Regeneration in the Rat by Exogenous Triiodothyronine. *Experimental Neurology,* vol. 39. pp. 389–394, 1973.

Gelfan, S., and S. Carter: Muscle Sense in Man. *Experimental Neurology,* vol. 18, pp. 469–473, 1967.

Guth, L.: Regeneration in the Mammalian Peripheral Nervous System. *Physiological Reviews,* vol. 36, pp. 441–478, 1956.

Moyer, E. K., and B. F. Kcliszewski: The Number of Nerve Fibers in Motor Spinal Nerve Roots of Young, Mature and Aged Cats. *Anatomical Record,* vol. 131, pp. 681–699, 1958.

Swash, M., and K. P. Fox: Muscle Spindle Innervation in Man. *Journal of Anatomy,* vol. 112. pp. 61–80, 1972.

Chapter 16

Central Nervous System

The brain and spinal cord (encephalon et medulla spinalis) are the principal components of the central nervous system (Fig. 16.1). Other closely related structures are the optic nerve, retina, and neurohypophysis. All arise embryologically from neural ectoderm, i.e., from an epithelium, a fact that can account for some of their interesting structural characteristics.

The central nervous system is highly cellular. Its cells take on many shapes, and all have processes. Cells and their processes of various length and form, including dendrites, telodendria of axons, and outstretched arms of the neuroglia, constitute the parenchyma of the brain and spinal cord.

A stroma of fibrous connective tissue, except in a few special regions, is found only along the main blood vessels entering or leaving the central nervous system. The smallest blood vessels lack an adventitia, and bare nonfenestrated endothelium makes contacts with the parenchymal cells with little interstitial ground substance intervening.

MEMBRANOUS COVERINGS

There are three membranes, or **meninges,** associated with the central nervous system; from deep to superficial, they are the pia mater, arachnoid, and dura mater. Actually, only two are prominent. Around the spinal cord and in a few places over the brain the arachnoid is a separate membrane, but elsewhere it is

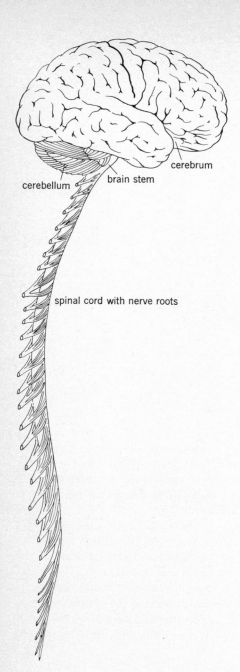

cerebrum

brain stem

cerebellum

spinal cord with nerve roots

Figure 16-1 Human brain and spinal cord, composing the main parts of the central nervous system. *(WEL)*

attached to the pia mater, and the two, together with the cerebrospinal fluid between them, form a cushion for the brain.

The **pia mater** proper is composed of fibrous connective tissue. There are a few nerves and many blood vessels, all larger than capillaries, in it. The vessels anastomose and give off branches at right angles to the surface of the brain to supply deeper parts of the central nervous system. As they enter the brain parenchyma, they are surrounded by a cuff of pia mater separated from their adventitia by a **perivascular space**. The pia mater and adventitia soon join, and from this point on into the brain no perivascular space exists (Fig. 16.2). However, shrinkage of the brain in fixing fluid usually produces an artifactitious space between the perivascular glial membrane and the adventitia.

Blood vessels entering the brain and spinal cord from the vascular pia mater are, functionally, end-arteries. Their occlusion results in destruction of that portion of the central nervous system to which they supply blood. Branches of pial arteries that enter the brain parenchyma regulate blood flow regionally. Smooth muscle cells in their walls provide for active constriction at three points. These are found in the main offshoots of pial arteries, in deeper parenchymal arterioles, and in anastomoses between the arterioles.

The pia mater invests the brain and spinal cord closely, following the various indentations, sulci, and fissures, and forming the connective-tissue cores of the choroid plexuses. It can be stripped away from the brain quite easily, because its connective-tissue fibers do not penetrate the brain tissue but are walled off by the external glial membrane. On its free surface, the pia mater is covered with flattened cells resembling simple squamous epithelium.

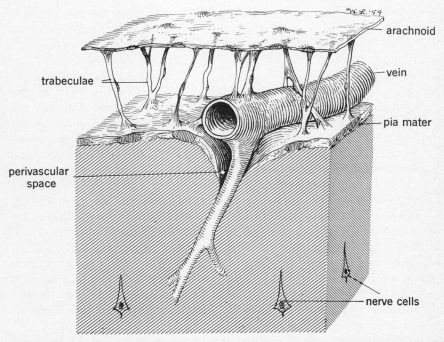

Figure 16-2 Diagram illustrating the relation of leptomeninges and a cerebral vein to the cerebral cortex. The perivascular space is limited to large vessels near the cortical surface. No perineuronal spaces exist. (Modified from Weed.) *(WEL)*

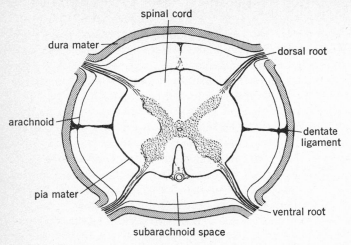

Figure 16-3 Diagram of the spinal meninges and spinal cord. *(WEL)*

The **arachnoid** is a gossamer-thin membrane of connective tissue covered on both sides with flattened cells. Innumerable delicate strands, the arachnoidal trabeculae, connect it with the pia mater proper over the surface of the brain (Fig. 16.2). The arachnoid is practically avascular.

Perhaps one should consider the arachnoid to be simply the outer part of the pia mater because it is so closely attached to the latter. The pia mater then may be said to be a spongy, vascular membrane traversed by large and small fluid-filled spaces, lined by flattened cells. The names "pia-archnoid" and "leptomeninx" are given to this combined membrane. The spaces in the pia-arachnoid become wider at sulci and other indentations which are bridged by the arachnoid proper. In this fashion, a number of **subarachnoid cisternae** are formed. The spaces coalesce to form a large **subarachnoid space** around the spinal cord (Fig. 16.3) and long spinal nerve roots of the **cauda equina**.[1] It is possible to insert a sharp cannula into this space caudal to the spinal cord (spinal puncture) to withdraw fluid for diagnostic tests.

Apertures in the thin roof of the fourth brain ventricle permit communication between the ventricular system of the brain and the subarachnoid space. Cerebrospinal fluid is contained in the subarachnoid space. It arises, for the most part, from the choroid plexuses of the ventricles and reaches the subarachnoid space through the apertures of the fourth ventricle of the brain.

The **dura mater** is a tough fibrous-connective-tissue membrane, sometimes called the "pachymeninx." Its inner surface is covered with simple squamous epithelium. In the cranium, the outer layer of the dura mater closely invests the bone and forms its periosteum. Folds of the inner layer form a number of partial septa between major subdivisions of the brain.

The membrane is supplied by blood vessels for its own nutrition, and con-

[1]So called because of its fancied resemblance to a horse's tail.

tains the large nonmuscular veins that drain blood from the brain to the jugular vein in the neck. These are the **venous sinuses** of the dura mater. In the spinal region, the outer and inner layers of the dura mater are separated by loose connective tissue containing adipose tissue and a plexus of veins. The inner layer, or dura mater proper, becomes attached to the pia mater of the spinal cord by longitudinal septa with scalloped inner edges, the "dentate ligaments" (Fig. 16.3).

Spinal and cranial nerve roots pierce the dura mater and carry along with them investments of its connective tissue which become the perineurium of the roots. The sheath of the optic nerve is an extension of the dura mater, blending with the sclera of the eyeball.

A subdural space is found between the dura mater and arachnoid. There is no communication between it and the subarachnoid space. It contains just enough fluid to moisten the surfaces of the membranes. Although the meninges lack lymphatic vessels, the two intermeningeal spaces effect slight communications with lymphatic vessels of the back.

INTERNAL STRUCTURE

The parenchyma of the central nervous system is packed with neuroglia cells, their processes, neurons, their processes, and the capillaries. There is less interstitial space than in connective tissue. The plasmolemma of one element lies next to that of another, with only the minimal 200-Å cleft between. Collectively, these clefts account for the interstitial fluid compartment in the brain and spinal cord. There is practically no ground substance in the parenchyma of the central nervous system. Regions where synaptic connections are prevalent constitute the **neuropil**.

The significance of all types of cell contact found in the neuropil is not known. Astrocytic processes are seen everywhere, and it seems likely that they constitute an elaborate transportation system for fluid and solutes en route from the blood plasma to the neurons or other cells and in the reverse direction. Direct transfer through capillary endothelium to neurons may take place in the newborn individual, before astrocytic processes attain full complexity. Capillaries nearly everywhere lie close to nerve cells. The neuropil contains a great many synapses. These have a characteristic appearance in electron micrographs. Those of the end-bulb type are shown in Fig. 14.11.

The principal cells of the central nervous system are neuron and neuroglia cells. Neurons are arranged in groups and layers, and their long axons, myelinated and unmyelinated, course from place to place in fiber tracts. The groups and layers of cells of the neuropil constitute the **gray matter,** while the fiber tracts make up the **white matter** (Figs. 16.4 and 16.5). Interspersed among nerve cells and fibers are the neuroglia cells and blood vessels. The cell bodies of most neurons are easily identified in routinely stained histologic sections. Neuroglia cells are more difficult to see, but they outnumber neurons by perhaps as many as four to one.

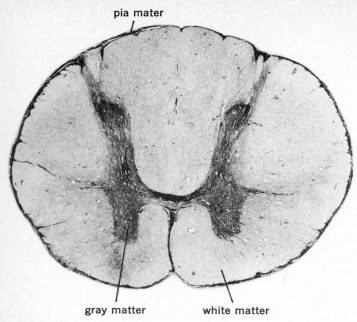

pia mater

gray matter   white matter

Figure 16-4 Human spinal cord from the thoracic region. Hematoxylin stain. Photomicrograph, × 10.

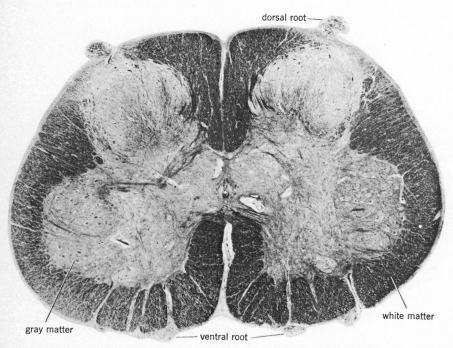

dorsal root

white matter

gray matter   ventral root

Figure 16-5 Human spinal cord from the sacral region; stained for myelinated nerve fibers. Photomicrograph, × 10.

Nerve Cells   The cell bodies of neurons were described in Chaps. 14 and 15. The difference between neurons of the brain and those of the peripheral ganglia and nerves is not one of fundamental intrinsic structure, but one of degree of variability in size and shape. Aside from this, the nerve cells of the central nervous system differ from those of the peripheral ganglia in respect to the type of cells that surround them and in the greater complexity of their interrelations. Surrounding elements of the neuropil are not clearly seen in preparations stained by analin dyes, although nuclei of neuroglia cells and capillaries are usually visible. Figure 16.6 shows a large nerve cell of the spinal-cord neuropil. Note a capillary in close proximity to it.

Neuroglia Cells   Neuroglia cells are sometimes spoken of collectively as "the neuroglia" (literally, nerve glue). Erroneously, they have been thought to constitute a type of connective tissue in the brain, but actually they provide little if any structural support. They are fitted in among the nerve cells and fibers, and the processes of some of them form a continuous thin membranelike layer between the blood vessels and fibrous connective tissue of the pia mater, on the one hand, and the neurons and other parenchymal elements, on the other. These cells take an active part in metabolism in the brain.

Neuroglia cells are of three types: astrocytes, oligodendrocytes, and ependymal cells. Microglia are often considered with neuroglia cells. All can be identified in hematoxylin and eosin preparations of the brain and spinal cord, although details of cytoplasmic structure are not seen, and one must depend upon nuclear differences to tell them apart (Figs. 16.7 and 16.8).

Astrocytes, as the name implies, are star-shaped cells with many cytoplasmic branches radiating about equidistantly. They are recognizable in ordinary preparations by relatively large, pale nuclei. Special methods reveal fibrils in

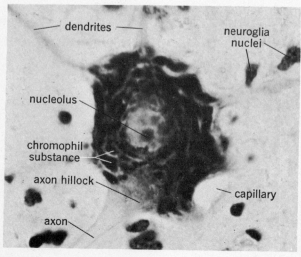

Figure 16-6 Multipolar nerve cell from the spinal cord of an adult cat. Thionine stain. Photomicrograph, × 600.

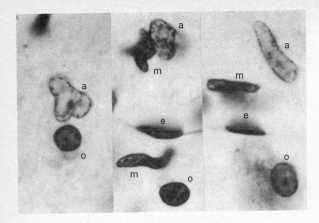

Figure 16-7 Nuclei of neuroglia and other nonnervous cells in the gray matter of the spinal cord: *a*, astrocyte; *e*, endothelial cell of capillary; *m*, microglia cell; *o*, oligodendrocyte. Composite photomicrograph, × 900. *(Contributed by J. Cammermeyer.)*

the cytoplasm around the nucleus and extending out into the processes of some astrocytes. The fibrils resemble those observed in the cytoplasm of neurons. Other astrocytes lack fibrils. Those with fibrils are called **fibrous astrocytes,** those without them, **protoplasmic astrocytes.** The fibrous astrocytes are prevalent among nerve fibers of the white matter. The protoplasmic astrocytes are more numerous in the gray matter. Special forms of astrocytes develop in the neurohypophysis and retina.

The living astrocyte in a tissue culture, shown in Fig. 16.9, closely resembles a fixed specimen stained by one of the special neuroglial methods. Its processes are so long that a very thin section, such as is required for transmission electron micrographs, seldom reveals any of them in continuity with the cell body. The processes are inserted among other cells of the central nervous parenchyma, and bits of them constitute the most numerous structures encountered in electron micrographs of the neuropil.

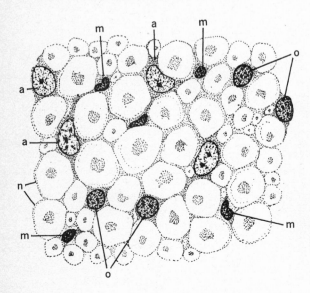

Figure 16-8 Nuclei of neuroglia and microglia cells among myelinated nerve fibers of the spinal cord; *a*, astrocyte; *m*, microglia cell; *n*, nerve fibers; *o*, oligodendrocytes. About × 900. *(JFN)*

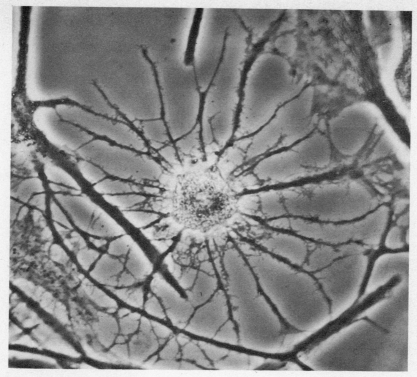

Figure 16-9 Astrocyte in tissue culture photographed with phase-contrast optics. Photomicrograph, × 900. *(Contributed by A. S. Rose.)*

The fibrils of astrocytes, which are the **gliofibrils** of light microscopy, appear to be conglomerates of the microfilaments and microtubules revealed in electron micrographs (Fig. 16.10). An astrocytic process in cross section is shown in Fig. 16.11 at high magnification.

The astrocytic processes often end in little expansions, or "foot plates," on the walls of the blood vessels (as shown in Fig. 16.12) and on the pia mater and its septa. They form a filamentous protoplasmic glial membrane around the vessels and under the pia mater, separating connective tissue from neurons and other parenchymal cells. The **perivascular glial membrane** and the external limiting, or **pia-glial membrane,** mark a boundary between connective tissue and nervous tissue in the adult brain and spinal cord. They are deficient in some species at birth, capillary endothelium with its basal lamina making direct contact with nerve cells or their processes. Astrocytes, under certain conditions, can engage in phagocytosis.

The perivascular glial membrane is one component of the **blood-brain barrier**. It and the nonfenestrated capillary endothelium with its basal lamina limit movement of substances between blood plasma and the central-nervous parenchyma. The blood-brain barrier plays a restrictive role, preventing elements of the immune system, for example, from reaching the parenchyma of the central nervous system. Large molecules normally cannot traverse it.

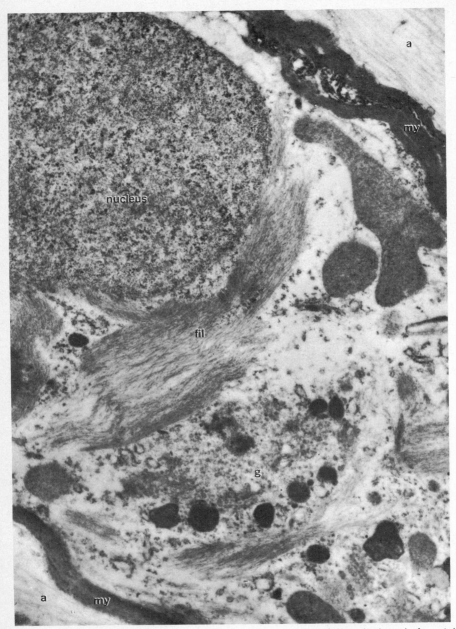

Figure 16-10   Part of a fibrous astrocyte, in the white matter of the spinal cord of a cat, lying between myelinated nerve fibers (upper right and lower left). A prominent compact bundle of microfilaments, *fil,* is seen between the nucleus and the golgi complex, *g.* Elsewhere the cytoplasmic matrix is clear and contains mitochondria, elements of the endoplasmic reticulum, and ribosomes. Axis cylinders, *a,* and myelin sheaths, *my,* of the nerve fibers are indicated. Electron micrograph, × 16,000. *(Contributed by Mary and R. P. Bunge.)*

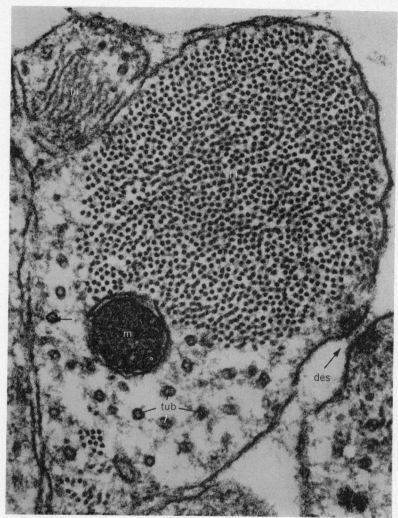

Figure 16-11 Astrocyte processes containing numerous microfilaments, *fil,* mitochondrion, *m,* and microtubules, *tub,* one with dark center (*small arrow*). Junction between processes marked by desmosome, *des.* Electron micrograph, ×140,000. *(Contributed by C. S. Raine.)*

After trauma and other forms of injury of the brain and spinal cord, fibrous astrocytes take part in healing by proliferating and constructing glial scar tissue. In so doing, they limit invasion by collagenous fibers, but at the same time they may block regeneration of the severed processes of neurons.

Oligodendrocytes are smaller than astrocytes and are the most numerous cells of the central nervous system. Subtypes, possibly representing different functional states, have been described. The nuclei of oligodendrocytes usually

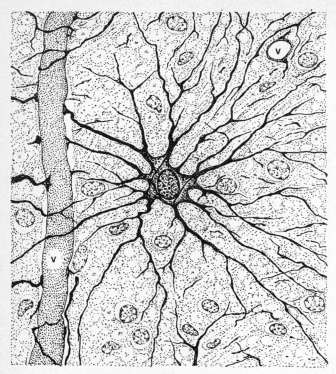

Figure 16-12 Fibrous astrocyte in the white matter of the brain. Note the attachment of two processes by foot plates to the wall of a small blood vessel, *v*. Other foot plates can be seen. Special stain. About × 900. *(JFN)*

appear a little darker and more rounded than those of astrocytes. It is difficult to stain the cytoplasm, which is scanty and extends out in a few, sparsely branched processes. These neuroglia cells often appear in groups around the cell bodies of large neurons, where they are referred to as "satellite" cells. In fiber tracts of the white matter, oligodendrocytes tend to be aligned in rows parallel to the nerve fibers and capillaries. Two in a living culture are shown in Fig. 16.13. An electron micrograph (Fig. 16.14) demonstrates the compact appearance of their cytoplasm.

Oligodendrocytes are active cells. In tissue culture photographed by time-lapse cinematography, their processes are seen to move constantly in a manner suggestive of pinocytosis. Oligodendrocytes have a higher metabolic rate than any elements of the central nervous system except neurons.

Some oligodendrocytes are associated with the process of myelination during development. They contribute myelin lamellae to the sheaths of axis cylinders of neurons in a manner comparable with that of the neurolemma cells in the peripheral nerves.

Ependymal cells line the ventricular system of the brain and spinal cord. They are direct descendants of the embryonic neural epithelium which formed the primitive neural tube. Ependymal cells resemble simple columnar epithelium of other organs (Fig. 16.15). Cilia may be seen on their exposed surface.

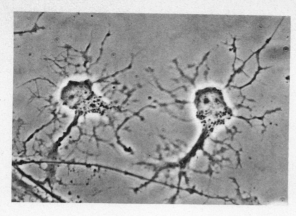

Figure 16-13 Oligodendrocytes in tissue culture under phase-contrast optics. Photomicrograph, × 900. *(Contributed by A. S. Rose.)*

Gliofibrils are demonstrable in the cytoplasm and in the one process which projects from the base of the cell into the subjacent tissue. In places where the pia mater or blood vessels are not too far away, a foot plate of the basal process takes part in the formation of the glial membrane. Ependymal cells appear to be closely related to the astrocytes in development.

Electron micrographs show numerous bundles of microfilaments sweeping through the cytoplasm and into the basal process. An internal limiting membrane is formed by a feltwork of neuroglial processes beneath the ependymal epithelium, but no basal lamina is seen there (Fig. 16-15*B*).

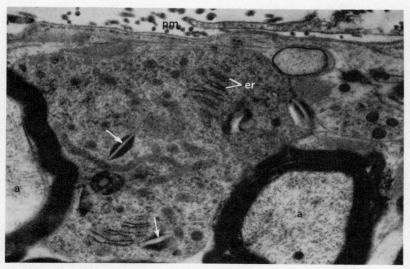

Figure 16-14 Part of an oligodendrocyte in the white matter of the spinal cord (cat). The section misses its nucleus, but the characteristics of the cytoplasm are well shown; parallel arrays of granular endoplasmic reticulum, *er,* are visible; matrix appears dense, owing to free ribosomes; mitochondria are present; several unidentified inclusion bodies with light centers (*arrow*) are seen. The oligodendrocyte lies just beneath the pia mater, *pm,* and is surrounded by myelinated nerve fibers, *a,* sheaths of which are black. Electron micrograph, × 16,000. *(Contributed by Mary and R. P. Bunge.)*

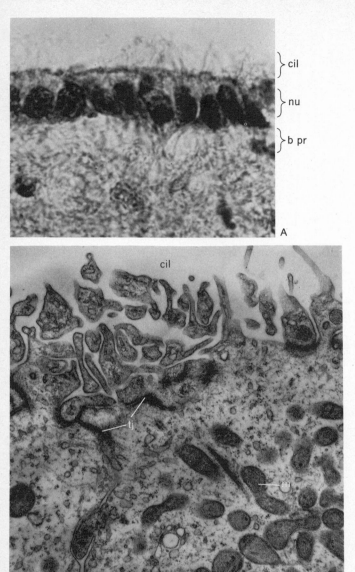

Figure 16-15 Ependymal cells. *A.* Lining of the central canal of human spinal cord; note cilia, *cil,* ependymal cell nuclei, *nu,* and the basal processes, *b pr,* extending into spinal cord parenchyma. Photomicrograph, × 900. *B.* Portions of adjoining ependymal cells (toad), showing cilia, *cil,* tight junctions, *tj,* and numerous mitochondria, *m.* Note pinocytotic vesicles in the cilia. Electron micrograph, × 35,000. *(Contributed by J. Rosenbluth.)*

cortical surface

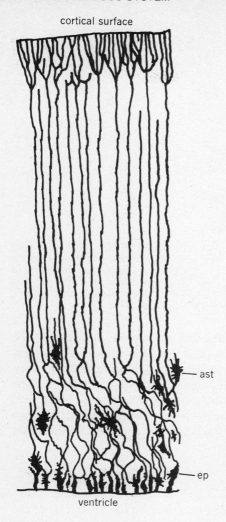

ventricle

Figure 16-16 Ependymal cells, *ep,* and astrocytes, *ast,* in the cerebral cortex of a rabbit several days old. The bodies of ependymal cells lie next to the ventricle; both types of cell send long processes to the cortical surface where they branch. *(Redrawn from Ramón y Cajal.) (CHP)*

Some neuroglia cells in the growing central nervous system extend long processes toward the surface of the brain. Their cell bodies may be found among the cells of the ependymal lining of the ventricles. Figure 16.16 illustrates a group of them in the cerebral cortex. These elongated neuroglia cells provide ladders, as it were, along which developing nerve cells can migrate away from the germinal layer to definitive locations in the growing brain.

Microglia Cells   The only parenchymal cell of the central nervous system arising from the embryonic mesoderm is the microglia cell. The small, dark nuclei of these cells can be identified in sections stained with hematoxylin and eosin (Fig. 16.7), but special silver methods are needed to stain their cytoplasm. These cells are found with outstretched protoplasmic processes

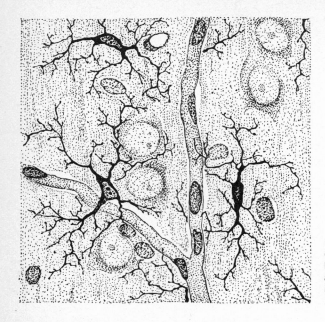

Figure 16-17 Three microglia cells in the gray matter of the brain. Capillaries, nerve cells, and nuclei of neuroglia cells are in the background. About × 900. *(JFN)*

among nerve cells and nerve fibers, like inactive phagocytic cells elsewhere (Fig. 16.17). They are the least numerous cells of the central nervous system—only about one microglia to ten neuroglia cells. During inflammatory processes and infections and after traumatic injuries of brain substance, they are thought to become active and appear as more compact cells, filled with phagocytized material. Other phagocytes arise from monocytes and lymphocytes of the blood and mobilize in and around the blood vessels of the brain when needed.

CHOROID PLEXUSES

Ependymal cells are modified structurally at four places in the ventricles of the brain.[2] There they are arranged in a low columnar epithelium over tufts of capillaries of the pia mater to form the choroid plexuses. These plexuses dip into the ventricles where they are bathed in the cerebrospinal fluid (Fig. 16.18).

The fine structure of the epithelium suggests an active role. The free surface has a striated border composed of club-shaped microvilli. The basal surface of the epithelial cells has an extensively folded plasmolemma, and there is a basal lamina beneath this.

The **cerebrospinal fluid** not only fills the ventricular system, but through communications between the fourth ventricle and a labyrinth of spaces between the pia mater and arachnoid membranes, the subarachnoid space, it surrounds the central nervous system and forms a hydraulic cushion for it. About one-tenth of a liter of fluid is present in these spaces.

[2] A somewhat similar modification occurs during development of the eye, leading to the formation of the epithelium of the nonvisual parts of the retina.

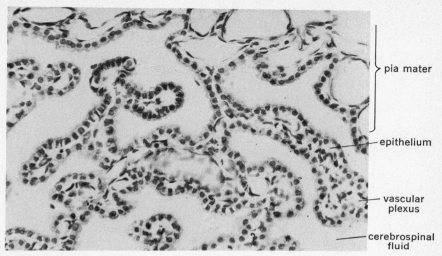

pia mater

epithelium

vascular plexus

cerebrospinal fluid

Figure 16-18 Choroid plexus of the lateral ventricle of an infant monkey. Thionine stain. Photomicrograph, × 300.

Cerebrospinal fluid is a special tissue fluid, not simply a transudate from blood plasma. It is formed largely by secretory activity of the epithelium of the choroid plexuses. The composition of cerebrospinal fluid is unlike interstitial fluid of other tissues of the body. It is about 99 percent water and contains little protein. Return of fluid to the blood is effected partly in the **arachnoidal villi,** which are short endothelium-covered fingers invaginating the large cranial venous sinuses. Cerebrospinal-fluid pressure is lower than capillary blood pressure in the choroid plexuses but higher than venous pressure in the cranial sinuses. There are no lymphatic vessels in the brain parenchyma.

FUNCTIONAL CONSIDERATIONS

The histologic structure of three parts of the central nervous system is illustrated in Figs. 16.19 to 16.21. The cerebrum, cerebellum, and spinal cord are chosen because they differ so widely in appearance. It would be misleading to declare that any one demonstrates a characteristic structural arrangement of elements of the central nervous system. Each is representative of only one particular region.

The study of the organization of nerve cells into groups, strata, and centers constitutes part of neuroanatomy, and will not be considered in detail in this book. In general, many neurons of similar structural characteristics tend to be organized into rather closely circumscribed groups in the gray matter for performance of some specific function. The motor-nerve nuclei[3] are examples of such circumscribed groups. Larger masses of diffuse arrangements of neurons

[3]"Nucleus" is a term used here to designate a collection of structurally or functionally similar nerve-cell bodies in the central nervous system.

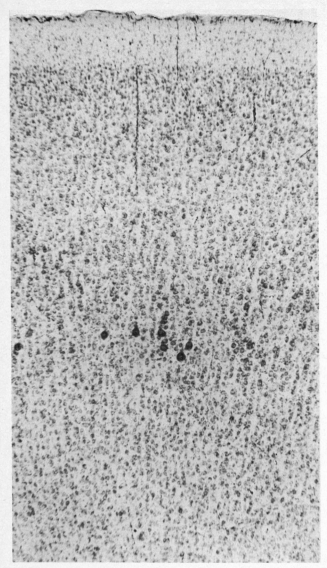

Figure 16-19 Cerebral cortex of an adult monkey. Thionine stain. Photomicrograph, × 80.

varying in size and shape usually have less specific functions. Such an arrangement is found in the cerebral cortex.

The brain and spinal cord are great synaptic centers. In the more circumscribed neuron groups of the central nervous system, the arrangement of synapses provides specificity of response. In some of the widely spread strata of neurons connections are duplicated and reduplicated, providing a broadside or avalanche type of activity. In certain places, it is possible to perceive an organization that favors precise timing for continuous conduction of impulses in

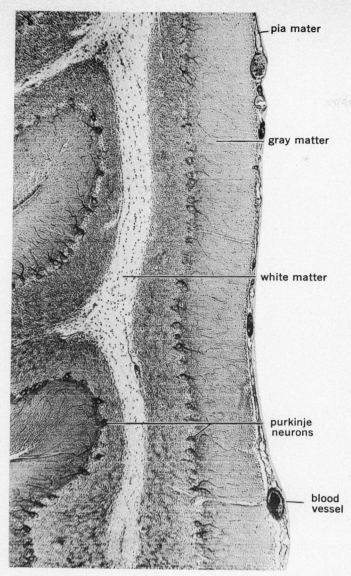

Figure 16-20   Cerebellar cortex of a dog. Silver stain. Photomicrograph, × 80.

circuits, some of which are structurally complicated. Some circuits facilitate or accelerate neuronal activity. Others are inhibitory. It is thought that imbalances between these types can lead to derangement of mental processes, but the changes in structure or function that may induce an imbalance between competing neuronal circuits are unknown. The number of neurons in the brain is immense, and the number of interconnections they make is almost infinite.

The internal environment of the parenchymal cells of the central nervous system is chemically different from the internal environment of cells of other

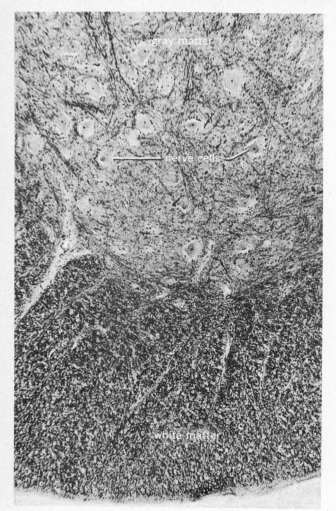

Figure 16-21   Human spinal cord, stained for myelin. Photomicrograph, × 80.

organs and is less subject to change. Nevertheless, activities are not independent of those of other organs. The contact with the circulatory system has been mentioned. The central nervous system initiates or regulates the actions of many organs through the peripheral nerves. Not only does it receive messages from the various sense organs and sensory nerve endings, which reach it over peripheral nerves, but it is also influenced by chemical messengers coming by way of the blood.

There is a close relationship between the central nervous and endocrine systems. Nerve impulses and, indeed, thought processes regulate endocrine secretions, and hormones, in turn, exert profound influence on nervous activity when presented to the brain by the blood. These interrelations are considered in Chap. 24.

REGENERATION AND AGING

Degenerative changes can be induced by disease and trauma. Some have been thought to occur as natural phenomena in aging. The brain and spinal cord exhibit fewer changes related to aging than do many other organs of the body. Those accompanying maturation during the early months and years of life are more striking than those seen in the declining years. The acquisition of myelin sheaths by nerve fibers of the white matter is incomplete at birth and goes steadily forward during infancy and childhood.

No neurons are believed to be added to the quota with which we are born. If there is a loss of neurons by natural processes, it is scarcely appreciable even in the brain of the aged. One of the few changes in nerve cells associated with old age is accumulation of lipofuscin pigment in the cytoplasm, and no important functional significance has been attached to this. A reduction is dendritic complexity with aging may occur. Neurons are good for the entire life-span, barring accidents and disease. Age changes in the blood vessels of the brain may be more marked than those in the neurons. Little is known at present about aging of neuroglia cells.

Disease and trauma account for most of the degenerative changes in the brain. Study of them falls to courses in pathology. We need mention only briefly the events that follow severance of nerve fibers of the central nervous system. These resemble the previously described changes after sectioning a peripheral nerve (Chap. 15). The neuron whose axon is cut undergoes chromatolysis. The distal portion of the axon, including its myelin sheath, degenerates, and the products of degeneration are removed by macrophages, but there are no neurolemma cells to proliferate and prepare a way for regenerative sprouts, as is the case in peripheral nerves. Neurolemma cells are absent in the central nervous system, and fibrous connective tissue is excluded from the nervous tissue by the perivascular and external glial membranes. When an axon of the brain is severed, attempts to form new sprouts must be made in an environment of neuroglia cell processes rather than within neurolemma membranes.

There are marked species differences in respect to adequacy of regeneration of severed nerve fibers in the central nervous system. One of the most baffling problems has been to learn why the severed spinal cord, for example, regenerates with great facility in fishes and certain amphibians, but so commonly fails to do so in mammals. Although the answer to that is as yet incomplete, it is now known that regeneration in the central nervous system of mammals is possible, both structurally and functionally.

Regeneration is merely a manifestation of perpetual growth of the neuron. When an axon in the spinal cord is severed, its distal segment degenerates, but, just as in a peripheral nerve, axoplasmic flow from the intact central portion proceeds to form an outgrowth, i.e., to regenerate.

Neurons normally have the potential for growth in length. Furthermore, their synaptic connections are less rigidly fixed than has been assumed. Fully satisfactory central regeneration in man is not related to a lack of intrinsic capacity of neurons to sprout new processes.

Successful regeneration in the severed spinal cord has been accomplished in experimental animals, notably the rat. The key to success lay in the inhibition of scar-tissue formation at the site of cord transection. Not only did nerve fibers then grow across the transection site, but, in time, motor and sensory functions were restored.

SUGGESTED READING

Axelrod, J.: Neurotransmitters. *Scientific American,* vol. 230, no. 6, pp. 59–71, June, 1974.

Brazier, M. A. B.: *The Electrical Activity of the Nervous System. A Textbook for Students,* 3d ed., Sir Isaac Pitman & Sons, Ltd., London, 1968.

Bundler, R. J., Jr., and J. P. Flynn: Neural Pathways from Thalamus Associated with Regulation of Aggressive Behavior. *Science,* vol. 183, pp. 96–99, 1974.

Buresorá, O., and J. Bures: Can the Brain Be Improved? *Endeavour,* vol. 28, pp. 139–145, 1969.

Eccles, J. C.: *The Understanding of the Brain.* McGraw-Hill Book Company, New York, 1974.

Evarts, E. V.: Brain Mechanisms in Movement. *Scientific American,* vol. 229, no. 1, pp. 96–103, July, 1973.

Fernstrom, J. D., and R. J. Wurtman: Nutrition and the Brain. *Scientific American,* vol. 230, no. 2, pp. 84–91, February, 1974.

Guth, L., and W. F. Windle: The Enigma of Central Nervous Regeneration. *Experimental Neurology, Suppl.* 5, pp. 1–43, 1970.

Llinás, R. R.: The Cortex of the Cerebellum. *Scientific American,* vol. 232, sec. 1, pp. 56–71, January 1975.

Rakic, P.: Mode of Cell Migration to the Superficial Layers of Fetal Monkey Neocortex. *Journal of Comparative Neurology,* vol. 145, pp. 61–84, 1972.

Ramón y Cajal, S.: *Degeneration and Regeneration of the Nervous System,* R. M. May (trans. and ed.) Oxford University Press, 1928. Reprinted by Hafner Publishing Company, Inc., New York, 1959.

Rutledge, L. T. T., C. Wright, and J. Duncan: Morphological Changes in Pyramidal Cells of Mammalian Neocortex Associated with Increased Use. *Experimental Neurology,* vol. 44, pp. 209–228, 1974.

Shuangshoti, S., and M. G. Netsky: Human Choroid Plexus: Morphologic and Histochemical Alterations with Age. *American Journal of Anatomy,* vol. 128, pp. 73–96, 1970.

Sperry, R. W.: Cerebral Organization and Behavior. *Science,* vol. 133, pp. 1749–1757, 1961.

Watson, W. E.: Physiology of Neuroglia. *Physiological Reviews,* vol. 54, pp. 245–271, 1974.

Windle, W. F. (ed.): *Biology of Neuroglia;* Charles C Thomas, Publisher, Springfield Ill., 1958.

Visual, Vestibular, and Auditory Organs

Sense organs receive and transfer to the brain information about changes in the environment. Only in the olfactory organ do dendritic processes of neurons come into direct contact with the elements. Specialized epithelial or connective-tissue cells intervene between dendrites and the environment and act in the capacity of transducers in many other sense organs.

Chemoreceptor, thermoreceptor, baroreceptor, and mechanoreceptor organs have been considered in other chapters. They have relatively simple structural characteristics. Three sense organs with much more complicated structure, the visual, vestibular, and auditory organs, remain to be described. The receptors for light and sound are especially noteworthy because more messages reach the brain from them than from all the other sensory receptors combined.

EYEBALL

The eye (oculus) has its genesis as an epithelial outpocketing of the forebrain of the embryo. This evagination of the neural tube forms the inner coat, including the retina of the adult eye. The retina and the optic nerve, which arises from it and connects it with the brain, thus are parts of the central nervous system.

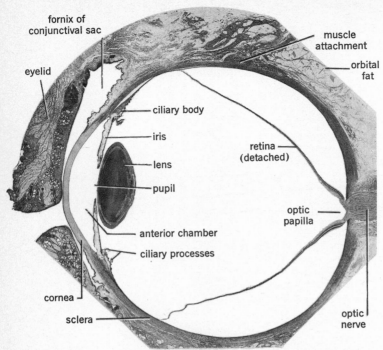

Figure 17-1 Human eyeball and eyelids sectioned sagittally through the pupil and optic papilla. This specimen was removed surgically for carcinoma of the lacrimal gland. Artifactitous detachment of the nervous portion of the retina demonstrates the progressive increase in thickness of that layer toward the optic papilla. The detachment occurs as far forward as the ora serrata, leaving the choroid intact. Photomicrograph, × 3. *(Contributed by L. L. Caulkins.)*

Like the rest of the central nervous system, they are covered with vascular and protective fibrous membranes. These coverings, derived from embryonic mesenchyme, are the middle vascular coat, comparable with the pia-arachnoid, and the outer fibrous coat, continuous with the dura mater. Another important component of the eye, the lens, arises separately from the surface ectoderm over the optic vesicle of the embryo. Spaces in front of the lens contain a special tissue fluid known as aqueous humor. Behind the lens is a jelly-like substance, the vitreous body. As in the brain, there are no lymphatic vessels in the nervous portion of the eyeball.[1]

The eyeball is remarkably like a camera, with its lenses, iris diaphragm, and photosensitive layer of tissue, the retina, in a black-pigmented compartment (Fig. 17.1). Transparency of the light-transmitting components of the eyeball is one of the most extraordinary features of the visual organ. This feature is not acquired but is maintained during development. In the early embryo all tissues are transparent.

[1]For that matter, no part of the eyeball except the corneal periphery at the junction with the conjunctiva has lymphatic vessels.

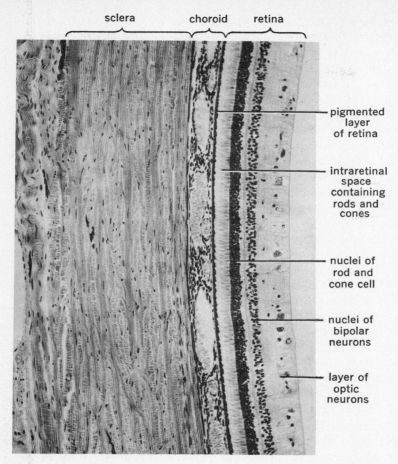

sclera   choroid   retina

— pigmented layer of retina

— intraretinal space containing rods and cones

— nuclei of rod and cone cell

— nuclei of bipolar neurons

— layer of optic neurons

Figure 17-2 Human eyeball. The section passes through all coats about 5 mm behind the ora serrata; exterior is toward the left. Photomicrograph, × 125.

Outer Coat The covering of the eye (tunica fibrosa bulbi) corresponding to the dura mater is dense fibrous connective tissue, even more compactly arranged than that around the brain. This is the layer that gives shape to the globe of the eyeball. Its two parts are the sclera and cornea.

The **sclera** forms the posterior five-sixths of the fibrous coat (Fig. 17.2). It is perforated behind by optic-nerve fibers and blends there with the fibrous-connective-tissue sheath of the optic nerve. In front, it joins the cornea and is covered at the white of the eye by part of the conjunctiva. The external layer of scleral connective tissue is more vascular than the inner portion. It is connected loosely to a dense fibrous capsule,[2] which adjoins the areolar tissue of the orbit. This lamellar arrangement of dense and loose tissues permits the eyeball to rotate freely.

Internally, at the junction of the sclera proper and the vascular coat of the

[2]Formerly called the "capsule of Tenon."

eyeball, numerous pigmented connective-tissue cells (melanocytes) are found. The inner aspect of the sclera presents an even surface to the vascular coat except at the sclerocorneal junction, where irregularities, shown in Fig. 17.5, occur. There, at the so-called **scleral spur** near the sclerocorneal junction, a prominent channel, the **scleral venous sinus,**[3] encircles the eyeball.

The eyeball lies in the bony orbit of the skull in a mass of loose connective tissue and orbital adipose tissue. The extraocular muscles that move the eyeball traverse the loose tissue of the orbit and are attached to the sclera. Arteries, veins, and nerves pass from the orbital tissue through the sclera to inner structures of the eyeball.

The **cornea,** forming the anterior one-sixth of the fibrous coat, has a greater curvature than the sclera, and this makes it protrude from the main part of the globe. The cornea is the most important element of the dioptric apparatus. It has two and one-half times the refracting power of the lens.

The dense fibrous connective tissue of the cornea is lamellated, and its fibrous as well as cellular constituents are transparent. In front, it is covered by stratified squamous epithelium, continuous with that of the conjunctiva. In back, it is lined by a single layer of squamous cells—mesothelium. Thick basement membranes, the **laminae limitans,** are seen beneath both epithelial layers. The anterior limiting lamina,[4] beneath the stratified epithelium, usually is more prominent than the posterior limiting lamina,[5] beneath the mesothelium. Both appear homogeneous in the usual preparations of light microscopy, but the electron microscope reveals fine fibrils of collagen arranged randomly in the anterior limiting lamina. The posterior limiting lamina is homogeneous and elastic. The lamina propria constitutes the main part of the cornea and consists of many layers of coarser collagenous fibrils running in different directions and passing from one layer to another. A matrix of ground substance permeates all layers. The structure of the cornea is illustrated in Fig. 17.3.

No blood vessels enter the cornea, but metabolism is provided for by diffusion from capillaries located at the junction of the corneal and conjunctival epithelium. Severe injury of the cornea may cause invasion by blood vessels from the conjunctiva, and this leads to opacity. Nerve fibers arising from free endings in the corneal epithelium are unmyelinated.

The **sclerocorneal junction** (Fig. 17.4) is a transition zone in which transparency of the cornea gives way to opacity of the sclera. The outer corneal epithelium thickens as it passes onto the vascular sclera at the white of the eye. The anterior limiting lamina ends at the border or **limbus** of the cornea. The posterior limiting lamina merges with some loose connective tissue mesial to the scleral spur and internal to the scleral venous sinus. This loose tissue contains tissue spaces,[6] some of which are prominent in histologic sections (Fig. 17.5).

Middle Coat   The middle coat of the eyeball (tunica vasculosa bulbi) is vascular and contains smooth muscle. This coat has a stroma of loose fibrous

[3]Formerly called the "canal of Schlemm."
[4]Formerly called the "membrane of Bowman."
[5]Formerly called the "membrane of Descemet."
[6]Formerly called the "spaces of Fontana."

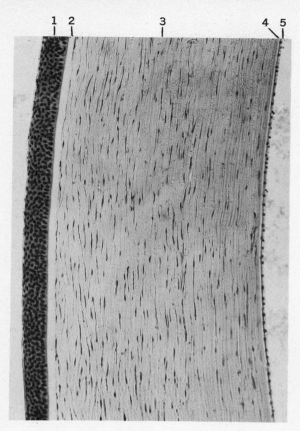

Figure 17-3 Human cornea. The corneal epithelium (*1*) and its anterior limiting lamina (*2*) are external to the transparent connective-tissue layer (*3*); the posterior limiting lamina (*4*) and simple squamous epithelium (*5*) are internal. Photomicrograph, × 125.

connective tissue firmly adherent to the inner coat, but only loosely attached to the outer one except at the point of exit of the optic nerve and at the sclerocorneal junction. A potential space between this coat and the sclera corresponds, in a way, to the subdural space. Three parts of the middle coat are designated the choroid, ciliary body, and iris.

The **choroid** lies between the sclera and the retina, extending only as far forward in the eyeball as the ora serrata of the retina. Its structure is demonstrated in Fig. 17.2. It contains a rich field of arterioles and venules in its external stratum and a thin bed of capillaries in the internal stratum. Its loose fibrous-connective-tissue stroma contains many melanocytes. The innermost part of the choroid forms the basement membrane of the pigmented epithelium of the retina, or **lamina basalis choroideae.**[7] Nutrition of photosensitive elements of the retina takes place through this lamina.

The **ciliary body** extends forward from the choroid at the ora serrata to a point just behind the sclerocorneal junction, i.e., to the scleral spur. It is the thickest portion of the middle coat, presenting a triangular appearance in meridional sections through the eyeball. It forms a fibromuscular ring to which is attached the suspensory "ligament" of the lens. The ciliary body is only

---

[7]Formerly called the "glassy membrane of Bruch."

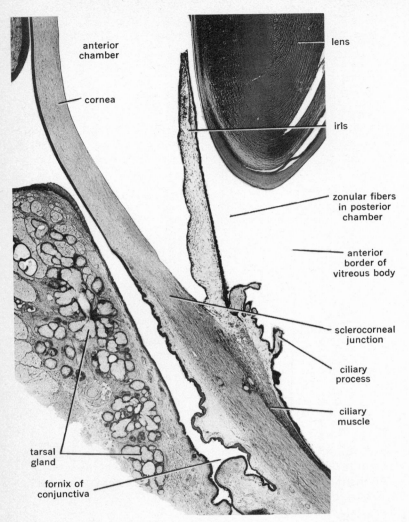

anterior
chamber

cornea

lens

iris

zonular fibers
in posterior
chamber

anterior
border of
vitreous body

sclerocorneal
junction

ciliary
process

ciliary
muscle

tarsal
gland

fornix of
conjunctiva

Figure 17-4 Human eye. The specimen is the same as in Fig. 17-1, showing iris, ciliary body, and other details. Photomicrograph, × 15.

slightly attached to the sclera except at the scleral spur, to which its muscle is firmly anchored. The inner surface of the ciliary body, covered by an epithelium continuous with the retina at the ora serrata, is thrown into 70 to 80 radiating folds. These folds are especially prominent at the free mesial edge of the ciliary body and are designated **ciliary processes.** In a gross specimen, they are accentuated by pigmentation of part of the epithelium between them (Fig. 17.7). The base of the iris adjoins the ciliary body as shown in Figs. 17.4 to 17.6.

The ciliary body contains all the elements of the choroid except the capillary layer. A significant addition is the **ciliary muscle** consisting of meridional, radial, and circular smooth-muscle fibers. The principal meridional fibers are attached to the sclera in front, especially to the scleral spur, and to the choroid behind. Their contraction puts tension on the choroid. Radial fibers are more mesial and pass from the sclera to the inner layers of the ciliary body. Near the base of the iris, the innermost bundles of fibers constitute a sphincterlike circular muscle. The ciliary muscle functions in accommodation of the eye for near vision.

The double layer of low simple columnar epithelium lining the ciliary body is the **pars ciliaris retinae.** The cells adjacent to the stroma of the ciliary body are heavily pigmented, whereas most of those constituting the layer on the inner surface are nonpigmented. A space is present between the two sheets of epithelium in the embryo but becomes obliterated during development.

The **iris** is the most anterior component of the middle coat. It is a thin annular plate of loose fibrous connective tissue, richly supplied with blood vessels, and lined on its posterior surface with nonnervous darkly pigmented epithelium known as the **pars iridica retinae.** The anterior surface is covered by a simple squamous epithelium, thinner than that on the posterior aspect of the cornea, with which it is continuous at the iris angle, as shown in Fig. 17.5. The iris lies on the anterior surface of the lens. The outer rim or root of the iris joins the vascular stroma of the ciliary body. The inner rim borders the **pupil,** which is the aperture admitting light to the visual compartment of the eyeball. Vascular rings are formed by arterioles in the root of the iris and in the stroma near the pupillary margin.

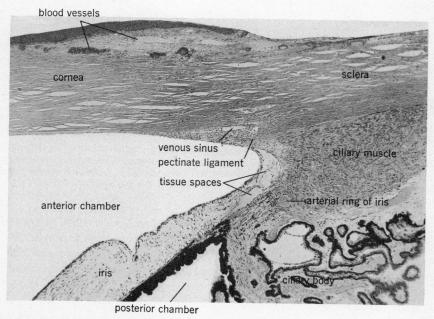

Figure 17-5   Iris angle of the human eye. Photomicrograph, × 40.

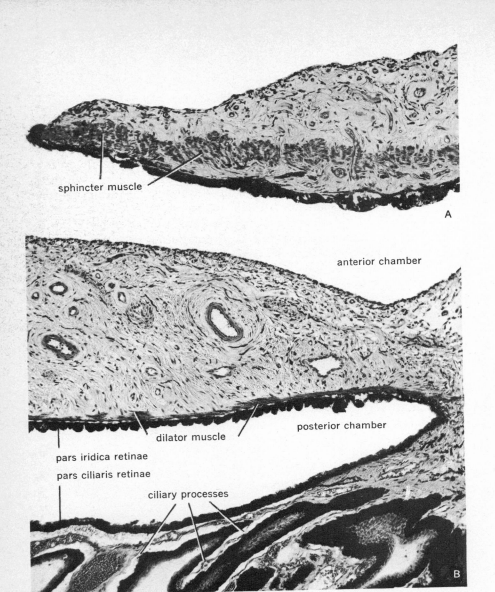

Figure 17-6 Human iris from a blue-eyed subject: *A*, inner rim of the iris showing its stroma, sphincter muscle, and pigmented epithelium on the posterior surface; *B*, peripheral one-third of the iris, posterior chamber, and ciliary processes. Note the arterioles with thick adventitia, the dilator muscle of the iris, and the pigmented epithelium of the pars iridica retinae. Photomicrographs, × 125.

A **sphincter muscle** is formed by circular bands of smooth-muscle fibers at the pupillary border of the iris, as shown in Fig. 17.6*A*. This muscle constricts the pupil. A **dilator muscle** is formed by myoepithelial cells arranged radially beneath the pars iridica retinae near the root of the iris. These can be observed in Fig. 17.6*B*. The muscles of the iris control the size of the pupil reflexly in response to changing brightness of light.

ora serrata

striae in
pars plana

fibers of
suspensory
ligament

ciliary
processes

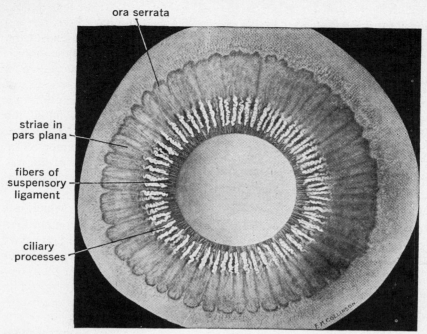

Figure 17-7 Ciliary body and lens of the human eye, viewed from behind; medial, to left; lateral, to right. *(From E. Wolff, The Anatomy of the Eye and Orbit, McGraw-Hill Book Company, New York, 1948.)*

The stroma of the iris contains a variable number of pigmented connective-tissue cells. Eye color depends upon their number. When many melanocytes are present, eyes are brown; when few, eyes are blue. Albinos not only have none in the stroma, but also have no pigment in the epithelium of the pars iridica retinae.

Inner Coat The inner coat of the eyeball (tunica interna bulbi) is the only one derived from the optic vesicle of the embryonic brain. The optic cup, formed by invagination of the optic vesicle, has two layers. The principal derivative of the outer wall of the optic cup is the **pigmented epithelium** of the retina. The inner wall of the optic cup forms the **nervous layer of the retina** proper. These two epithelial layers are easily separable in the adult eye because a potential **intraretinal space** exists between them as far forward as the ora serrata. In the specimen shown in Fig. 17.1, the retina had become detached at this space. Retinal detachment in the living person is a cause of partial blindness. The intraretinal space represents the original optic-vesicular cavity, an extension of the ventricular system of the embryonic brain. Indeed, even in the adult it contains tissue fluid comparable to cerebrospinal fluid, albeit in minute quantity.

The nonnervous part of the retina has been mentioned in the description of the middle coat. It is a forward continuation of the inner coat of the eyeball, beginning at the **ora serrata** as a double layer of simple columnar epithelium and passing over the inner surface of the ciliary body and the iris to end at the pupillary border of the iris. Its pupillary border represents the lip of the embryonic optic cup. The inner, nonpigmented layer of the **pars ciliaris retinae** is formed by simple columnar epithelium, some cells of which resemble cells of the choroid plexuses of the brain. They may be responsible for secretion of a fluid comparable with cerebrospinal fluid, the **aqueous humor,** filling the chambers of the eyeball in front of the vitreous body and lens. The outer epithelial cells of the **pars iridica retinae** have lost their deep pigmentation. From them are derived the myoepithelial elements of the muscles of the iris. The inner layer of the pars iridica retinae, unlike that of the pars ciliaris retinae, is intensely pigmented (Fig. 17.8*A*).

The **pars optica retinae** is composed of the pigmented layer, which is a low simple columnar epithelium adjacent to the choroid, and the retina proper, which is a thin sheet of nervous tissue. The cells of the pigmented layer have basal folds of the plasmolemma on a pronounced basal lamina that is continuous with the basal lamina of the choroid. Villous processes from their free border extend into the intraretinal space among the visual elements (Fig. 17.8*B*). The pars optica retinae is thin, measuring only 0.4 mm at the posterior pole of the eyeball and 0.1 mm at the ora serrata.

Like other parts of the central nervous system, the retina proper is composed of neurons and neuroglia cells walled off from fibrous connective tissue and blood vessels by two glial membranes, known here as the **external limiting membrane** and the **internal limiting membrane.** The cells whose processes form

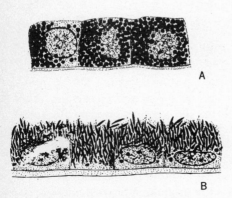

Figure 17-8 Pigmented epithelia from rabbit eye: *A,* heavily pigmented cells of pars iridica retinae; *B,* pigmented layer of retina proper showing a ragged surface (above), indicative of cell processes that protrude into the interretinal space. There is a thick basal lamina constituting a basement membrane (below). About × 1,200. *(JFN)*

these membranes are modified astrocytes arranged with their long axes at right angles to the retinal surface. The internal limiting membrane is thin and difficult to see; it forms the retinal surface that is presented to the vitreous body. The external limiting membrane is more prominent; it borders the intraretinal space.

The retina proper, exclusive of its pigmented epithelium, has three distinct layers of nuclei. These belong to the three principal types of cell composing it: **visual cells, bipolar neurons,** and **optic neurons.**[8] Nonnucleated layers in the retina will be noted. Synapses occur in the nonnucleated layers between visual cells and bipolar neurons and between bipolar neurons and optic neurons. The innermost layer, seen at the top of Fig. 17.9, is formed by the unmyelinated

[8]Actually there are more than three types of neuron in the retina, but others are omitted from this description in the interest of simplicity and brevity.

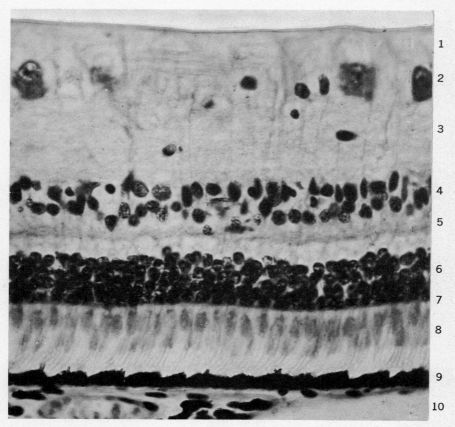

1
2
3
4
5
6
7
8
9
10

Figure 17-9 Human retina; a detail from Fig. 17-2 at higher magnification. The upper surface is internal. Numerals indicate the layers: *1*, nerve fiber layer; *2*, optic neurons; *3*, inner synaptic layer; *4*, bipolar neurons; *5*, outer synaptic layer; *6*, rod and cone nuclei; *7*, external limiting membrane; *8*, rods and cones; *9*, pigmented epithelium; *10*, choroid. Photomicrograph, −600.

axons of the optic neurons coursing parallel to the surface of the retina. These converge upon a point in the eyeball about 3 mm medial to its posterior pole. At this point, the **optic disc** or blind spot, the axons pass through perforations in the sclera to form the fascicles of the **optic nerve.** The nerve fibers acquire myelin sheaths at the optic disc. Converging axons pile up around the optic disc, forming a raised area, called the **optic papilla.** Other retinal elements are absent at the optic disc, as will be seen in Fig. 17.10.

At the center of the thick portion of the retina, near the posterior pole of the eyeball, there is a central depression called the **fovea centralis.** Few retinal elements except the outer portions of visual cells are present in the fovea (Fig. 17.11). The other cells and the nerve fibers accumulate around this depression to form the **macula;** its thick annular ridge sometimes has a yellowish coloration

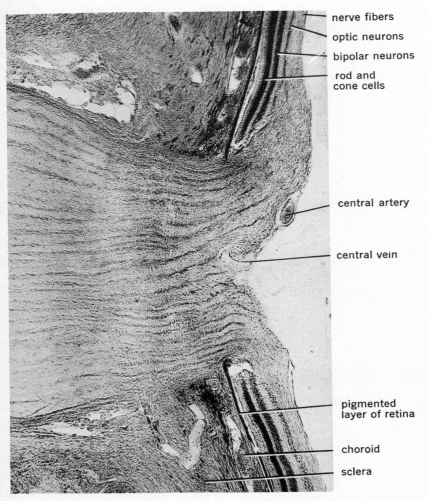

nerve fibers

optic neurons

bipolar neurons

rod and cone cells

central artery

central vein

pigmented layer of retina

choroid

sclera

Figure 17-10 Optic papilla and optic nerve of a human eye. Photomicrograph, × 40.

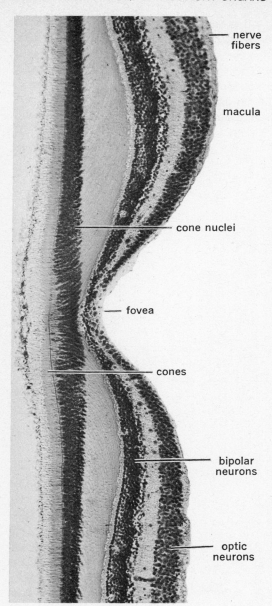

nerve
fibers

macula

cone nuclei

fovea

cones

bipolar
neurons

optic
neurons

Figure 17-11 Macula and fovea of a detached human retina. The cones, seen on the left, have pulled away from the pigmented epithelium, cleavage taking place in the intraretinal space. Compare the thickness of each layer in the macula with the same layers in Fig. 17-2. Photomicrograph, ×125.

in the living eye. Light rays can reach the layer of photoreceptors at the fovea centralis without traversing all the other layers of the retina. In consequence of this, the fovea is the point of greatest visual acuity. Everything that one views directly and critically comes to focus upon it.

The photoreceptors are of two kinds: the **rod cells** and the **cone cells.** They are neuroepithelial cells lying partly inside the nervous stratum of the retina and partly in the intraretinal space. The nucleated portions of the cells and their

basal processes are found in the former location, while the outer, highly specialized, light-sensitive processes pierce the external limiting membrane of the retina and lie in the intraretinal space. These specialized processes of the visual
cells are the rods and cones proper. They are seen in Fig. 17.9.

Rods are about 60 μm long, twice as long as **cones,** but are only 2 μm thick,
while the cones measure about 7 μm in diameter. Each consists of an inner,
thick segment and an outer, thin one, but the outer segment of the cone is much
shorter than that of the rod (Fig. 17.12*A*).

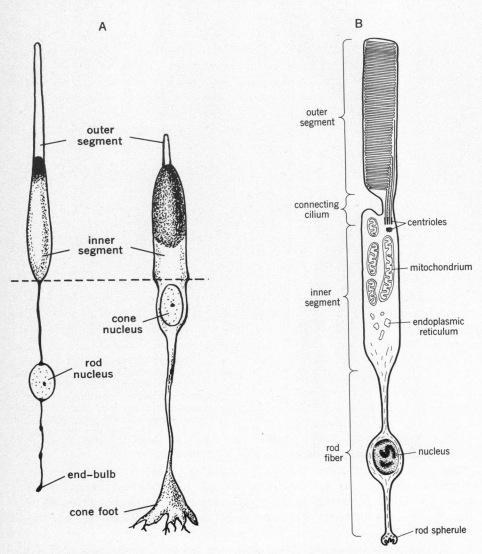

Figure 17-12 *A.* Diagram of human rod cell (right) and cone cell (left). The broken line marks
the external limiting membrane. *(WEL). B.* Diagrammatic representation of a rod cell based on
electron microscopic findings. The outer segment, filled with stacked membranes, has been
foreshortened in the diagram. *(CHP)*

The body of the rod cell is thin and is called a "rod fiber." It contains the nucleus. The rod proper has a remarkably fine structure. Its thicker inner segment contains mitochondria, endoplasmic reticulum, and, at the junction of the two segments, a prominent basal body with centrioles. A cilium springs from one and connects the inner and outer segments (Fig. 17.12B). Most of the outer segment is composed of a stack of disclike unit membranes derived from infoldings of the plasmolemma. The fine structure of cones is similar, but of different proportions.

The only photoreceptors in the fovea centralis are cones. Elsewhere the rods outnumber cones about 20 to 1. Rods function in dim-light vision; cones are concerned with bright-light and color vision. In bright light, the pigment granules of the epithelial cells extend into the protoplasmic processes that lie in the intraretinal space among the outer rod segments. These processes with pigment granules retract in dim light and permit more light rays to reach the rods.

At the fovea centralis, each cone cell synapses with a single bipolar neuron which, in turn, synapses with one optic neuron. All rod cells and some cone cells in other parts of the retina are grouped in relation to a bipolar neuron. The macula, containing the nervous elements for cone cells of the fovea centralis, gives rise to one-third of all the neurons of the optic nerve. This is remarkable, for the fovea is a tiny spot, occupying no more than one-twentieth of the area of the retina.

The rods and cones are not supplied directly by blood vessels, the intraretinal space in which they lie being avascular. Substances diffuse into this space from the choroid. The retina proper has its own blood supply, the **central artery** and **central vein** that enter and leave the eye through the optic nerve and optic disc. These blood vessels ramify over the inner surface of the retina, where they penetrate only into the layer of bipolar cell nuclei. Their branches avoid the fovea centralis. The central artery is an end-artery, inasmuch as it has no important anastomoses with other arteries, and its branches do not anastomose with one another. Occlusion of one central artery results in blindness in that eye. Occlusion of one of the major branches of the artery causes defective vision with blindness in one part of the retinal field.

Optic Nerve   The optic nerves are fiber tracts connecting the retinae with the brain after executing a partial decussation in the **optic chiasma.** In human beings, each nerve contains more than 1 million nerve fibers, all of which are myelinated. They exceed in number the sum of all other sensory nerve fibers that reach the central nervous system. The optic nerves are sheathed in connective-tissue membranes that are prolongations of the membranes of the brain. The pial sheath sends septa into the nerve, resembling perineurial septa.

Chambers of the Eyeball   The greatest part of the space within the eyeball is occupied by the vitreous body. A space bounded by this body, the lens, and the posterior surface of the iris is known as the **posterior chamber** of the eye (Fig. 17.4). The space is filled with tissue fluid of special type, probably a secretion of the epithelial cells of the ciliary processes. This fluid passes freely between the lens and the iris to enter the **anterior chamber** of the eye, bounded by the iris and lens posteriorly and by the cornea anteriorly. Flow is unidirectional, the iris' apposition to the front of the lens acting as a valve.

The **aqueous humor** filling the two chambers of the eyeball is maintained at a pressure of about 28 mmHg, which helps keep the eyeball spherical. Transudation of aqueous humor through various soft tissues, but especially through the loose connective tissue at the iris angle (Fig. 17.5), into tissue spaces and thence into the scleral venous sinus permits a constant slow removal to the blood stream and accounts for its circulation from posterior to anterior chambers of the eyeball.

Light rays pass through the cornea, lens, vitreous body, and layers of the retina to reach the intraretinal space containing the photosensitive rods and cones. Clear normal vision is maintained only so long as these structures remain transparent. Aging may impair their transparency or may discolor them.

The **vitreous body** fills the posterior four-fifths of the eyeball. A slightly viscid intercellular matrix substance, it adheres to the retina proper but is not firmly attached to structures anterior to the ora serrata. It is not replaced in the adult when lost during surgery. The vitreous body is traversed by the **hyaloid canal,** marking the site of the artery by that name that supplied the lens in fetal life. Involution of the vascular supply occurs normally in the late fetal life, but an oversupply of oxygen can jeopardize the process and result in a condition known as "retrolental fibroplasia" and infantile blindness.

Lens   The lens is an epithelial structure that has undergone interesting specialization. It begins as a thickening, then an invagination of the surface ectoderm over the optic vesicle of the embryo. A lens vesicle is formed and is pinched off within the optic cup. Only the posterior wall of the lens vesicle becomes specialized. The anterior wall remains as a single layer of low columnar or squamous cells. The posterior epithelial cells become exceedingly tall; in fact, they become the concentrically arranged **lens fibers,** many attaining a length of 10 mm. A transparent homogeneous lamina, the **lens capsule,** encloses the lens. The center of the lens is denser than the periphery and is the oldest part. The peripheral layers of the lens gradually harden with aging. As the elasticity of the lens diminishes, its usefulness in accommodation declines, and the condition known as "presbyopia" results as a normal phenomenon of aging.

The suspensory "ligament" of the lens is formed by many delicate **zonular fibers** connecting the lens capsule at the periphery or equator of the lens with the ciliary body. These fibers hold the lens under slight tension which decreases its anterior-posterior diameter, a condition favorable for effortless focusing of images of distant objects onto the retina. When the ciliary muscle, especially the meridional fibers, contracts, it pulls the choroid of the eyeball forward ever so slightly. This action slackens the zonular fibers, relieving the tension on the lens, and the lens then assumes a greater convexity. In other words, the lens then becomes thicker at the center and permits images of nearby objects to be focused upon the retina. When the elasticity of the lens is lost with aging, it becomes impossible to accommodate for near vision, and spectacles must be worn for reading.

CONJUNCTIVA AND ASSOCIATED STRUCTURES

The anterior aspect of the eyeball, especially the cornea, is exposed to the external environment. Several accessory structures perform important protective functions. Among these are the conjunctiva, eyelid, lacrimal glands, and tear ducts.

The **conjunctiva** is a mucous membrane of simple construction. It consists of a layer of stratified squamous epithelium of the noncornified variety on a basal lamina, beneath which is found fibrous connective tissue containing blood vessels, lymphatic vessels, and nerves. The mucous membrane is continuous with the skin at the edges of the eyelids. It lines the posterior surface of the eyelids, folds back upon itself at the fornix, and covers the anterior surface of the eyeball to its continuation with the corneal epithelium at the sclerocorneal junction. The conjunctival sac is opened and closed by the eyelids. As is demonstrated in Fig. 17.13, the conjunctiva provides smooth surfaces on the eyelids but is wrinkled and thrown into folds in the fornices. The most marked irregularity is found at the medial aspect of the eye, where the conjunctiva is elevated by the **lacrimal caruncle.**

The stratified squamous epithelium of the conjunctiva beomes thin and is reduced to a double layer of cells in some regions of the posterior surface of the eyelids. In the fornix, mucous cells are encountered. The epithelium is tightly bound to the tarsal plates of the eyelids and to the surface of the eyeball by dense fibrous connective tissue. Elsewhere it is loosely attached by areolar tissue containing clumps of lymphocytes and some small tubuloacinous serous glands, the ducts of which open on the anterior wall of the fornix.

The major gland in relation to the conjunctiva is the **lacrimal gland,** lying in the orbit above the eyelid and opening into the conjunctival sac in front of the superior fornix by 10 to 14 ducts. The lacrimal gland is a compound tubuloacinous serous gland (Fig. 17.14). Its secretion of tears is under nervous control. A constant flow of secretion from the gland provides the conjunctiva and cornea with a film of moisture. Excess secretion is collected at the medial ends of the eyelid margins, where there are two little papillae, each containing an opening of one of the **lacrimal canaliculi.** These two ducts are lined with stratified squamous epithelium. They empty into the **lacrimal sac,** and the secretion carried by them is ultimately conveyed to the nose by means of the **nasolacrimal duct.**

The **eyelids** (palpebrae) are simply folds of thin skin. These structures are illustrated in Figs. 17.13 and 17.15. A **tarsal plate** of dense fibrous connective tissue gives form to each eyelid. In this plate are embedded the **tarsal glands,** which are branched acinous glands of the holocrine variety, i.e., modified sebaceous glands. The ducts of the tarsal glands open onto the margins of the eyelids. Their secretion prevents the eyelids from sticking together and helps confine the tears to the conjunctival sac.

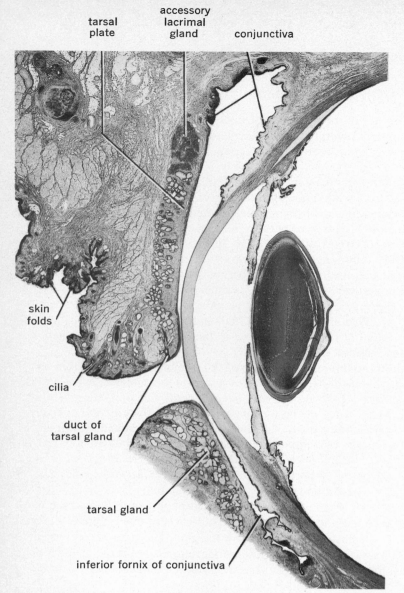

tarsal plate · accessory lacrimal gland · conjunctiva · skin folds · cilia · duct of tarsal gland · tarsal gland · inferior fornix of conjunctiva

Figure 17-13 Conjunctiva, eyelids, and anterior segment of the eyeball; the same specimen as in Figs. 17-1 and 17-4. The dark region in the upper left is a neoplasm. Photomicrograph, × 7.

Skeletal-muscle fibers of the **orbicularis oculi** muscle form a prominent layer in the eyelid in front of the tarsal plate. Their action closes the lids. The upper eyelid is raised by action of another muscle that lies outside the eyelid in the orbit; its tendon inserts into the dense fibrous connective tissue of the tarsal plate as well as into the skin. Smooth-muscle fibers, forming the **tarsal muscle,** occur above the tarsal plate of the upper eyelid.

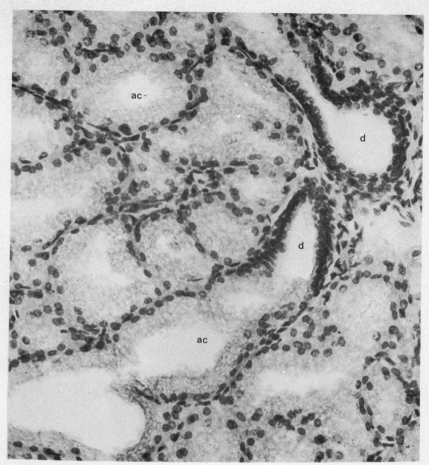

Figure 17-14 Human lacrimal gland. The junction of secreting acini, *ac,* with ducts, *d,* is seen. The frothy appearance of acinar cells and dilated lumens indicates active secretion. Photomicrograph, × 600.

The edges of the eyelids are bordered by the **cilia,** or eyelashes, forming two or three irregular rows placed close together. They are strong outwardly curving hairs whose follicles are buried deeply in the border of the eyelid. These hair follicles lack the usual arrector muscles but have sebaceous glands. A row of modified sweat glands, the **ciliary glands,** is found between the follicles.

EXTERNAL AND MIDDLE EAR

The external ear is made up of the auricle and external auditory meatus. The **auricles** are useful for catching sound waves and have aesthetic value. Each is formed of thin skin, containing scanty and small sweat glands, covering an irregularly shaped plate of elastic cartilage. The auricle opens into a cartilaginous and bony canal, called the **external auditory meatus,** lined with skin and containing ceruminous glands which secrete earwax.

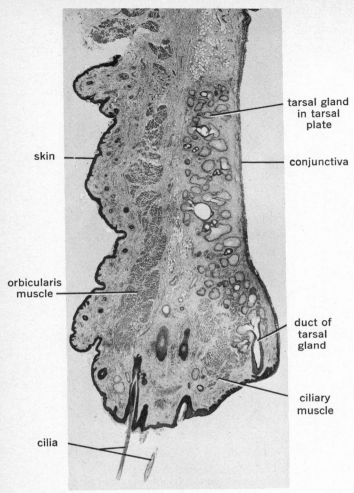

skin

tarsal gland
in tarsal
plate

conjunctiva

orbicularis
muscle

duct of
tarsal
gland

ciliary
muscle

cilia

Figure 17-15 Human eyelid. Photomicrograph, × 20.

The middle ear is a bony space, separating the deeply embedded auditory organ proper from the outside world. It consists of the **tympanic cavity** and a variable number of interconnecting air sinuses, called "mastoid cells." It opens into the nasopharynx by way of the **auditory tube.**[9]

The **tympanic membrane,** or eardrum, separates the middle ear from the external auditory meatus. It is a thin membrane made up of three layers. The outermost is composed of stratified squamous epithelium; the middle layer, of radial collagenous fibers; and the inner layer, simple squamous or cuboidal cells of the mucous membrane lining the tympanic cavity.

The **auditory ossicles** bridge the tympanic cavity from the tympanic

[9]Formerly called the "Eustachian tube."

membrane to the oval window. They are three tiny bones: the **malleus,** partly embedded in the tympanic membrane; the **stapes,** whose base fits into the oval window; and a third ossicle, the **incus,** connecting the other two. The ossicles are covered by the mucous membrane. Vibrations of the tympanic membrane can be transmitted by the ossicles to the internal ear. Function of this system may become impaired by sclerosis with aging.

Two "windows" of the bony labyrinth of the inner ear are found on the medial wall of the tympanic cavity. These are not open communications, for the **oval window** (fenestra vestibuli), lying adjacent to the vestibule, is partly filled by a bone, the freely movable footplate of the stapes, and the **round window** (fenestra cochleae) is closed by a fibrous membrane.

There are two muscles in the middle ear that help control the amount of sound reaching the inner ear. One, called the **tensor tympani,** is attached to the malleus and is innervated by the trigeminal nerve. The other is called the **stapedius** and is innervated by the facial nerve. Relationships of the components of the ear are shown in Fig. 17.16.

INTERNAL EAR

The internal ear is enclosed in the dense petrous portion of the temporal bone. It is suspended in a fluid-filled tubular space. The complex manner in which this tube winds its way through the bone has given rise to the term "labyrinth." The

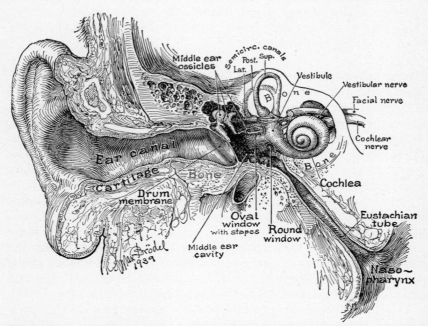

Figure 17-16 The human ear; a schematic drawing. *(From M. Brödel, Three Unpublished Drawings of the Anatomy of the Human Ear, W. B. Saunders Company, Philadelphia, 1946.)*

space, called the **osseous labyrinth,** is filled with a liquid, **perilymph,** surrounding the internal ear proper. Perilymph is similar to cerebrospinal fluid, and the perilymph space is continuous with the subarachnoid space through a channel that is partially filled with fibrous tissue. This channel is called the **perilymphatic aqueduct.** The wall of the bony labyrinth is deficient at the oval and round windows, which are closed by the stapes and a fibrous membrane, respectively.

A complicated system of fluid-filled tubes is suspended in the perilymph of the osseous labyrinth. This system, with its dilatations, constitutes the **membranous labyrinth.** Its epithelial lining is derived from the embryonic ectodermal otic vesicle. The fluid in the membranous labyrinth is called **endolymph,** chemically differing from perilymph by its high K^+ and low Na^+. The membranous labyrinth does not have a close association with the middle ear. All parts of the membranous labyrinth intercommunicate, but no part communicates with any other space.

The term "membranous labyrinth" is not synonymous with organ of hearing but refers to the system of tubes and vesicles in which the vestibular as well as the auditory sensory receptors are located. The only part concerned with hearing is the **cochlear duct**—the rest serves for balance and orientation. Other subdivisions of the membranous labyrinth are the three **semicircular canals** with **ampullae;** the **utriculus,** into which the semicircular canals and ampullae open; the **sacculus,** interposed between the utriculus and the cochlear duct; and the narrow interconnecting channels, including a terminal dilatation of one of them, called the **endolymphatic sac.** The semicircular canals occupy separate bony channels in three spatial planes. The utriculus and sacculus together occupy the one bony vestibule. The relationships of these various subdivisions of the membranous labyrinth are illustrated in Figs. 17.17 and 17.18.

Vestibular Labyrinth   The walls of the sacculus, utriculus, and semicircular canals are structurally alike. They are composed of dense fibrous connective tissue lined with simple squamous epithelium except in regions where patches of special neuroepithelium occur. One such patch is found in each ampulla, one in the sacculus, and one in the utriculus. The sensory regions of the ampullae are the **cristae,** little ridges transverse to the long axis of the canal. The sensory parts of the sacculus and utriculus are called **maculae.** All have similar structure, as illustrated in Figs. 17.19 and 17.20.

The wall of the labyrinth is locally thickened at the cristae and maculae. The epithelium increases in height, becomes columnar and then pseudostratified, and rests upon a basal lamina. Among the tall columnar cells are some shorter cells, located at the surface of the epithelium, which do not reach the basal lamina. They have tufts of long modified microvilli and one cilium, giving them the name **hair cells.** The tufts extend into the endolymph and support a layer of gelatinous substance that forms the **cupula** of the cristae (Fig. 17.19). In the maculae, this substance forms the **otolithic membrane** with little crystalline particles, called **statoconia,** embedded in it (Fig. 17.20).

Hair cells are of two types, one columnar and the other flask-shaped. They

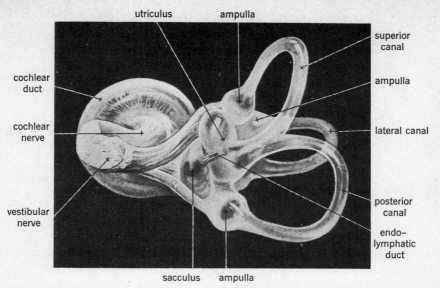

utriculus   ampulla

superior
canal

cochlear
duct

ampulla

cochlear
nerve

lateral canal

posterior
canal

vestibular
nerve

endo–
lymphatic
duct

sacculus   ampulla

Figure 17-17   Model of human membranous labyrinth. *(From W. Spalteholz, Handatlas der Anatomie des Menschen, 10th ed., S. Hirzel Verlag KG, Stuttgart, 1921.)*

are components of the sensory end organs. The flask-shaped hair cells, prevalent on the apex of each crista, are embraced by dendrites of sensory nerve fibers. Other nerve endings are efferent and resemble small presynaptic endings of neurons. Synaptic vesicles are present in endings of efferent telodendria on both types of hair cell. Stimulation of the hair cells by movement of the head or changing its position initiates afferent nerve impulses.

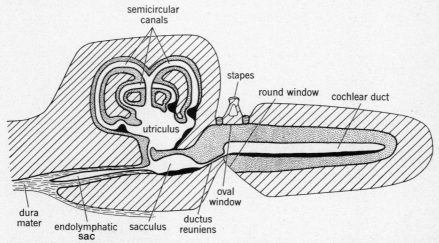

semicircular
canals

stapes

round window   cochlear duct

utriculus

oval
window

dura
mater

endolymphatic   sacculus   ductus
sac   reuniens

Figure 17-18   Diagram of the relations of components of the labyrinths, with the spiral cochlea uncoiled. Bone is shown crosshatched; perilymph, stippled; endolymph, clear; and patches of neuroepithelium, solid black. *(CHP)*

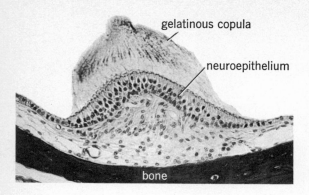

Figure 17-19 Ampullary crista of the posterior semicircular canal; guinea pig labyrinth. The gelatinous mass containing process of hair cells has shrunk in fixation of the tissues. Photomicrograph, × 90.

The fibrous connective tissue beneath the epithelium of the maculae and cristae is thickened and contains **vestibular nerve** (pars vestibularis nervi statoacoustici) fibers which, after arising from dendrites about the hair cells, pierce the basal lamina and become myelinated.

Cochlea   The auditory part of the bony labyrinth is the cochlea. It is a spiral channel 25 to 35 mm long, making two and one-half turns in the human ear. When viewed in mesial section from base to apex, as in Fig. 17.21, a central bony stalk, the **modiolus,** will be seen. A spiral shelf of bone winds up the modiolus like spiral stairs around a central pillar. This shelf, or **osseous spiral lamina,** partly subdivides the bony cochlea.

The cochlea, like other parts of the bony labyrinth, is lined with fibrous connective tissue forming its periosteum. This layer varies in thickness on different parts of the cochlear wall. It is especially thick, spongy, and vascular on the outer wall, where it is called the **spiral ligament.**

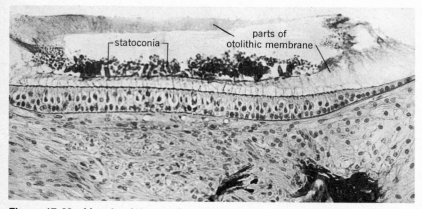

Figure 17-20   Macula of the utricle; guinea pig labyrinth. The otolithic membrane has been deformed in preservation of the tissues; statoconia are present. Photomicrograph, × 90.

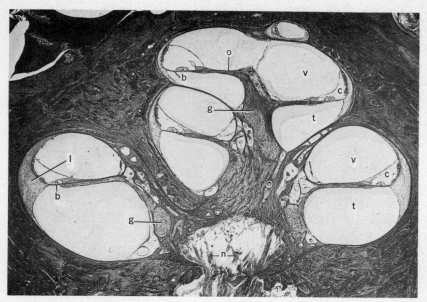

Figure 17-21 Human cochlea sectioned through the modiolus: *b*, basilar membrane (compare width in lower and upper turns); *c*, cochlear duct; *g*, spiral ganglion; *l*, spiral ligament; *n*, cochlear nerve bundles; *o*, osseous spiral lamina; *t*, scala tympani; *v*, scala vestibuli. Connective-tissue stain; photomicrograph, × 15.

The **cochlear duct** is the membranous labyrinth of the cochlea. It has blind ends (Fig. 17.18) but communicates at its lower turn with the sacculus by a very narrow tube, the **ductus reuniens.** Through this tube, the endolymph of the cochlear duct is continuous with that of the membranous vestibular labyrinth. The wall of the cochlear duct is made of fibrous connective tissue, lined with epithelium, a small part of which is neuroepithelium. In this respect, it resembles other parts of the membranous labyrinth; but here the similarity ends, for the cochlear duct has become remarkably specialized.

Instead of being loosely suspended in the bony labyrinth by trabeculae of fibrous connective tissue, as is the case of the membranous vestibular labyrinth, the cochlear duct is fused with the spiral ligament on the outside and with the osseous spiral lamina mesially. These attachments cause it to assume a triangular shape in cross section. The connective tissue of its upper wall is thin. That of its lower wall is stout and forms the **basilar membrane** which is stretched between spiral ligament and osseous spiral lamina as a ribbon of dense fibrous connective tissue. As seen in Fig. 17.21, the basilar membrane is narrowest in the lower turn and widest in the upper turn of the cochlea.

The thin upper wall of the cochlear duct is lined with simple squamous epithelium and is called the **vestibular membrane.**[10] The spongy outer wall, at-

---

[10]Formerly, "Reissner's membrane."

taching to the spiral ligament, is lined with pseudostratified epithelium, forming the **stria vascularis,** so called because it contains capillaries from the subjacent connective tissue.[11] Columnar cells, particularly those of the stria vascularis, may secrete endolymph. The epithelium of the basal wall of the cochlear duct is columnar but presents a remarkable appearance where it is adapted to receive vibrations and transduce them into nerve impulses. There it forms the spiral organ.

The **spiral organ**[12] is an avascular structure consisting of modified columnar epithelium on the outer rim of the osseous spiral lamina and on the basilar membrane. It contains small fluid-filled tissue spaces. The most prominent of these is triangular and is called the **tunnel.** This is bounded by an inner and an outer **pillar cell** united at their free surfaces, where they are capped by a cuticular plate. The base of the inner pillar is on the bony lip; that of the outer, on the basilar membrane. The rest of the epithelium of the spiral organ consists of **supporting cells,** of several shapes and named for their discoverers, and the sensory receptor cells, or **hair cells.** The latter are found on either side of the tunnel. A single row of hair cells is present on the inner side, three or four rows on the outer side. Neither inner nor outer hair cell reaches the basal lamina, but the supporting cells do. The free surface of the hair cells is covered by a cuticle, with modified microvilli projecting into the lumen of the cochlear duct. Upon their tips rests a delicate gelatinous structure, the **tectorial membrane.** This peculiar structure is possibly a product of more mesially placed epithelial cells on the **spiral limbus,** which is a mass of connective tissue on the spiral lamina. The structure of the spiral organ is illustrated in Fig. 17.21.

The hair cells of the spiral organ are clasped by the dendrites of the **cochlear nerve** (pars cochlearis nervi statoacoustici). The afferent nerve fibers pierce the osseous spiral lamina and run to the **spiral ganglion,** where bipolar cell bodies occur on them. The ganglion lies in the spiral canal of the modiolus, as seen in Figs. 17.21 and 17.22. Efferent nerve fibers come from the brain. Upon reaching the basal lamina, their myelin sheaths are lost, and the axons enter the epithelium of the spiral organ, traversing fluid-filled tissue spaces to reach the hair cells. Their telodendria are found there, forming synaptic endings on the hair cells.

The cochlear duct and osseous spiral lamina together subdivide the cochlea. Above and below them lie perilymph spaces that communicate with each other at the apex, where the cochlear duct ends blindly. These perilymph spaces are given special names in the cochlea. That above the cochlear duct is the **scala vestibuli;** that below is the **scala tympani.** The scala vestibuli communicates freely with the perilymph spaces of the vestibule surrounding the sacculus. The scala tympani ends at the round window, which is covered by a thin fibrous membrane separating it from the middle ear. Both scalae are lined by a little connective tissue and simple squamous epithelium, as in other perilymph spaces.

[11]This is an exception to the rule that there are no blood vessels in epithelia.
[12]Still commonly called "organ of Corti."

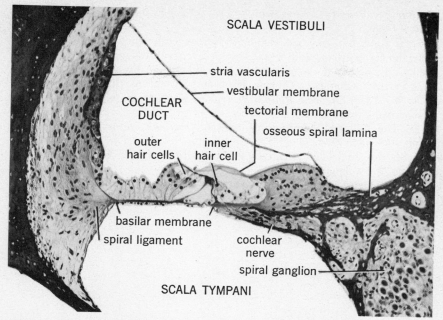

SCALA VESTIBULI

stria vascularis

vestibular membrane

COCHLEAR DUCT

tectorial membrane

osseous spiral lamina

outer hair cells

inner hair cell

basilar membrane

spiral ligament

cochlear nerve

spiral ganglion

SCALA TYMPANI

Figure 17-22 Cochlear duct with spiral organ; guinea pig. Photomicrograph, × 125.

Sound vibrations are transmitted to the fluids of the inner ear by the ossicles. They impinge upon the scala vestibuli through the oval window and set up force waves in the perilymph. How the hair cells are stimulated is not known. The basilar membrane may be caused to vibrate. Its lower and narrower portion responds to higher frequencies of vibrations than its upper and wider portion. This appears to be part of the mechanism for selective sound analysis: high tones at the lower end of the cochlear duct, low tones at the higher.

SUGGESTED READING

Fine, B. S., and M. Yanoff: *Ocular Histology. A Text and Atlas,* Harper & Row, Publishers, Incorporated, New York, 1972.

Flock, A.: Sensory Transduction in Hair Cells, pp. 396–441, in W. R. Loewenstein (ed.), *Handbook of Sensory Physiology,* vol. 1, *Principles of Receptor Physiology;* Springer-Verlag, OHG, Berlin, 1971.

Godfrey, A. J.: A study of the Ultrastructure of Visual Cell Outer Segment Membranes. *Journal of Ultrastructure Research,* vol. 43, pp. 228–246, 1973.

Hogan, M. J., J. A. Alvarado, and J. E. Weddell: *Histology of the Human Eye. An Atlas and Textbook;* W. B. Saunders Company, Philadelphia, 1971.

Hollenberg, M. J., and A. W. Spira: Human Retinal Development: Ultrastructure of the Outer Retina. *American Journal of Anatomy,* vol. 137, pp. 357–385, 1973.

Mann, I.: *The Development of the Human Eye,* 3d ed. British Medical Association, London; 1964.

Okisaka, S., T. Kuwabara, and S. I. Rapoport: Selective Destruction of the Pigmented Epithelium in the Ciliary Body of the Eye. *Science,* vol. 184, pp. 1298–1299, 1974.

Rasmussen, G. L., and W. F. Windle (eds.): *Neural Mechanisms of Auditory and Vestibular Systems,* Charles C Thomas, Publisher, Springfield, Ill., 1960.

Rodieck, R. W.: *The Vertebrate Retina. Principles of Structure and Function.* W. H. Freeman and Company, San Francisco, 1974.

Ross, M. D.: The Tectorial Membrane of the Rat. *American Journal of Anatomy,* vol. 139, pp. 449–481, 1974.

Werblin, F. S.: The Control of Sensitivity in the Retina. *Scientific American,* vol. 228, no. 1, pp. 70–79, January, 1973.

Young, R.: Visual Cells, *Scientific American,* vol. 223, no. 4, pp. 80–91, October, 1970.

Chapter 18

Integument

The integument is the skin with its appendages, the hair, nails, and cutaneous glands. It is a large organ, covering the body and protecting it from drying and other adverse factors of the external environment. Its total weight is estimated to be 3 to 5 kg, and its surface area in the adult is 1.75 m^2, more or less. From birth to maturity, integument surface increases sevenfold, while body weight increases twentyfold.

The importance of the integument goes beyond its protective role. Regulation of body temperature, control of blood volume, and synthesis of vitamin D are among its functions. A considerable amount of body heat is dissipated through its surface during physical exercise and when environmental temperature is high. Moreover, the integument functions in reception of messages from the environment, making it the largest sense organ of the body.

SKIN

The main part of the integument is the skin. Although it appears to form a relatively impervious barrier, many substances pass through it. Being on the outside of the body, it is prone to abrasions, cuts, and burns, but its self-healing property is notable.

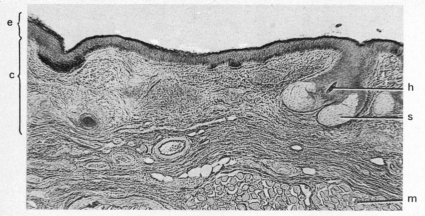

Figure 18-1 Thin skin of the human upper eyelid. This is one of the least highly developed types, consisting of narrow epidermis, *e,* and dermis or corium, *c.* The stratum corneum is a thin dark line on the surface. A sebaceous gland, *s,* and part of a hair follicle, *h,* are visible. The muscle of the eyelid, *m,* appears at the bottom on the right. Photomicrograph, × 50.

The basic structure of the skin consists of stratified squamous epithelium on its outer part, the **epidermis,** and a fibrous-connective-tissue inner layer, called **dermis** or **corium.**[1] Skin thickness, especially that of the dermis, varies from place to place. Skin is thinnest on the eyelid and thickest on the back.

Epidermis The stratified squamous epithelium is cornified. Its thickness and structural complexity lead to subdivision of the skin into two types, known simply as "thick skin" and "thin skin." The thickest epidermis is found on palmer and plantar surfaces. It may show only two clearly defined strata where it is thin (Figs. 18.1 and 18.2), but four distinct strata where it is thick (Fig. 18.7).

The inner or basal layer of the epidermis is the **stratum germinativum.** It rests on the dermis, into which it sends projections or folds that are more prominent in thick than in thin skin (compare Figs. 18.2 and 18.3). The row of basal columnar or cuboidal cells resting on the dermis is concerned with epithelial growth. Each cell has submicroscopic basal processes, numerous mitochondria, and a high concentration of ribosomes. The cytoplasm is basophilic. Basal cells undergo mitosis and thus provide replacement cells that are moved slowly outward through the epidermis (Fig. 18.4). A basal lamina beneath the cells can be seen in electron micrographs. In dark-skinned individuals melanin pigment granules are prominent in basal cells (Figs. 18.5 and 18.6).

Above the basal cells are stacked polyhedral cells of the so-called "prickle" layer.[2] These are so-called because they appear to be covered with little spines, some of which seem to pass from one cell to another (Fig. 3.7). Electron micrographs show the spines to be heavy condensations of microfila-

[1]*Nomina Anatomica* (1966) admits the more widely used term "dermis" as an alternative to the official, accepted "corium."
[2]Basal and polyhedral cells together form the "Malpighian layer."

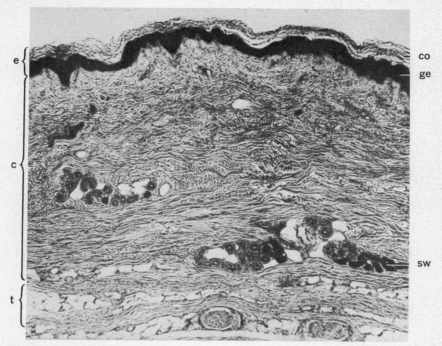

Figure 18-2   Thin skin of human wrist over the radial artery. This is thicker than that shown in Fig. 18-1 and has a wider epidermis, *e,* and dermis or corium, *c.* Two layers, stratum corneum, *co,* and stratum germinativum, *ge,* compose the epidermis. Sweat glands, *sw,* in the dermis show lighter, secreting, and darker, duct, portions. Subcutaneous tissue is indicated at *t.* Photomicrograph, × 50.

ments converging on prominent desmosomes along the plasma membranes of the cells at points of greatest adhesion. Masses of microfilaments form the tonofibrils of light microscopy and represent a stage in development of the structural protein of keratin.

As cells move outward toward the cornified layer, they lose water and gradually flatten. They also lose their basophilia, and most organelles disappear as they become keratinized (Figs. 3.8, 18.6, and 18.7).

Above the polyhedral cells, the **stratum granulosum** is identified as a single or multiple row of flattened cells with cytoplasm that contains darkly stained keratohyalin granules (Figs. 3.9, 18.4, and 18.7). In electron micrographs, these granules appear to be inclusions closely associated with condensations of microfilaments.

The **stratum lucidum** is encountered in thick epidermis of friction surfaces. It is seldom clearly seen in thin skin. It appears as a brilliant homogeneous and slightly acidophilic band between granular and cornified layers. The stratum lucidum is composed of several rows of squamous cells packed with keratohyalin and filaments but with only an occasional pyknotic nucleus (Fig. 18.7). Individual cell boundaries are indistinct or invisible.

The outer layer of the epidermis is the **stratum corneum.** Its thickness is more variable than in other strata; compare it in Figs. 18.2 to 18.3. It is com-

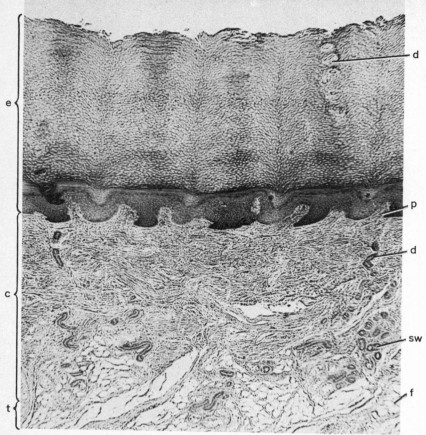

Figure 18-3 Thick skin from palmar surface of a human finger. This shows a heavy multilayered epidermis, *e*, the dermis or corium, *c*, and a small part of the subcutaneous tissue, *t*. Other abbreviations are *d*, duct of a sweat gland; *f*, lipocytes; *p*, papilla of the dermis; *sw*, sweat gland. Compare with Figs. 18-1 and 18-2. Photomicrograph, × 50.

posed entirely of dead scalelike cells that stick together but are continually being sloughed from the free surface of the skin. Keratin forms the main component of these cells. It is made up of microfilaments about 80 Å in diameter filling the cytoplasm, all other organelles having disappeared.

The stratum corneum is thickest on the friction surfaces of palms and soles. It is ridged on thick skin, as shown in Figs. 18.3 and 18.16, each ridge coinciding with a papillary ridge on the dermis. The ridges of the epidermis form patterns, known as dermatoglyphics, with details that differ from one person to another. Dermatoglyphics make fingerprints.

Dermis (Corium)   This fibrous-connective-tissue layer of the skin consists of an outer **papillary body** adjacent to the epidermis and a deeper **reticular body** that blends with underlying subcutaneous connective tissue. The papillary body consists of fine fibers, in contrast with the reticular body which is made up

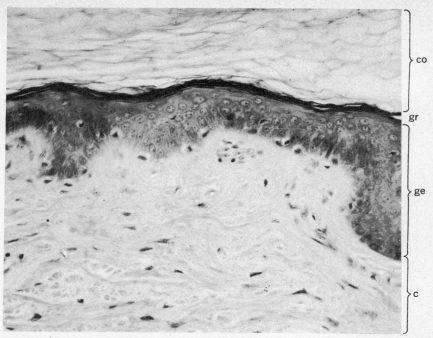

Figure 18-4 Skin of the wrist, showing stratum corneum, *co;* stratum germinativum, *ge;* and part of the dermis, *c*. A single row of cells, *gr*, composes the stratum granulosum. There is an imperfect stratum lucidum in the dark band. Photomicrograph, × 300.

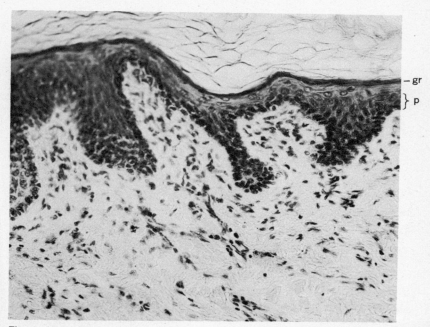

Figure 18-5 Female genital skin. Basal and polyhebral cells of the stratum germinativum are pigmented, *p*. There is a narrow stratum granulosum, *gr*. Photomicrograph, × 300.

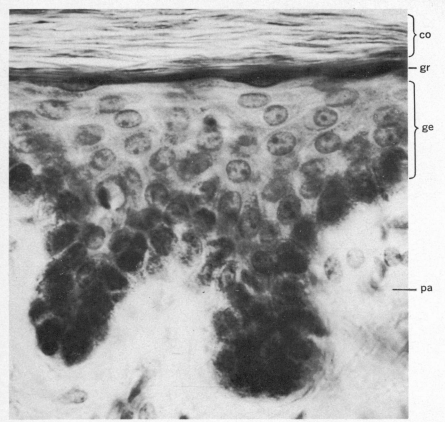

co

gr

ge

pa

Figure 18-6 Pigmented thin skin of the scalp of a black person. The layers seen are *co*, stratum cornium; *gr*, stratum granulosum; *ge*, stratum germinativum with pigmented basal cells; *pa*, papilla of the dermis. Photomicrograph, × 900.

of coarse ones. It is usually difficult to tell where the dermis ends and the subcutaneous tissue begins.

The fine elastic and reticular fibers in the papillary body make contact with the thin basal lamina of the stratum germinativum. The papillary body derives its name from the fact that it is thrown into projections, the **papillae of the dermis,** which fit into the basal surface of the epidermis, alternating with inward projections of the epithelium. In histologic sections of thick skin of the palms and soles, the papillae appear to be arranged in a regular pattern, the epidermis being laid down in parallel ridges, as shown in Fig. 18.3. This, however, is a false impression; in split-skin preparations, the underside of the epidermis has a sculpturing that differs in the various parts of the body.

The papillae of the dermis may be simple or complex, with several small secondary projections into the epidermis. Most papillae contain capillary loops. Some have specialized sensory end organs, such as the tactile corpuscles, one of which can be seen in Fig. 18.7. The latter are numerous on the fingers.

The reticular body of the dermis consists of coarse bundles of fibrous con-

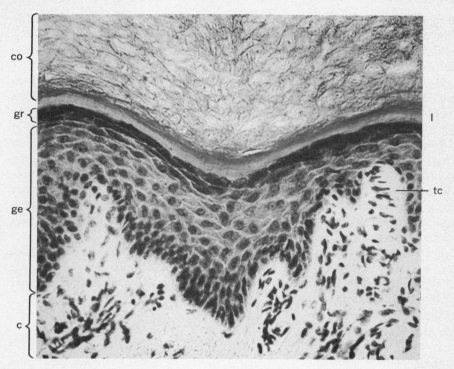

Figure 18-7 Portion of thick skin of a human finger showing all layers of the epidermis with two papillae of the dermis. The papilla on the left is vascular; the one on the right contains a tactile corpuscle, *tc*. The layers shown are *co*, cornified layer; *l*, stratum lucidum; *gr*, stratum granulosum; *ge*, stratum germinativum; *c*, dermis or corium. Photomicrograph, × 300.

nective tissue. The collagenous fiber bundles of the dermis are arranged both tangential and parallel to the surface of the skin, according to the specific regions. Blood vessels and nerves, as well as sweat glands and hair follicles, are found in this layer. Smooth-muscle bundles are present in the scrotum (Fig. 25.11).

Skin Color Color is imparted to the skin by pigment in cells of the epidermis and by blood in the superficial vessels of the dermis. The stratum corneum has an inherent yellowish color due to the presence of a small amount of the pigment carotene. However, the main coloration of skin is produced by melanin, found in the cells of the deep part of the stratum germinativum (Fig. 18.6). All individuals except albinos have some melanin pigment in their skin. Those with fair complexions have little pigment, and it is confined to the basal cells. In dark-skinned people, it is found in all parts of the germinative layer and may appear even in the stratum granulosum and stratum corneum. A few stellate cells, melanocytes, among and beneath the basal cells produce melanin in the form of granules (melanosomes) which are transferred to the basal cells. Cells moving out from the basal row gradually lose melanin. The pigment is deficient in palmar and plantar skin and occurs in increased amounts in genital, circumanal, and axillary skin, as well as in that of the areola and nipple of the breast. Freckles are small spots of increased melanin pigmentation. A physiologic increase in melanin production occurs in the skin after exposure to ultraviolet light of the sun.

It is noteworthy that ultraviolet radiation also results in synthesis of vitamin D by cells of the deep epidermis. Excessive pigmentation tends to prevent the rays from producing this effect.

Tela Subcutanea   This layer of fibrous-connective and adipose tissues is not part of the skin. It is the "superficial fascia" seen in gross anatomy. In some places, the loose construction of this layer permits movement of the skin over the underlying structures. The adipose-tissue component varies in thickness in different places and in different people. Sex differences in body contours become apparent after puberty as the distribution of adipose tissue in the tela subcutanea changes.

Portions of sweat glands and hair follicles, as well as blood vessels, lymphatic vessels, nerves, and some sensory end organs lie in the tela subcutanea. Skeletal muscle fibers are present in it in a few regions, such as the face, and extend into the skin proper.

HAIR AND NAILS

Hair   The proverbial hairlessness of human beings is more apparent than real. Close inspection will show that most of their bodies have numerous, but fine, soft, and inconspicuous, hairs. The few places lacking hair, the palms, soles, and dorsal aspects of terminal portions of the digits, are glabrous. Other hairless regions are the red lip borders, portions of both male and female genitalia, nipples and areolae of the breasts, and the umbilicus. The fine hair of the body is much the same in both sexes, but at puberty, coarse hair develops in the axillary and pubic regions of both, as well as on the face and other parts of the body of the male. Special hairs on the eyelids of both sexes were mentioned in Chap. 17.

Hair forms an important protective coat and heat insulator in most mammals, but it is impossible to make a good case for it in human beings, except perhaps for the hair of the scalp. The role of hairs in tactile perception is noteworthy, although large tactile vibrissae, present in certain other animals, are missing in the human species. The **hair follicles,** lying in the deep layer of the dermis and in the subcutaneous tissue, are of considerable importance for regeneration of epidermis denuded by surface lacerations and burns, regeneration taking place from the epithelium of which the deeply placed follicles are composed.

A hair follicle (folliculus pili) develops in the embryo from a bud of epithelium growing into the underlying mesenchymal precursor of the dermis of the skin and the subcutaneous connective tissue. A hair consists of a free shaft and a root embedded in the hair follicle, from which it arises. The shaft is formed by cornified cells like the cells of the stratum corneum of the skin. The cells on the surface of the hair shaft are flat and form a layer called the "cuticle"

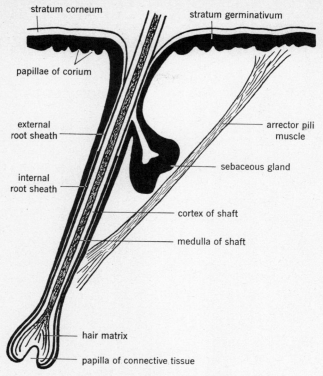

Figure 18-8   Diagram of a hair follicle. *(MWS)*

of the hair.[3] The inner cornified cells of the shaft are elongated. Actively dividing cells in the bulb of the hair follicle give rise to the cornified cells of the shaft. They are comparable with those of the germinative layer of the epidermis.

A hair follicle sectioned longitudinally (Fig. 18.8) resembles a thin invagination of skin into the subcutaneous tissue. All skin layers turn inward. The stratum corneum and stratum granulosum disappear at about the level of the openings of sebaceous glands. The stratum germinativum continues down the follicle as the outer root sheath of the hair and merges with germinative cells of the bulb of the follicle. The two layers of the dermis lie external to the outer root sheath with a basement or "vitreous" membrane between the connective-tissue sheath and root sheath. The papillary body of the dermis passes up into the bulb to form a dermal papilla, like those invaginating the stratum germinativum of the epidermis. Certain cells, formed by the germinative cells of the bulb, move outward with the hair between its surface and the outer root sheath. They compose the inner root sheath. This sheath is not found above the level of sebaceous-gland ducts. Figures 18.9 to 18.11 illustrate a number of these features.

Smooth muscles (musculi arrectores pilorum) are attached to the bulge of the hair follicles on the "leeward" side of the hair slant. These extend

[3] This is not a true cuticle (Chap. 3).

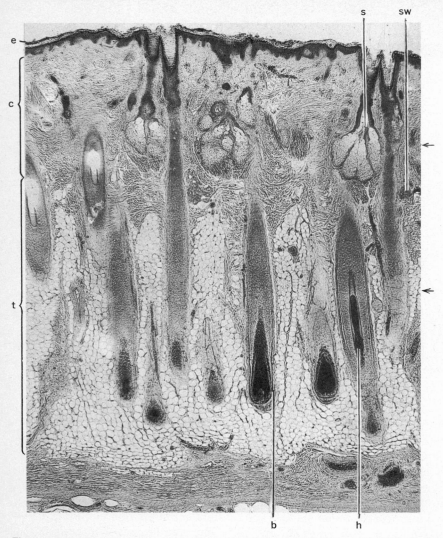

Figure 18-9 Human scalp; compare with skin sections (Figs. 18-1 to 18-3), but note that the magnification is less. Designated structures are *b,* bulb of hair follicle; *c,* dermis; *e,* epidermis; *h,* hair shaft, *s,* neck of a sebaceous gland; *sw,* sweat gland; *t,* subcutaneous tissue. *Arrows* refer to the two levels of Fig. 18-10. Photomicrograph, × 30.

diagonally past the sebaceous glands to insert into the papillary body of the dermis. Contraction of these muscles elevates the hairs, compresses the sebaceous glands, and depresses the skin near the hairs to form "goose pimples." The muscles are innervated by autonomic nerve fibers and contract reflexly in response to cold and emotional stimuli. By elevating the hairs, a more efficient blanket for insulation of the skin of the furred animals is created.

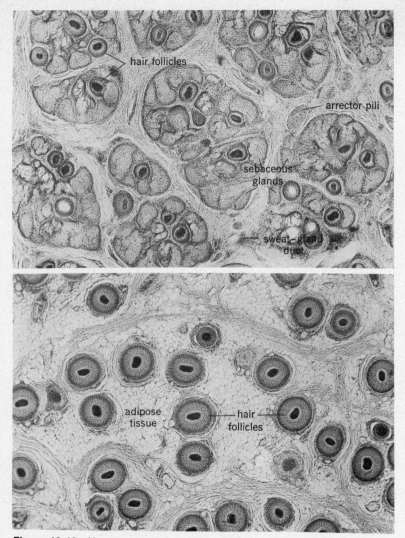

Figure 18-10 Human scalp, sectioned parallel to surface. Upper figure represents a section through level of upper arrow in Fig. 18-9. Lower, a section through level of lower arrow in Fig. 18-9. Photomicrograph, × 30.

Shedding of hair is seasonal in some animals but not in human beings. Their hairs are lost and replaced gradually, those of the scalp having the longest life, which may be as great as 9 years. Proliferation of cells of the bulb matrix stops. The base of the hair becomes club-shaped and keratinized, and the entire follicle is then rudimentary. Later, a vestigial hair germ in the vicinity of the

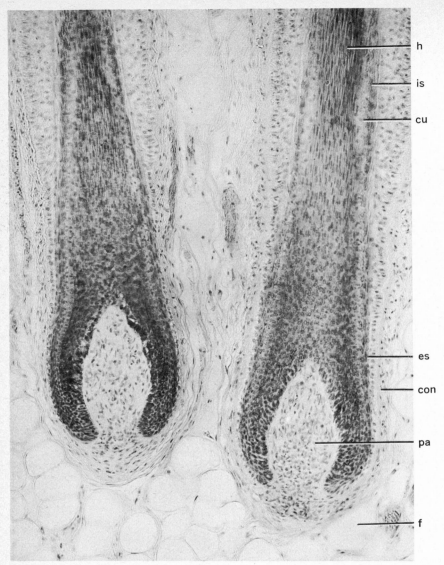

Figure 18-11 Human scalp, showing bulbs of two hair follicles with indenting connective-tissue papillae. Abbreviations: *con*, connective tissue continuous with the dermis; *cu*, hair "cuticle"; *es*, external root sheath; *f*, lipocytes; *h*, hair shaft; *is*, inner root sheath; *pa*, papilla. Photomicrograph, × 150.

papilla proliferates and forms the outer root sheath, much as it did in the fetus. The newly developed hair is often present on one side of the old one which is shed.[4]

[4]Myths and superstitions concerning human hair are believed by many seemingly informed persons. Among those common ones that can be branded as false are that baldness is a sign of virility; that shaving stimulates hair growth; that intense emotional experiences may cause hair to turn white overnight; and that the beard continues to grow after the body is laid to rest in the grave!

Nails Like claws and hoofs, these are a modification of the stratum corneum of the epidermis on the dorsal aspect of the terminal phalanges of the digits. A nail is rooted in the nail groove, an invagination of the integument surrounded by a crescentic rim of skin, the nail fold. The stratum germinativum and stratum corneum of the proximal nail fold continue back above the root of the nail into the groove, but the stratum germinativum alone returns along the underside of the root. The projecting crescentic fold of the stratum corneum is called the **eponychium.** Beneath the proximal part of the nail, the stratum germinativum is thickened and is called the matrix in the root, where active cell proliferation occurs. The nail is the modified stratum lucidum and stratum corneum of the part of the integument constituting the nail bed. The epidermis of the nail bed is grooved by longitudinal, more or less parallel, ridges. Transverse sections through the proximal parts of the digits show these ridges (Fig. 18.13), but longitudinal sections do not (Fig. 18.12).

Proliferation of the cells of the matrix causes the nail to grow outward. The dividing cells move outward and distally to become cornified and incorporated into the nail.

GLANDS

All cutaneous glands develop by growth of buds of epithelium into underlying mesenchyme. There are four main types of gland: sebaceous; eccrine sudariferous (sweat); apocrine (scent); and mammary glands.

Sebaceous Glands Most sebaceous glands develop from solid buds of the epithelium in the necks of hair follicles. They are holocrine glands of a simple

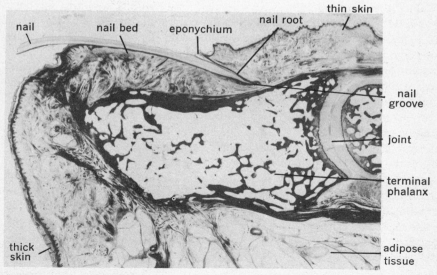

Figure 18-12 Fingernail sectioned longitudinally. Photomicrograph, × 6.

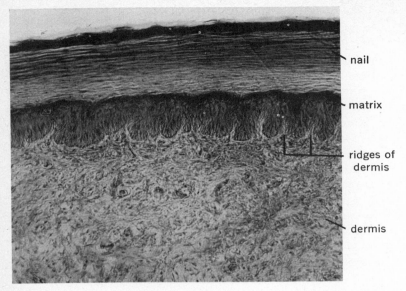

nail

matrix

ridges of
dermis

dermis

Figure 18-13 Fingernail sectioned transversely to show the ridges of the dermis; compare with skin (Fig. 18-3). Photomicrograph, × 150.

or branched alveolar type, opening by means of short ducts into the distal portion of hair follicles. Their secretion, sebum, is discharged into the infundibulum of the hair follicles and flows through it onto the skin.

The secreting portion of the sebaceous gland consists of one or more ovoid masses of epithelial cells (Fig. 18.1, 18.9, and 18.10). The cells on the rim of each lobule resemble the basal cells of the germinative stratum of the epidermis and produce the secreting cells. They rest on a basal lamina adjoining the connective tissue of the dermis. The inner cells, corresponding to the polyhedral cells of the stratum germinativum, are swollen with lipid droplets. These cells later undergo degeneration. They are displaced toward the duct of the gland, their nuclei become pyknotic and disappear (Fig. 18.14), and the cells disintegrate, forming the secretion of the gland. Cells lost in secretion are largely replaced by cells from the peripheral layer of the lobule.

Large compound sebaceous glands are found in the skin of the entire facial disc and the external auditory meatus. The hairs with which they are associated are fine and often go unobserved. Elongated sebaceous glands are found in the eyelids on the tarsal plate, the tarsal glands[5] (Fig. 17.15). Sebaceous glands not associated with hair follicles are found along the borders of hairless skin, and are particularly large in the labia minora of the female genitalia. The thick skin of the palms and soles lacks sebaceous glands.

Sebum consists of the oily secretion mixed with protein constituents of the disintegrated gland cells. The exact way in which sebum is secreted is not known.

[5]Meibomian glands.

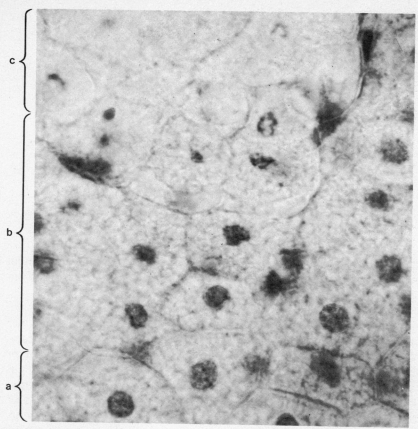

Figure 18-14 Sebaceous gland from human scalp: *a*, upper limit of large living cells swollen with secretion droplets; *b*, zone of dying cells with dark nuclei; *c*, disintegrating cells. Photomicrograph, ×900.

Eccrine Sudoriferous Glands Sweat glands are simple coiled tubules located in most areas of skin, absent only in the skin of the nipple, margins of the lips, concave surfaces of the external ear, and portions of the genital skin. In some locations, they are less numerous than in others. Some are even found on the eyelids. There are about 90 glands per square centimeter on the leg, almost 400 per square centimeter on the palms and soles, and even greater numbers on the finger tips.

The coiled portions of sweat glands are located deep in the reticular body of the dermis, although some glands may extend to the tela subcutanea. The glands have an undulating duct that extends from the tightly coiled knot deep in the dermis to the epidermis. The knots, or glomeruli, are about 0.1 to 0.5 mm in diameter. The greater part of each glomerular coil is made up of the secreting portion of the tubule. About one-fourth of the coiled portion is an excretory duct. Sweat glands may be seen in Figs. 18.2 and 18.3.

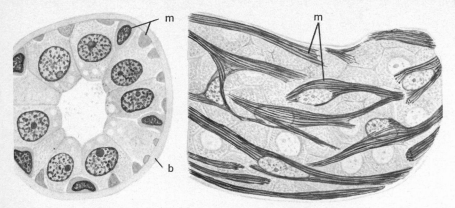

Figure 18-15 Secreting portions of a human sweat gland, showing myoepithelial cells, *m*, and basal lamina, *b*. × 600. *(JFN)*

The secretory part of the tubule is formed by simple columnar or cuboidal epithelium on a basal lamina. Spindle-shaped myoepithelial cells are located between the epithelium and basal lamina (Fig. 18.15).

Three parts of a sweat-gland duct can be distinguished. The deep part, coiled with the secretory part, begins abruptly. The myoepithelial cells end, and the columnar secreting cells give way to a double or triple layer of lower columnar epithelial cells with darker cytoplasm than the secreting cells. The diameter of the duct is smaller than that of the secretory tubule. Sometimes a slight hyalinized surface of the cells next to the lumen can be observed. The second part of the duct runs toward the epidermis, with which its cells blend (Fig. 18.3). The third part, especially where it traverses the thickened stratum corneum of the palms and soles, is twisted like a corkscrew (Fig. 18.16). As the duct enters the epidermis, its cells are lost among those of the stratum germinativum. The basal lamina blends with that of the epidermis. The lumen is all that is left, and it runs through the epithelium as a twisted cleft.

Ciliary glands[6] of the eyelid margins, and ceruminous glands of the external auditory meatus, are modified sweat glands. The ciliary glands have relatively straight, simple, or branched tubules. The ceruminous glands, larger than most others, have branched, coiled secretory portions and often have branched duct systems; their secretion is thick, filled with yellow pigment, and solidifies upon exposure to the air, forming the earwax.

The importance of the sweat glands can scarcely be overemphasized, although they are not indispensable. Occasionally they are deficient or even largely absent. Their secretion is a watery fluid containing some solutes, mainly sodium chloride. A certain amount of moisture escapes directly from the skin, and evaporation of this imperceptible perspiration is sufficient to meet ordinary needs of the skin. The secretion of the sweat glands is essential in the regulation of body temperature during unusually warm weather and during exercise. An

[6]Glands of Moll.

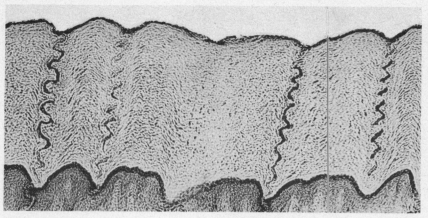

Figure 18-16 Ducts of sweat glands traversing the stratum corneum of a human finger. Photomicrograph, × 50.

adult person may lose 10 to 12 liters of water per day in perspiration. Under abnormal conditions of exercise and high environmental temperature, the body can give off more sodium in a few hours than is taken in by mouth.

Apocrine Glands These are scent glands, located principally in the skin of the axilla, mons pubis, and circumanal region. They are larger than sweat glands and are set deeper in the subcutaneous tissues (Fig. 18.17). Their thin ducts empty into hair follicles instead of onto the surface of the skin. Their myoepithelial cells are well-developed. The mode of formation of secretion of the apocrine glands differs from that of sweat glands, as was described in Chap. 3. The glands secrete small amounts of a viscous substance that, when degraded by surface bacteria, attains the characteristic axillary odor. The apocrine glands undergo hypertrophy at about 8 years and assume their functions in early puberty.

Mammary Glands These are the largest cutaneous glands, secreting portions of which are located in the subcutaneous tissue of the chest. Their ducts traverse the dermis to reach the skin surface of the nipple. Embedded in adipose and connective tissues, they form the female breasts.

Mammary glands are alike in both sexes at birth. Those of the male attain maximum development in about 20 years, resembling at the end of that time the female glands of early puberty. The female mammary glands undergo rapid development at puberty, but are not fully formed until the end of pregnancy.

The glandular part of the breast consists of 15 or 20 lobes, each with its own duct system. The lobes lie in adipose and fibrous connective tissue of the superficial fascia. Branching tubules of mammary lobules are embedded in loose fibrous connective tissue lacking lipocytes. The breast is covered with thin skin, which assumes special characteristics on the areola and nipple.

Simple columnar epithelium, tall in most places and alternating with

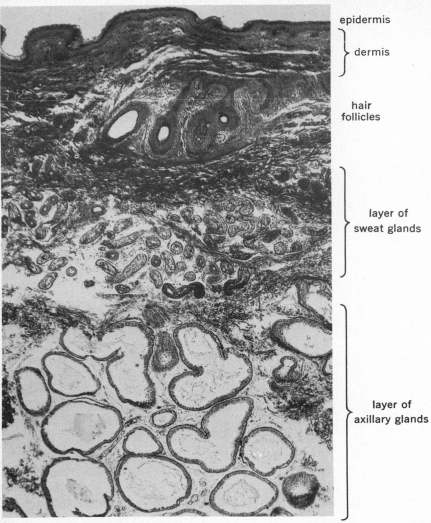

epidermis

} dermis

hair
follicles

layer of
} sweat glands

layer of
} axillary glands

Figure 18-17 Skin and subcutaneous tissue of the human axilla. Apocrine scent glands lie deeper than the eccrine sweat glands. Photomicrograph, × 50.

patches of pseudostratified epithelium here and there, lines the **lactiferous ducts.** Toward the nipple, the epithelium becomes stratified squamous as the ducts end in small pores upon the nipple. In their course, the ducts are much wider than their openings, and their walls are folded longitudinally. A dilatation in each duct is called a **lactiferous sinus.** The epithelium of the duct has a basal lamina. Much of the subepithelial connective tissue is arranged circularly.

The structure of the mammary gland changes with age and varying functional states. During the early days or even weeks after birth, each branching lactiferous duct is seen to be divided into small tubules, dilated at their ends to form acini. These are lined with simple columnar epithelium in which secretory

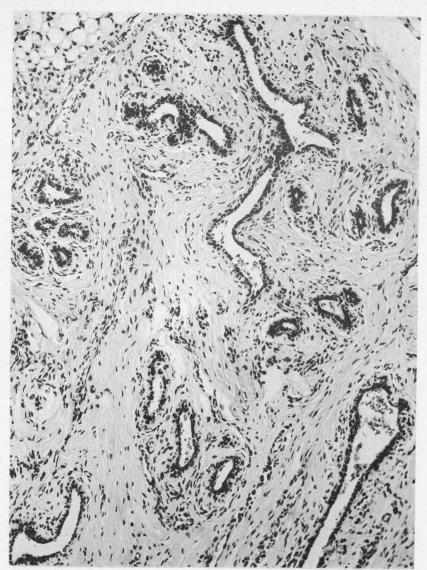

Figure 18-18 Mammary gland with lactiferous ducts, from a human infant soon after birth. The gland still shows some of the hypertrophy induced by maternal hormone. Photomicrograph, × 150.

activity may be observed. The acini and ducts contain some of the secretion; free cells are present in the secretion as they are at the beginning of lactation in the adult gland. Figure 18.18 illustrates the structure during this period.

The mammary glands during childhood are rudimentary. Lying beneath the nipple, they measure only about 10 mm in diameter. Each lobule consists of ducts with blind ends and no secretory epithelium. Just before puberty the female glands begin to enlarge, causing the areola of the breast to become

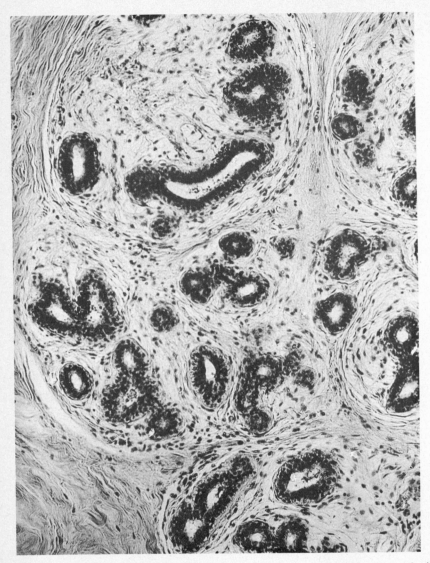

Figure 18-19 Mammary gland of a nonpregnant woman. In this resting stage, the branching tubules occupy islands of loose fibrous connective tissue. Photomicrograph, × 150.

elevated. Growth of the duct system, reappearance of acini, and accumulation of adipose tissue between glandular lobes gradually develop the breast during adolescence. Such growth occurs cyclically and is stimulated by newly functioning ovaries.

The resting adult mammary glands, before the first pregnancy, consist of many groups of branching tubules or cords of cells and immature acini connected with each lactiferous duct. These are embedded in islands of loose intralobular connective tissue, more cellular than that forming the main stroma (Fig. 18.19). The ducts and acini are lined with simple low columnar epithelium on a basal lamina and are clasped by myoepithelial cells, much like those of sweat glands.

With pregnancy, marked changes culminating in lactation take place. Terminal ducts and acini increase in number, and the latter grow in size. Groups of them crowd the intralobular connective tissue so that it becomes no longer visible. The coarser connective tissue forms capsules for the lobules of the glands. The skin over the breast becomes stretched.

Cells of the columnar epithelium of the acini display droplets of secretion in their cytoplasm during the eighth month of gestation. These droplets run together to form larger drops near the outer pole of the cells. They are extruded by bulging from the free surface and pinching off as they enter the lumen. Macrophages make their way into the lumen and phagocytize some of the droplets of secretion. The macrophages become much enlarged and are known as "colostrum corpuscles." Ducts and the lactiferous sinuses fill with milk, containing these corpuscles and other cells and cell fragments.

Active lactation begins after labor. It is stimulated by a hormone, prolactin, from the adenohypophysis. The first secretion is called **colostrum.** Fat content of the mammary-gland secretion soon increases, and true **milk** replaces colostrum. Secretion takes place at different times in different acini. Each undergoes periods of secretion alternating with periods of inactivity. During lactation, the glands are made up very largely of hypertrophied acini, and the connective tissue is reduced in amount. Figure 18.20 shows the lactating gland.

Ejection of milk from the lactating mammary glands is facilitated reflexly. For example, the infant's cries may be associated with increased pressure in the mother's lactiferous ducts, apparently through contraction of myoepithelial cells around milk-filled acini. This "milk-ejection reflex" appears to be stimulated by release of the hypophyseal hormone, oxytocin (Fig. 18.21).

Lactation continues so long as milk is drawn from the glands, but structural regression gradually occurs when nursing is stopped. The acini then cease to function and become reduced in size and number, some however remaining for considerable time, even until the next pregnancy. The intralobular connective tissue reappears, and the interlobar adipose tissue increases in amount.

Involution of the mammary glands occurs after the menopause. This, too, is a gradual process. The acini disappear, lobes diminish in size, and the ducts become atrophic.[7] In old age, there is a trend toward the prepubertal structure. The condition seen in Fig. 18.22 is one of advanced atrophy.

Areola and Nipple   The nipple and areola are covered by thin skin. The dermis of the nipple invaginates the epidermis with many vascular papillae. Hair and true sweat glands are absent, but peripherally arranged areolar glands[8]

---

[7]However, old women who receive estrogens rejuvenate these glands.
[8]Glands of Montgomery.

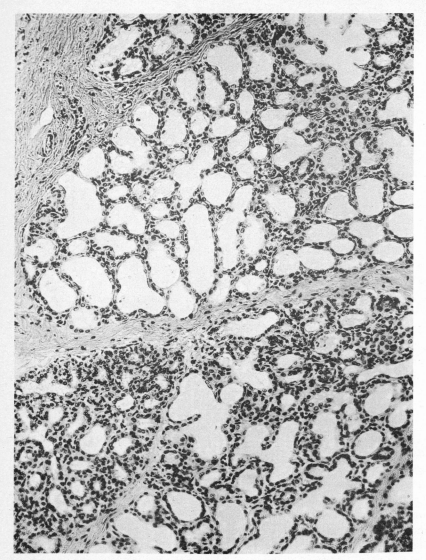

Figure 18-20   Lactating human mammary gland, showing portions of several lobules in different stages of secretory activity. Photomicrograph, × 150.

are noteworthy. They are modified mammary glands. The deep layers of the dermis contain smooth muscle arranged circularly and vertically. The areola is pigmented, especially in dark-complexioned women. Pigmentation increases with the advent of pregnancy and decreases afterward. Adipose tissue is absent from the dermis of the areola and the nipple. A rich supply of sensory nerve endings is present.

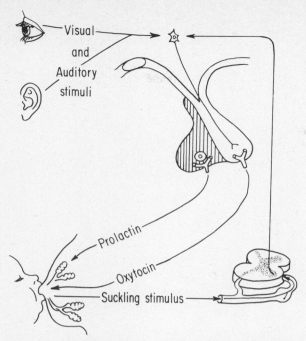

Visual
and
Auditory
stimuli

Prolactin

Oxytocin

Suckling stimulus

Figure 18-21 Neuroendocrine control of lactation and milk ejection. Neurovascular pathways involve hypothalamoadenohypophyseal regulation of prolactin release, and hypothalamoneurohypophyseal production of oxytocin. *(Modified from C. Ezrin, J. O. Godden, R. Volpé, and R. Wilson,* Systematic Endocrinology, *Harper & Row, Publishers, Incorporated, New York, 1973.) (CHP)*

VESSELS AND NERVES OF THE INTEGUMENT

The arteries entering the skin from the subcutaneous connective tissue first form an anastomosing network, the cutaneous plexus in the reticular body of the dermis. Small branches pass toward the surface from this plexus into the papillary body, where another anastomosing network is located. This is the papillary plexus; it gives rise to the capillary tufts of the papillae of the dermis as well as the little vessels that supply the sebaceous glands and upper portions of the hair follicles. The sweat glands and deeper parts of hair follicles are supplied by branches from the cutaneous plexus. Arteriovenous anastomoses are found in many locations, especially in the skin of the palms, finger tips, and nail bed and in the lips.

Venules collecting blood from capillaries of the papillae of the dermis form a papillary plexus. These flow into a network of larger venules between papillary and reticular bodies of the dermis. A third plexus is formed by the larger subcutaneous veins, and this receives tributaries from all parts of the skin.

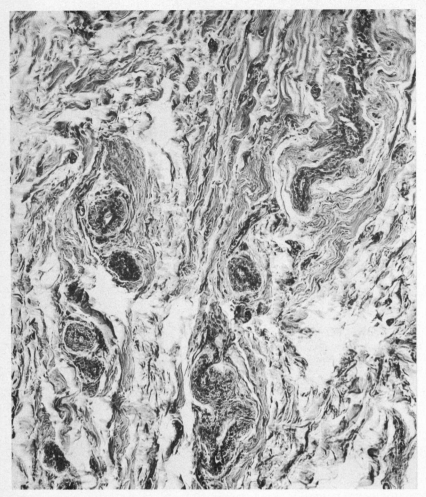

Figure 18-22 Atrophic mammary gland of a 66-year-old woman. The tubules are surrounded by dark (acidophilic) bands, the remnants of intralobular connective tissue. Interlobular connective tissue is dense and shows much artifactitious shrinkage. Photomicrograph, × 150.

Lymphatic capillaries are numerous in the papillary body. Collecting lymphatics are found more deeply, especially in the superficial fascia. They are not present in great numbers in deep fascia. Lymphatic vessels of the breast are noteworthy because they provide routes for metastasizing cancer cells to reach lymph nodes.

The integument is well supplied with nerves and sensory end organs. Not all the nerve fibers are sensory. Many motor nerve fibers enter the skin and supply the smooth muscle of blood vessels. Others end upon the smooth muscles of the hair follicles and myoepithelial cells in the secretory tubules of the sweat glands.

The sensory end organs of the integument have been described in Chap. 15. Although one of the main functions of the skin is reception of stimuli resulting from changes in the external environment, not all regions are equally receptive. Specialized bulbous and corpuscular end organs occur in thick skin, especially that of the finger tips, but are not found in the thin skin of the general body surface. There they are of a less specialized type.

SUGGESTED READING

Bell, M.: A Comparative Study of Sebaceous Gland Ultrastructure in Subhuman Primates. *Anatomical Record,* vol. 170, pp. 331–342, 1971.

Corvie, A. T., and J. S. Tindal: *The Physiology of Lactation.* Edward Arnold (Publishers) Ltd., London, 1971.

Cummings, H., and C. Midlo: *Finger Prints, Palms and Soles.* Dover Publications, Inc., New York, 1961.

Folley, S. J.: The Milk-Ejection Reflex: A Neuroendocrine Theme in Biology, Myth and Art. The Sir Henry Dale Lecture for 1969. *Journal of Endocrinology,* vol. 44, pp. x–xx, 1969.

Hellgren, L.: *Tatooing.* Almquist & Wiksell, Stockholm, 1967.

Montagna, W.: The Skin. *Scientific American,* vol. 212, no. 2, pp. 56–66, February, 1965.

——— and P. F. Parakkal: *The Structure and Function of Skin,* 3d ed. Academic Press, Inc., New York, 1974.

Ross, R.: Wound Healing. *Scientific American,* vol. 220, no. 6, pp. 40–50, June, 1969.

Spearman, R. I. C.: *The Integument: A Textbook of Skin Biology.* Cambridge University Press, London, 1973.

Vorherr, H.: *The Breast. Morphology, Physiology, and Lactation.* Academic Press, Inc., New York, pp. xii and 282, 1974.

Wooding, F. B. P.: Formation of Milk Fat Globule Membrane without Participation of the Plasmalemma. *Journal of Cell Science,* vol. 13, pp. 221–235, 1973.

Chapter 19

Mouth and Pharynx

The digestive system consists of the alimentary tract and associated structures. It is essentially a long tube, the lumen of which is an extension of the exterior. It differs structurally from the integument, with which its lining epithelium is continuous. It is primarily engaged in assimilating substances entering it from the exterior, rather than in guarding the body from adverse factors in the environment. However, its tonsilar tissue and gastric acid do serve in protection against bacterial invasion.

The process of digestion begins in the mouth. There food is mashed by the teeth and softened and lubricated by secretions from many glands opening into the mouth. After chewing has moistened dry food and reduced its coarseness, it is passed into the pharynx by the tongue. Swallowing is initiated in the oral pharynx, the vestibule of the esophagus. The mouth is more than a convenient starting point for a pleasant meal. Because of the roles it plays in speech and breathing and because the battle against invading microorganisms and toxins starts in the mouth, its lining membrane assumes considerable importance.

MUCOUS MEMBRANES

The entire digestive tract is lined by a **tunica mucosa**, or mucous membrane[1]
with regional variations in structure. The simplest form of mucous membrane is
an epithelium on a basal lamina and a layer of connective tissue. The epithelium
may be columnar or, as in the mouth, stratified squamous. The connective tissue may be largely reticular, as in the intestines, or rather dense collagenous,
such as that encountered in the gums. The connective-tissue layer is the **lamina
propria** of the mucous membrane. A lamina basalis separates it from the lamina
epithelialis.

The lamina propria contains the blood and lymphatic vessels and the
nerves. Smooth muscle is found in it in many regions. Lymphatic tissue is abundant, for the mucous membrane is the first barrier to antigens, and lymphocytes
assemble there.

The mucosa of the mouth and pharynx has stratified squamous epithelium,
adhering to muscle, dense fibrous connective tissue, or bone in most places. It
is loosely attached to deep structures in a few places by a **tela submucosa** of
connective tissue. Some small glands are found in the lamina propria, but larger
ones lie in the submucosa and empty onto the surface of the mucous membrane
by ducts. The largest glands, such as the parotid, are found some distance away
from the mucous membrane and send their ducts through both submucosa and
lamina propria to the epithelial surface.

ORAL CAVITY

The oral cavity may be divided into a **vestibule**, in front of the teeth and gums,
and the **mouth proper**, behind them. The tongue lies in the floor of the mouth
proper; the tonsils are located at the rear, where the mouth and oral pharynx
join; the palate forms the roof of the oral cavity (Fig. 19.1).

The oral mucosa resembles skin. It has a stratified squamous epithelium,
thicker than that of most skin and cornified in only a few places. The lamina
propria projects into the epithelium to form connective-tissue papillae, similar
to those of the dermis. These papillae contain loops of capillaries, as well as
nerve fibers.

Lips and Cheeks   The lips and cheeks are formed principally by skeletal
muscles and fibrous connective tissue covered on the outside with thin skin and
on the inside by the oral mucous membrane.

A sharp transition between skin and mucous membrane occurs at the red
part of the lip. The stratified squamous epithelium gradually becomes thicker.
The outer cells, in the process of cornification, are continually moistened. This
renders them translucent and permits the vascular lamina propria to be seen

---

[1]The term "mucous membrane" does not imply that mucus is always secreted by the
membrane or is even associated with it. The mucous membrane of the urinary bladder is an example of one that secretes no mucus.

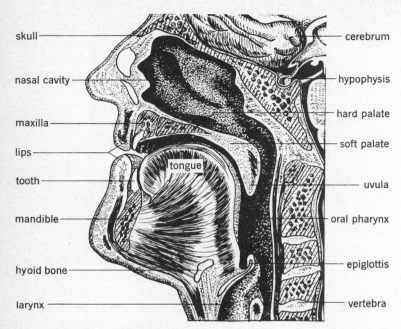

skull — cerebrum

nasal cavity — hypophysis

— hard palate

maxilla — soft palate

lips —

tongue

tooth — uvula

mandible — oral pharynx

— epiglottis

hyoid bone —

— vertebra

larynx —

Figure 19-1 Mouth and pharynx in relation to other parts of the head; midsagittal section; nasal septum removed. *(CHP)*

through them, imparting the red color to the lip. Hair and sweat glands stop abruptly at the outer margin, but a few sebaceous glands without hair follicles may be present there. Figure 19.2 shows the lip.

The inner surface of the lip is formed by a mucous membrane with noncornified epithelium like that lining the cheek. Its lamina propria forms especially prominent papillae. The mucous membrane of lips and cheeks blends with submucous connective tissue, dense strands of which attach the mucous membrane to underlying muscles and thus prevent it from getting in the way of the teeth during chewing.

Glands of the lips and cheeks are numerous. **Labial glands** form a ring about the oral opening at the inner border of the red part of the lip. They are principally tubuloacinous mucous glands, although a few groups of serous cells are present. Glands of the cheeks are called **buccal glands** in the submucosa and **molar glands** outside the muscle of the cheek near the parotid duct. Both are predominantly mucous.

Gums   The gums (gingivae) are illustrated in Fig. 19.9. They are formed by mucous membranes reflected onto the alveolar portions of the mandible and maxilla from the lips, cheeks, floor of the mouth, and palate. The basal cell layer of the gingival epithelium may be pigmented in dark-skinned individuals. The superficial squamous cells are often cornified, and a stratum granulosum

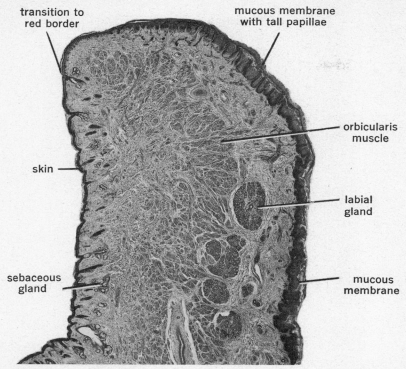

transition to red border

mucous membrane with tall papillae

orbicularis muscle

skin

labial gland

sebaceous gland

mucous membrane

Figure 19-2 Human lip, showing the transition from skin to mucous membrane. The red lip border has prominent connective-tissue papillae. Photomicrograph, × 15.

may be present. Cornification is related to abrasion by coarse food. The epithelium turns downward at the margin along the teeth, lining one side of a potential cleft, the other side of which is formed by tooth enamel in youth and cementum in the aged. The gingival lamina propria is dense and firmly anchored to subjacent periosteum. Its connective-tissue papillae are tall. No glands are present in the gums.

Palate The roof of the mouth is formed by the palate. The mucous membrane of the hard palate is continuous with that covering the gums of the upper jaw and is firmly attached to the subjacent periosteum. Irregular transverse ridges characterize the anterior part of the **hard palate;** its epithelium, with cornified surface cells, resembles that of the gums. Numerous **palatine glands,** composed of mucous acini with small ducts, are found beneath the mucous membrane.

The **soft palate** is formed by mucous membranes on two sides of a layer composed of skeletal muscle, fibrous connective tissue, and glands, as seen in Fig. 19.3. At the place where the mucous membrane folds over the free surface, a prolongation of the palate hangs down into the oral cavity. This is the **uvula.**

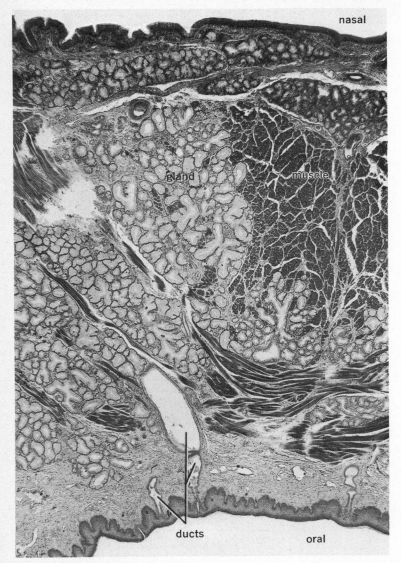

Figure 19-3 Soft palate, showing the oral surface below and the nasal surface above. Photomicrograph, × 40.

The oral side of the soft palate and uvula is covered with noncornified stratified squamous epithelium. The pharyngeal side resembles the oral side for a little way beyond the border but then becomes lined with ciliated pseudostratified epithelium containing goblet cells. The lamina propria of the palate is connected with the deeper layer of mucous glands by many elastic fibers. Lymphocytic infiltration is encountered in the lamina propria and epithelium of the soft palate.

Tongue The tongue (lingua) is not only a device for speech and a tool for moving food, but is the great tester of substances that enter the mouth, accepting or rejecting the materials to be submitted to the digestive organs. The tongue is an important sense organ, richly supplied with tactile endings as well as those for taste and chemical sense.

The tongue has extrinsic and intrinsic skeletal muscles. The extrinsic muscles attach the tongue to skeletal structures, whereas the intrinsic muscles form its bulk. A layer of dense fibrous connective tissue forms the **lingual septum**, dividing the tongue longitudinally into halves. The intrinsic muscle fibers are arranged in longitudinal, vertical, and transverse planes on either side of the septum. Fibers of the intrinsic muscles attach to the septum and to the lamina propria of the lingual mucous membrane. A transverse section through the tongue will show some muscle fibers cut across and others parallel to the cut surface. The interlacing of muscles is illustrated in Fig. 19.4. Fibrous connective tissue separates muscle bundles and conducts blood vessels, lymphatic

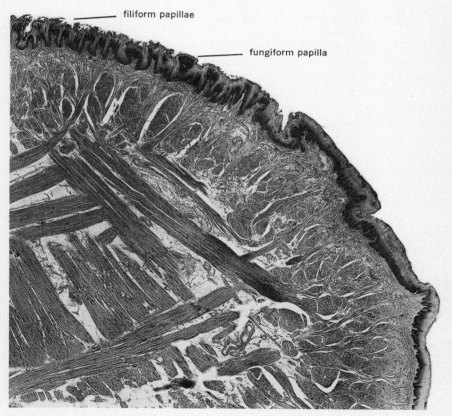

— filiform papillae

— fungiform papilla

Figure 19-4 Human tongue, showing the junction of the rough papillary dorsal surface with the smooth lateral surface. Note the interlacing muscle bundles running in three planes. Photomicrograph, × 7.

vessels, and nerves through the substance of the tongue. The connective tissue is loose at the root of the tongue, permitting it to move freely.

The mucous membrane of the tongue is closely adherent to the subjacent skeletal muscle. A submucosa is present only on part of its lower surface, where the mucosa is thin and loose. This is especially evident at the **frenulum** of the tongue, where the mucosa joins that of the floor of the mouth.

The mucous membrane of the undersurface is quite smooth. That of the borders and anterior two-thirds of the upper surface is roughened by many fine projections, the tiny **lingual papillae,** giving this "papillary area" a plushlike appearance. The posterior one-third of the dorsal surface of the tongue has an irregularly bumpy appearance and lacks the fine plush of the anterior two-thirds. It is characterized by lymphatic follicles in the lamina propria and is called the "lymphatic area." The boundary between these two portions of the mucosa is marked by a V-shaped sulcus in the infant. The sulcus disappears, and the row of vallate papillae lies near the boundary in the adult.

The papillary area of the lingual mucous membrane is beset by the lingual papillae, some of which are illustrated in Fig. 19.4. **Conical** and threadlike **filiform papillae,** many with brushes of secondary papillae on their tops, are most numerous. The papillae tend to occur in multiple rows, parallel to the V-shaped sulcus, and radiating outward and forward from the midline of the tongue. Some conical papillae may project as much as 3 mm from the surface. Epithelial cells on the papillae are flattened, although not cornified in man. The lamina propria extends into the base of each papilla a little way.

Fungiform papillae, less numerous than filiform and conical papillae, are small, mushroom-shaped projections scattered over the lingual surface. They are visible as little red spots, because the lamina propria with its capillaries comes close to the upper surface where the epithelium is thin. These papillae are lower and thicker than the conical papillae. Some of them have taste buds in the epithelium.

The **vallate papillae** are the largest of all the lingual papillae (Fig. 19.5). There are 7 to 11 of these arranged in a V-shaped line at the rear of the papillary area, each measuring 1 to 2 mm across the free surface. They do not rise above the level of the other lingual papillae, but each is surrounded by a moat, 1 to 1.5 mm deep. A ring-shaped wall of mucous membrane, nearly free of filiform projections, encircles each vallate papilla. Taste buds are always numerous in the epithelium lining the moat. Ducts of the serous gustatory lingual glands empty into the bottom of the moat, keeping it full of clear fluid which serves as a solvent for particles of food substances to be tasted.

Foliate papillae may be found at the side of the tongue, just in front of the anterior palantine arch. They are rudimentary in man but well developed in some animals. When present, they appear as parallel vertical folds of the mucosa.

Taste buds are small, ovoid bodies embedded in the stratified squamous epithelium of the tongue. Each occupies the entire thickness of epithelium from the lamina propria to a little opening, the pore canal, on its free surface. Taste

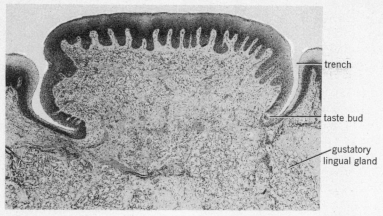

trench

taste bud

gustatory
lingual gland

Figure 19-5   Vallate papilla, human tongue. Photomicrograph, × 40.

buds are widely distributed but are most numerous in the walls of the moat surrounding each vallate papilla. They are not confined to the tongue, having been
found in the palate, the pharynx, and even the epiglottis. Their number is greatest at birth. Taste buds in a trench between foliate papillae of a rabbit are
shown in Fig. 19.6.

Each taste bud is formed by a number of tall columnar epithelial cells
bunched together something like segments of an orange. An occasional low
basal cell may be seen. The tall cells have long microvilli that project into the
pore of the taste bud. Their bases are clasped by the dendrites of special sensory nerve fibers. The integrity of the taste bud depends on the nerve fibers being
intact. Figure 19.7 illustrates the structure of a taste bud.

Taste buds are often classified among organs of special sense. The
neuroepithelial cells are chemoreceptors that are stimulated by substances dissolved in the saliva. In the vallate papillae, diffusion takes place into the serous
fluid of the moats surrounding them. The neuroepithelial cells function as transducers to initiate impulses in the dendrites of afferent nerve fibers clasping
them.

There are four qualities of taste, namely sweet, salt, bitter, and sour. All
are able to stimulate taste buds on the tip of the tongue. The dorsum is most
sensitive to sweet and salt; the borders, to sour; and the base to bitter.

The lymphatic area of the lingual mucous membrane is coarsely roughened
by subjacent lymphatic follicles, arranged around tubular depressions or crypts
of the surface epithelium. The lymphatic follicles and their epithelial crypts
form the **lingual tonsils.** These bodies resemble the palatine tonsils but are
simpler. The epithelium is heavily invaded by lymphocytes from the underlying
lymphatic tissue of the lamina propria.

There are three groups of glands embedded in the connective tissue among
muscle bundles. All are small tubuloacinous glands with numerous small ducts.
Their secretion is added to that of the major salivary glands of the mouth. The

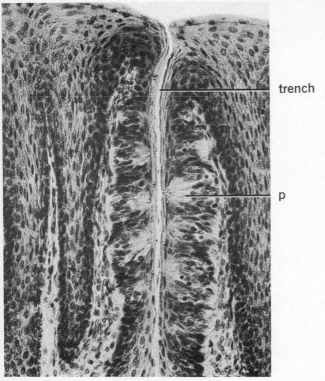

Figure 19-6   Taste buds lining a trench between foliate papillae (rabbit); one shows a pore canal, *p*. Photomicrograph, × 300.

anterior lingual glands occur in groups, measuring about 8 by 16 mm in diameter, on either side of the frenulum beneath the tip of the tongue. Their mixed mucous and serous acini lie deep among muscle bundles and open by about five ducts on either side of the oral cavity. The **posterior lingual glands** are found just in front of the most medial vallate papilla, along the margins of the tongue near its root, and under the mucosa of the lymphatic area. They are mucous glands with numerous ducts, and some of them empty into the crypts of the lingual tonsils. The **gustatory lingual glands** are purely serous glands lying deep among muscle bundles in the vicinity of the vallate papillae. Their ducts open into the moats surrounding the papillae.

TEETH

Teeth (dentes) are unusual products of living cells, being constructed in part by a flintlike material, the hardest substance in the body. Teeth are actually elaborate papillae of the lamina propria, as will be readily appreciated in considering their development.

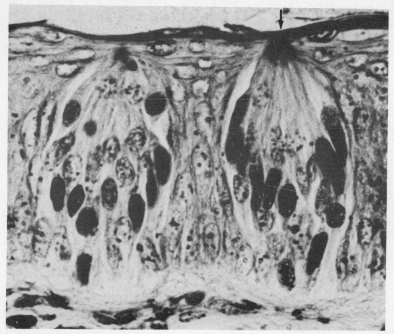

Figure 19-7   Taste buds in the stratified epithelium of a circumvallate papilla (rat), stained with iron hematoxylin. The pore in the right bud is indicated by an *arrow*. Photomicrograph, × 900. *(Contributed by L. Guth.)*

The crown, or projecting portion, of each tooth is capped with **enamel,** the product of ectodermal cells. The main body of the tooth, including its roots extending below the level of the gums, is of mesodermal origin and is composed of ivorylike **dentine.** Encasing the dentine below the neck of the tooth at the gingival border is a thin layer of bonelike cementum. Figure 19.8 illustrates the main parts of a tooth.

Outside the root, anchoring the tooth in its socket in the alveolar processes of the jaws, is a layer of dense fibrous connective tissue, forming the **peridontal membrane.** The center of the dentine has a hollow pulp cavity in the dry tooth, but in life this is filled with a loose type of connective tissue, the **pulp.** At the tip of each root, the pulp merges with the connective tissue of the peridontal membrane through a minute apical foramen. Blood vessels and nerves make the peridontal membrane and pulp vital parts of a tooth.

Pulp   The loose connective tissue of the pulp contains delicate reticular and collagenous fibers in a mucoid ground substance which exhibits a slightly basophilic staining reaction. It also contains many stellate cells, resembling those of mesenchyme, as well as a few macrophages and occasionally other cells encountered in areolar tissue.

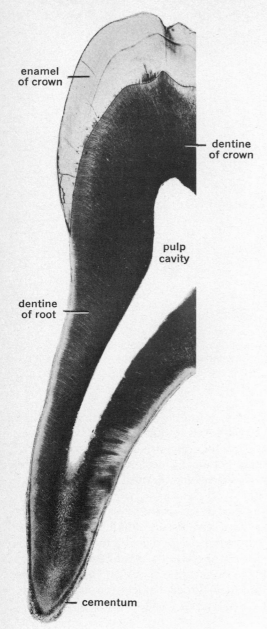

enamel
of crown

dentine
of crown

pulp
cavity

dentine
of root

cementum

Figure 19-8 Human molar tooth; part of
a ground and polished dry section. Photomicrograph, ×8.

Around the periphery, at the junction of pulp with dentine, there is a single
layer of specialized pulp cells resembling simple columnar epithelium. These
peripheral cells are called **odontoblasts.** Each odontoblast extends short basal
processes into the pulp and one or two long apical processes into the dentine.

The long processes, called dentinal fibers,[2] occupy minute canals in the dentine. The odontoblasts take part in formation of dentine, just as osteoblasts take part in formation of bone. However, the odontoblasts avoid becoming trapped during deposition of the dentine by orderly retreat into the pulp, leaving only their extended dentinal fibers. Dentine formation by odontoblasts does not cease with full development of a tooth but slows considerably. Irritation of dentine in later life may lead to renewal of activity with construction of secondary dentine. The amount of pulp in a tooth decreases with age as additional dentine is produced. Cellularity of the pulp likewise decreases and the proportion of collagenous fibers increases in the course of time.

Usually one arteriole and one or two venules enter the foramen of each root canal. An extensive capillary network is formed in the pulp, especially next to the layer of odontoblasts. Lymphatic vessels occur in the pulp.

Small nerves accompany the arterioles into the root canals. Unmyelinated nerve fibers are distributed to smooth muscle in the wall of the arterioles. Small myelinated nerve fibers with free endings among the odontoblasts provide the sensory innervation of the pulp. It is thought that odontoblasts act as neuroepithelial receptors, functioning as transducers to initiate painful afferent impulses in the dendrites around them.

Dentine The major part of the tooth consists of dentine, a substance containing about 70 percent inorganic material. Dentine is somewhat harder than most bone and has no cells embedded in it—only the long processes of odontoblasts. Like bone, the calcified dentine matrix contains collagenous fibrils, but these are invisible in ordinary histologic preparations. Collagenous fibrils tend to course parallel to one another and appear as closely packed wavy lines in ground sections of the dentine. Some canaliculi branch along their course through the dentine, and most of them divide into several terminal branches at their outer ends (Fig. 19.10). The number of canaliculi per unit area is about four times as great on the pulpal surface as it is near the enamel surface of the dentine. It is estimated that there are 30,000 to 75,000 canaliculi per square millimeter of pulpal surface.

When dentine is laid sown, the process begins at the cusp of a tooth, one conical increment being added within another at an average rate of approximately 6 μm per day. Rhythmical growth differences account for **incremental lines,** often faintly seen coursing at right angles to the dentinal canaliculi (Fig. 19.9).

Variations in degree of calcification of dentine are encountered in small local regions, especially in the crown. An outer layer of dentine lacking parallel canaliculi but with many tiny spaces and fine canaliculi running in all directions is often seen in the root of the tooth next to the cementum. This is called the granular layer because of its appearance in ground sections.

---

[2]These are called "Tomes' fibers" by dental histologists. Names of many other early writers, commonly used in describing elements in the teeth, have been omitted in this brief descriptive account.

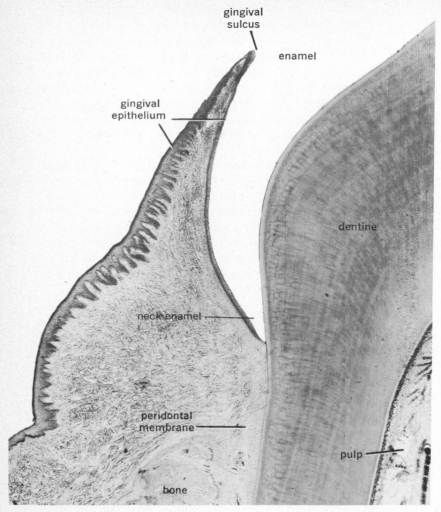

Figure 19-9 Junction of gum and tooth of a child. The enamel was dissolved in preparing the tissue, leaving a clear space. The dentine exhibits incremental lines faintly. Photomicrograph, × 40.

The vital components of the dentine are **dentinal fibers,** which, in life, fill the dentinal canaliculi. Inorganic substances are actively exchanged between the blood and the dentine. Some exchange takes place between the dentine and the enamel. Diffusion probably occurs via the canaliculi.

Aging is accompanied by formation of dentine of irregular structure, bordering the pulp. This leads to reduction of size of the pulp space and root canals. When the enamel wears down and the dentine is exposed, the odontoblast processes die or recede, and the dentinal canaliculi are filled with cal-

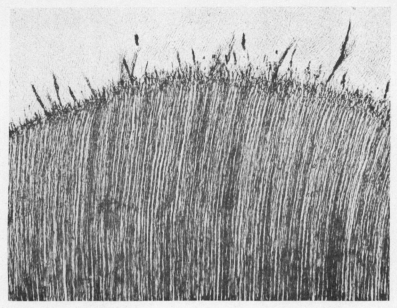

Figure 19-10 Dentine-enamel junction of a human tooth; a ground and polished dry section. Note the parallel dentinal tubules extending upward toward the enamel, the light upper part, and their branching. Photomicrograph, × 150.

cified matrix, forming a more homogeneous and less sensitive dentine. Young dentine, in which the dentinal fibers extend well out toward the enamel, is very sensitive to pain. Old dentine, from which dentinal fibers have receded, is less sensitive.

Enamel The enamel contains 96 percent inorganic solids, mainly calcium and phosphorus in a crystalline arrangement, and less than 2 percent organic substances, the balance being water. Consequently, practically nothing is left of it when it is decalcified with acid. Enamel forms the highly resistant covering or crown of the tooth. It attains a thickness of about 2 mm on the cusps of molar teeth, becomes thinner over the sides, and ends at the neck of the tooth. In young individuals, the enamel at the neck of the tooth is covered by the gums, as shown in Fig. 19.9. As the gingival border recedes with aging, the enamel of the neck and part of the cementum or dentine below the neck are exposed.

Enamel is a cuticle formed on the surface of epithelial cells of the enamel organ during development of the tooth. Each cell produces a thin columnar **enamel prism.** Adjacent prisms are held together by a minute quantity of organic cement substance. Horizontal striations on the prisms indicate a rhythmical formation of this material. In cross section, the prisms of enamel look somewhat like minute fish scales with irregular outlines. Few are perfectly hexagonal (Fig. 19.11).

The enamel prisms do not run straight through the enamel but pursue irreg-

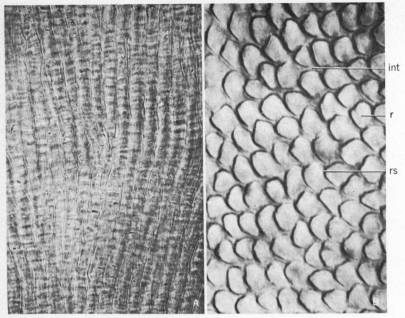

Figure 19-11 Enamel of tooth: *A,* ground longitudinal section showing cross striations of enamel prisms; *B,* decalcified cross section of enamel prisms; *int,* interrod substance; *r,* rod; *rs,* rod sheath. Photomicrographs. *(Contributed by B. Orban.)*

ular courses. Most of them begin as parallel columns perpendicular to the surface of the dentine, then curve in complex spirals through the middle of the enamel, and finally run perpendicular to the surface of the tooth. There is a certain amount of intertwining of prisms, especially on the cusps and edges of the teeth, forming gnarled enamel.

Concentric **incremental lines** in the enamel are often more pronounced than those seen in ground sections of dentine. At the places where the lines reach the surface of the tooth, slight depressions can be observed.

The surface of a newly erupted tooth is covered with a layer, about 1 μm thick, of slightly different composition from the rest of the enamel. A somewhat thicker outer layer of keratinlike substance represents a last contribution to the crown by the enamel organ. Both are worn away on the incisal edges of the teeth, but they persist for many years in places protected from abrasion.

Cementum The roots of the teeth are covered by a thin layer of cementum which helps anchor them in their sockets and protects the dentine of the roots of the teeth. Of all the tooth components, it most clearly resembles compact bone. Cementum consists of a calcified ground substance into which collagenous fibers penetrate from the surrounding peridontal membrane. Like compact bone, cementum contains about 45 percent inorganic material.

Cementum is thickest around the apex of the root to which it often adds appreciable length in old teeth. Except in the vicinity of the apex, the cementum encasing the root is usually noncellular. Layers of a cellular variety of this tissue tend to be superimposed on the noncellular cementum at the apex. Lacunae with canaliculi are present there (Fig. 19.12). In the living tooth, the lacunae contain **cementocytes** with processes radiating out into the canaliculi. At the junction of cementum and dentine of the root, canaliculi of the cementum may communicate with the dentinal tubules. Haversian systems are usually absent, and nourishment is provided by blood vessels in the surrounding peridontal membrane.

Peridontal Membrane The peridontal membrane is simply the dense fibrous connective tissue around the root of a tooth. It is the periosteum of the alveolar processes of the tooth socket and the **pericementum** of the tooth root. Some of its fibers are continuous with those of the gingival lamina propria. The peridontal membrane lacks elastic fibers, and its collagenous fibers are arranged in coarse compact bundles, many of which penetrate the matrix of the cementum.

Indifferent cells in the peridontal membrane give rise to osteoblasts of the

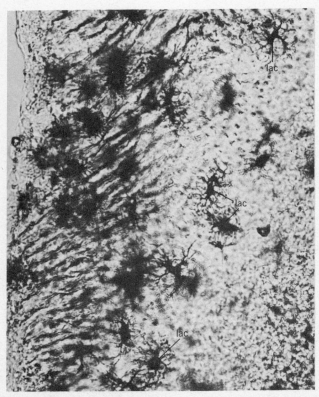

Figure 19-12 Cementum with lacunae, *lac,* of stellate cementocytes; a ground and polished dry section. The dentine is toward the left; the peridontal membrane is toward the right. Photomicrograph, × 300.

alveolar bone and **cementoblasts** on the roots of the teeth. There is no significant cytologic difference between the two cells. Osteoclasts are present during resorption of deciduous teeth. Where they occur in relation to cementum and dentine, they receive the name **odontoclasts.**

A vitalizing plexus of small blood and lymphatic vessels courses through the peridontal membrane. Small nerves distribute myelinated fibers, some arising from proprioceptive pressure end organs which serve reflexly to regulate the strength of the bite. Others come from tactile receptors. Unmyelinated fibers are vasomotor.

Groups of epithelioid cells are sometimes encountered in the peridontal membrane. These seem to be remnants of the epithelial root sheath of the developing tooth. Occasionally they give rise to cysts and tumors.

Development of Teeth   Teeth form beneath the epithelium of the gums in prenatal life, but none pierces the epithelium to erupt into the mouth cavity until about 6 months after birth. Initiation of primordia of teeth is a progressive phenomenon starting in the second fetal month and continuing until about the fifth postnatal year. Eruption and the accompanying growth extend over a longer period of time, being incomplete even at puberty (Fig. 19.13). Two sets of teeth are formed. The child is provided with deciduous, or "milk," teeth which erupt during the first 2 years. These are replaced by permanent teeth, beginning about the sixth year. Development is similar in both dentitions.

The first indications of tooth formation in human embryos is a thickening of oral ectoderm in each jaw to form a curved dental lamina, just inside the primordium of the lip furrow. Buds of epithelial cells from this lamina invaginate the subjacent mesenchyme. Unequal growth in the bud results in first a cap-shaped and then a bell-shaped epithelial structure enclosing a **dental papilla** of mesenchyme; this represents the primordium of the tooth pulp and later gives rise to the dentine. The wall of the bell is a double epithelial layer constituting the **enamel organ.** The handle of the bell attaches the enamel organ to the dental lamina in early stages, but breaks occur in it later, and the enamel organ is left unattached to the lamina. Ten enamel organs are formed in each jaw for development of the deciduous teeth.

While the enamel organs for deciduous teeth are developing, a second series of buds arises from the dental lamina, one just behind each of the first series. These are the primordia of the permanent dentition (Fig. 19.14). Extension of the dental lamina to the more distal parts of the developing jaws provides other buds from which enamel organs of the permanent molar teeth develop later.

Each enamel organ consists of an inner and an outer layer of epithelial cells. Those of the inner layer form a tall simple columnar epithelium and are called **ameloblasts.** These cells produce the enamel prisms. The outer layer of cells is a low simple columnar epithelium. Between the two epithelia of the enamel organ other epithelial cells derived from the bud are transformed into stellate cells, resembling those of reticular connective tissue. They constitute

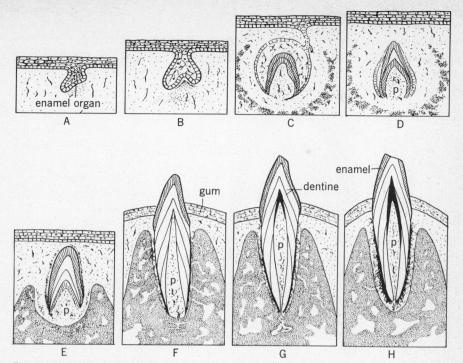

Figure 19-13 Diagram illustrating the development of a tooth. *A, B,* and *C* show its early development from bud to bell stages; at *D* and *E* dentine and enamel are forming; *p* indicates pulp; the progress of eruption is illustrated in *E* and *F*; attrition of enamel with secondary dentine formation (black) is seen in *G* and *H*. Bone is stippled heavily; cementum is black. *(Redrawn from B. Orban.) (WEL)*

the **enamel pulp,** which is avascular and is nourished by capillaries of the mesenchyme outside the outer epithelium of the enamel organ (Fig. 19.15).

While ameloblasts are developing in the enamel organ, the outer cells of the pulp mesenchyme in the dental papilla form a columnar epitheliumlike layer of odontoblasts. Dentine formation starts from this layer at the cusp of the tooth and proceeds in ever-widening conical layers toward the root. Ameloblasts do not begin forming enamel so long as they lie close to a source of nourishment from the capillaries of the odontoblast layer of the dental papilla. When the first dentine cuts them off from their blood supply, they begin to lay down the first enamel. Thus, enamel deposition follows that of dentine, being laid down on the latter. Enamel production extends only to the neck of the tooth.

The double layer of enamel epithelium continues down over the dental papilla after enamel has reached the neck and becomes the **epithelial root sheath.** As a rule, no enamel is formed by the inner cells of this sheath, which are of low columnar type, but induction of development of odontoblasts from mesenchymal cells of the dental papilla beneath the root sheath continues, and this results in formation of the dentine of the root.

The mesenchyme external to the outer epithelium of the enamel organ and epithelial root sheath gives rise to the peridontal membrane. Continuity with

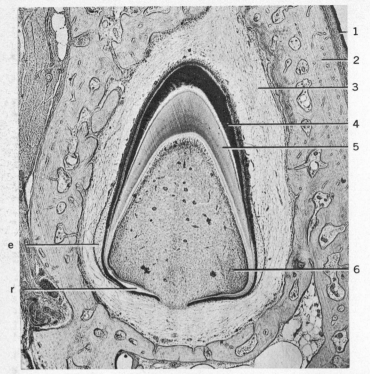

Figure 19-14   Developing tooth: an unerupted tooth in its alveolar space showing the following: *1*, gum; *2*, bone; *3*, connective tissue; *4*, enamel; *5*, dentine; *6*, pulp; *e*, remnant of enamel organ; *r*, epithelial root sheath. Photomicrograph, approximately × 20.

the tooth pulp is effected at the apex of the root, where the epithelial root sheath is deficient at the lip of the bell-shaped enamel organ. This can be seen in Fig. 19.14.

As the jaws grow, the deciduous teeth enlarge and shift forward and outward to maintain a superficial position in respect to the bones. Maturation of the crown and growth of the root develop pressures that effect the changes in bony structure necessary for eruption. Growth of the enamel organ of the permanent tooth behind and beneath the deciduous tooth contributes to the process. Even before the deciduous tooth has erupted to its full extent, the enlarging permanent tooth and its enamel organ crowd it, and erosion of the deciduous root begins. Osteoclasts and odontoclasts develop in the peridontal membrane and are often numerous along the sites of active erosion. Gradually the outward shift of the tooth and the erosion of its roots loosen it and cause it to be shed before the permanent crown is visible above the surface of the gums.

Eruption of the permanent teeth is likewise a slow, continuing process. Even after all teeth have appeared, in fact, in later life, a gradual outward movement brings the neck of the tooth closer and closer to the gingival border and in old age may carry it well beyond that line, so that some of the cementum or dentine of the root itself becomes visible.

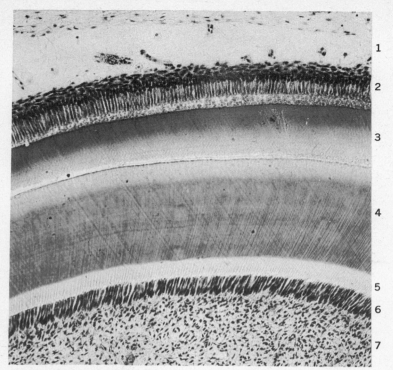

Figure 19-15 Developing tooth: a small portion of an unerupted tooth showing the following layers from above downward: *1,* enamel pulp; *2,* ameloblasts; *3,* enamel; *4,* calcified dentine; *5,* noncalcified dentine; *6,* odontoblasts; *7,* pulp. Photomicrograph × 150.

GLANDS

Numerous small glands, lacking extensive duct systems, take part in production of saliva. They are branched tubular and tubuloacinous glands with mucous, serous, or mixed secreting portions. The small salivary glands have been described. Three large glands are the **parotid, submandibular,** and **sublingual.** Each consists of secreting acini, tubules, and duct systems, which constitute the parenchyma of the organ, and a supporting framework of fibrous connective tissue, the stroma. A definite fibrous-connective-tissue capsule is present in the parotid and submandibular glands but is lacking in the sublingual gland. Septa of connective tissue subdivide the parenchyma into lobes and lobules. Blood vessels, nerves, and the major subdivisions of the ducts traverse these septa.

Each gland contains a branching system of ducts carrying the secretion to the mouth. These are called **excretory ducts.** The main excretory duct, in each instance, is lined with stratified squamous epithelium at the point of its opening into the mouth. Elsewhere it is formed by a two-layer stratified columnar epithelium or a pseudostratified epithelium. Figure 19.16 shows the parotid duct. As it branches into smaller subdivisions, the duct becomes lined with simple columnar epithelium. The excretory ducts have dense fibrous-connec-

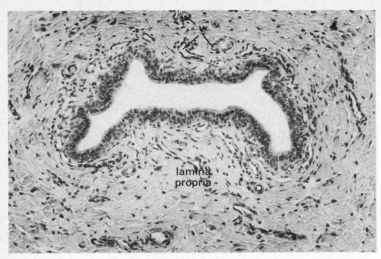

Figure 19-16 Human parotid duct. The mucous membrane is formed by a multilayered epithelium which is stratified columnar in some places and pseudostratified in others; near the oral end it becomes stratified squamous. The lamina propria consists of dense fibrous connective tissue, containing small blood vessels, *v.* Photomicrograph, × 150.

tive-tissue walls, and the largest, notably the main duct of the submandibular gland, may contain a few smooth-muscle cells. The smaller subdivisions of the excretory ducts enter the lobules of the glands and are divided further into **secretory ducts.**

The secretory ducts are formed of simple columnar epithelium. The cells appear striated, indicative of some secretory activity. In the parotid and submandibular glands, the secretory ducts branch into much smaller **intercalated ducts,** made up of flattened or low columnar epithelial cells. These, in turn, open into the secreting tubules or acini. Figure 19.17*A* and *B* show secretory and intercalated ducts.

The secreting acini of the salivary glands are composed of pyramidal cells of a simple columnar epithelium on a basal lamina. Between the pyramidal cells and the basal lamina are a few stellate cells resembling the myoepithelial cells of the sweat glands. The secreting cells are of two types, serous and mucous, described in Chap. 3.

Parotid Gland The only purely serous glands in the mouth are the gustatory lingual (Fig. 19.5) and parotid glands (Fig. 19.18). The parotid gland, located in front of the ear in relation to the ramus of the mandible, is the largest of the salivary glands. It possesses a single large duct opening into the vestibule of the mouth opposite the upper second molar tooth.

The secreting tubules and acini of the parotid gland are elongated and branched. They empty into the narrow intercalated ducts; these are numerous and relatively long in the parotid gland. The intercalated ducts enter secretory ducts lined with simple columnar epithelium.

The fibrous-connective-tissue septa of the parotid gland contains lipo-

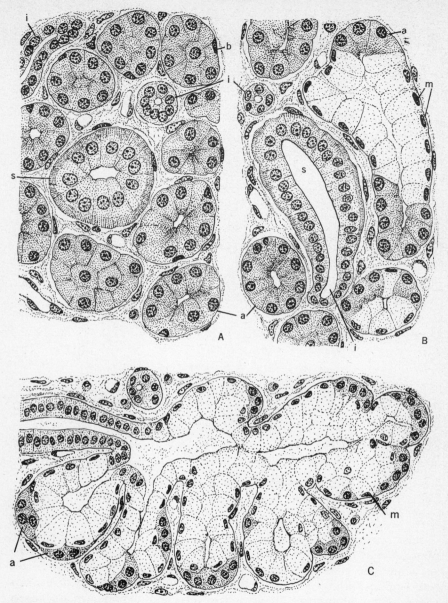

Figure 19-17 Human salivary glands: *A*, parotid; *B*, submandibular; *C*, sublingual; *a*, serous acini and serous cells; *b*, myoepithelial cell; *m*, mucous cell nuclei; *i*, intercalated duct; *s*, secretory duct. × 600. *(JFN)*

cytes, imparting a characteristic vacuolated appearance to histologic sections of this organ. The amount of fat increases with age.

Submandibular Gland The name "submaxillary" was formerly used for this large mixed gland. Its acini are largely serous in human beings, although

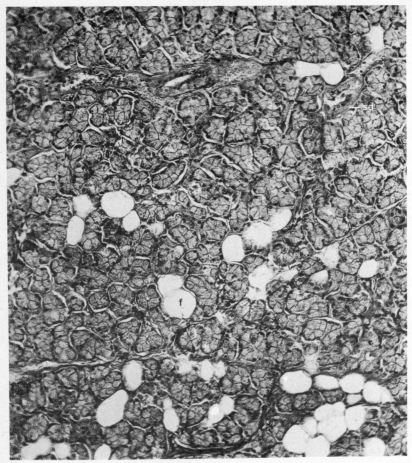

Figure 19-18 Human parotid gland. Note the lipocytes, *f*, and secretory duct, *sd*, among serous acini. Photomicrograph, × 150.

the submandibular glands of some other species of animals contain many mucous acini. The gland is located behind the mandible in the floor of the mouth. It empties through a single main duct into the mouth cavity at the side of the frenulum of the tongue. The excretory duct and its branches are similar to those of the parotid gland.

The secretory ducts of the submandibular gland are more numerous and are longer than those of the parotid gland. On the other hand, the intercalated ducts are short and difficult to observe. Mucus-secreting tubules and acini, when present, are distinct from the predominating serous variety. Some of them are capped with serous cells, which appear in sections as semilunar groups, the demilunes. These groups of serous cells open into the same lumen with the mucous cells. Figure 19.19 illustrates the structure of the human submandibular gland.

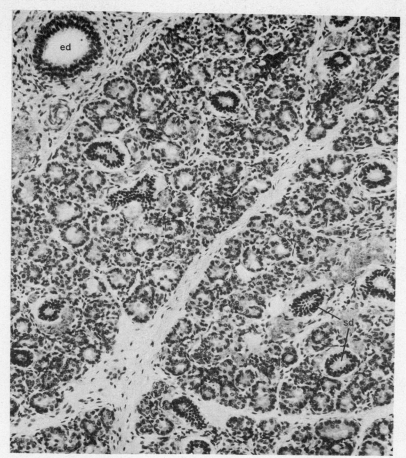

Figure 19-19 Human submandibular gland, predominantly serous. Note one large duct in the stroma at the upper left, *ed*, and many small intralobular ducts, *sd*. Photomicrograph, × 150.

Sublingual Gland   The sublingual gland is a mixed gland in the forward part of the mouth just beneath the mucous membrane. Its structure varies from lobe to lobe. As a matter of fact, it is made up of a group of glands with several separate ducts emptying into the anterior part of the mouth beneath the tongue.

Mucous tubules and acini predominate, and most serous cells occur in demilunes upon the mucous acini and the sublingual gland. Few, if any, intercalated ducts will be found, the secretory ducts becoming directly continuous with the tubules and acini. The duct system is less prominent in the sublingual gland than in the other major salivary glands. Figure 19.20 shows the structure of the human sublingual gland.

Saliva   The mixed secretion of all the glands of the oral cavity is saliva, a fluid containing some cellular debris and lymphocytes. Secretion by the major

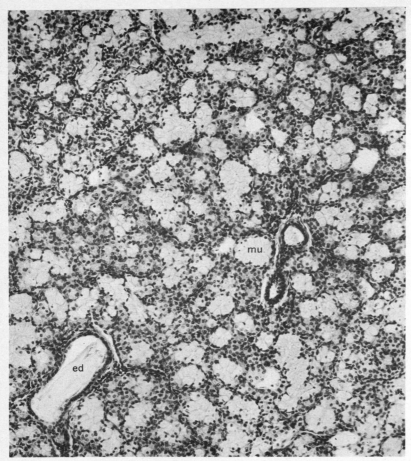

Figure 19-20 Human sublingual gland. Note the predominance of mucous acini, *mu;* ducts, *ed,* are few and contain mucus. Photomicrograph, × 150.

salivary glands is controlled reflexly. The amount produced by the human salivary glands has been estimated as about 1.5 liters per day. Saliva contains enzymes that probably have little to do with digestion of food in the mouth because of the short time it remains there. However, salivary amylase in the interior of a bolus of carbohydrate may continue to be active in the stomach so long as it is protected from the action of gastric acid. The main functions of saliva are to keep the mouth wet and to moisten and lubricate the food so that it can be swallowed.

PHARYNX

The mouth opens into the oral pharynx at the palatine arches, which are folds of mucous membrane formed at the sides of the free posterior borders of the soft palate (Fig. 19.1). The oral pharynx joins the nasal pharynx above and the laryngeal pharynx below. It plays an important part in the act of swallowing.

The pharynx is the throat. It is a musculofibrous sac, lined by a mucous membrane similar to that of the mouth. Its wall has an outer layer formed by the pharyngeal constrictors and associated muscles, all of which are the skeletal variety. Dense fibrous connective tissue containing many elastic fibers forms a submucous layer between muscularis and mucosa.

The mucous membrane consists of epithelium and lamina propria. The epithelium is stratified squamous, continuous above in the nasal pharynx with the pseudostratified variety. The lamina propria is formed of reticular and loose fibrous connective tissue. An abundance of lymphatic tissue characterizes the mucous membrane of the pharynx. This lymphatic tissue is diffuse in some places and compact in others, with many lymphatic follicles occuring in aggregates.

The aggregates of lymphatic follicles form tonsils, the principal ones being the palatine tonsils. Pharyngeal, tubal, and lingual tonsils are found in the posterior wall of the pharynx, around the opening of the auditory tubes, and at the root of the tongue. All these are lymphatic organs and, as such, play an important role in the immune system.

SUGGESTED READING

Almeida, O. P., and L. Bozzo: Morphology of the Nerve Fibers in Both Normal and Inflamed Human Dental Pulp. *Acta Anatomica,* vol. 84, pp. 597–607, 1973.

Bernick, S.: Innervation of the Human Tooth. *Anatomical Record,* vol. 101, pp. 81–107, 1948.

Kagayama, M.: The Fine Structure of the Monkey Submandibular Gland with a Special Reference to Intra-acinar Nerve Endings. *American Journal of Anatomy,* vol. 131, pp. 185–196, 1971.

Mattern, C. F. T., and N. Paran: Evidence of a Contractile Mechanism in the Taste Bud of the Mouse Fungiform Papilla. *Experimental Neurology,* vol. 44, pp. 461–469, 1974.

Palay, S. L.: Morphology of Secretion, pp. 305–342, in S. L. Palay (ed.), *Frontiers in Cytology.* Yale University Press, New Haven, 1958.

Permar, D.: *Oral Embryology and Microscopic Anatomy. A Textbook for Students of Dental Hygiene,* 5th ed. Lea & Febiger, Philadelphia, 1972.

Sicher, H., and S. N. Bhaskar: *Orban's Oral Histology and Embryology.* The C. V. Mosby Company, St. Louis, 1972.

Tandler, B., and R. A. Erlandson: Ultrastructure of the Human Submaxillary Gland. IV. Serous Granules. *American Journal of Anatomy,* vol. 135, pp. 419–434, 1972.

Weinstock, A., and C. P. Leblond: Elaboration of the Matrix Glycoprotein of Enamel by the Secretory Ameloblasts of the Rat Incisor as Revealed by Radioautography after Galactose-^{3}H Injection. *Journal of Cell Biology,* vol. 51, pp. 26–51, 1971.

Chapter 20

Alimentary Tract

The alimentary tract, or canal, is a tubular and sacular structure, 9 or 10 m long, extending from the mouth to the anus. Its upper parts, the mouth and pharynx, are considered in the preceding chapter. The remaining components are the esophagus, stomach, small and large intestines, and anal canal. Table 20.1 compares the principal tubular digestive organs. A variety of substances from the external environment, many of nutritional value, pass into these organs.

The function of the alimentary tract is threefold. It involves digestion, i.e., the mechanical and chemical disintegration of food and its solution in digestive secretions; absorption of dissolved and altered usable material; and excretion of the unusable residue. Many water-soluble or emulsifiable substances, other than food, are also readily absorbed. Advantage is taken of this fact by the physician who prescribes drugs to be administered by mouth.

STRUCTURAL PLAN

The digestive tube consists of various arrangements of three principal layers, called tunics: the mucosa, muscularis, and adventitia or serosa. The accompanying low-power photomicrograph of a section through the esophagus (Fig. 20.1) illustrates this general structural plan.

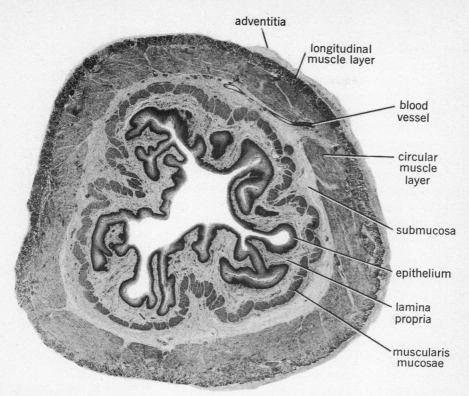

Figure 20-1 Human esophagus, illustrating the general plan of the tubular digestive organs. The section is from the upper one-third of the esophagus; the outer layer of muscle is mainly skeletal. Photomicrograph, × 12.

The **tunica mucosa** is the mucous membrane. Its three components are the epithelium, lamina propria mucosae, and lamina muscularis mucosae. Below the esophagus, the epithelium is beset with innumerable pits and glands. In some places, where absorption takes place, the epithelium and lamina propria are thrown into folds and fingerlike villi that protrude into the lumen. Variations in the structure and arrangement of the epithelium characterize different portions of the digestive tube. A basal lamina underlies the epithelium.

The lamina propria fills the space between pits and glands. It consists of areolar and reticular tissue, filled with lymphocytes, which transform it into diffuse lymphatic tissue in many places. Single and aggregate lymphatic follicles, as well as many small glands, occur in it, and lymphatic vessels, blood vessels, and nerves course through this layer.

The muscularis mucosae is a thin layer or two of smooth muscle, marking the outer boundary of the mucosa.

The tela submucosa is the fibrous connective tissue beneath the mucous membrane. Through it course larger vessels as well as plexuses of autonomic nerve fibers containing groups of nerve cells.

The **tunica muscularis** consists of two principal layers. Throughout most of the digestive tract, these are composed of smooth muscle. The inner layer is called circular, but is arranged in a helical manner. The outer is longitudinal, thickest in the esophagus and thinnest in the colon where it is reduced to three longitudinal bands. The circular muscle is thickened in several places to form sphincters. A small amount of fibrous connective tissue, containing blood vessels and nerves, permeates the layers of smooth muscle. A ganglionated autonomic nerve plexus is found between the circular and the longitudinal layers.

The **tunica adventitia** is the outermost coat of the digestive tube. It is formed of fibrous connective tissue blending with that of the surrounding structures in the esophagus and rectum. The portions of the alimentary tract lying in the abdominal cavity have a layer of mesothelium over the surface of the adventitia. This transforms the tunica adventitia into a **tunica serosa**, which is the visceral peritoneum. A tela subserosa is present beneath it.

ESOPHAGUS

The esophagus is insignificant in digestive processes, for it is nothing more than a short tube connecting the pharynx with the stomach and conveying the food bolus and fluids to the latter organ. Its lining is lubricated mainly by secretions of glands in the mouth and pharynx. The esophagus has great elasticity and can be dilated considerably during the act of swallowing, in which it functions involuntarily. When no food is passing, its lumen is collapsed, and its mucous membrane is thrown into irregular longitudinal folds.

Liquids trickle down the esophagus very quickly. Solid food takes 5 or 6 seconds to be passed by peristaltic action of the tunica muscularis. Gravity plays a part. Food passes more slowly when swallowed while the swallower is reclining than while sitting or standing.

Mucosa and Glands The mucous membrane of the esophagus is lined with stratified squamous epithelium of the noncornified variety in human beings and most other mammals. It becomes cornified in those animals that swallow rough vegetable matter. The thick layer of epithelium is deeply indented by papillae of the subjacent lamina propria (Fig. 20.2). The stratified squamous epithelium ends abruptly, and simple columnar epithelium begins at the line of junction of the esophagus with the cardiac end of the stomach (Fig. 20.3).

Few glands are found along most of the esophagus, but a number of them are present near the lower end. Superficial and deep **esophageal glands** secrete mucus which is emptied onto the surface epithelium by means of short ducts. The main ducts are rather wide and are lined with stratified squamous epithelium. Their small branches are formed by simple columnar epithelium. The deep esophageal glands are of the tubuloacinous type and are found in the submucosa as well as the lamina propria of the mucous membrane. The superficial esophageal glands are branched tubular glands, restricted to the lamina propria and resembling cardiac glands of the stomach. Although the superficial glands are most numerous near the stomach, they may be encountered farther up the esophagus.

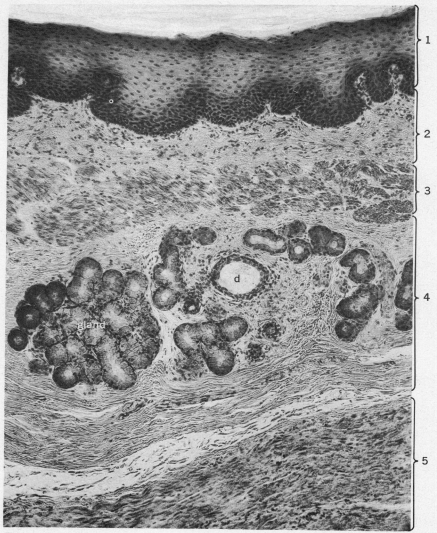

Figure 20-2 Human esophagus; a detail showing the following layers: *1*, stratified squamous epithelium; *2*, lamina propria; *3*, muscularis mucosae; *4*, submucosa containing a deep esophageal gland with a duct, *d*, in cross section; *5*, inner circular layer of the muscularis. Photomicrograph, × 125.

The lamina propria of the esophagus contains less lymphatic tissue than that of other parts of the digestive tract. Occasionally, lymphatic follicles are encountered in the vicinity of the ducts of glands.

The muscularis mucosae is a prominent layer in the lower portion of the esophagus, but it is often indistinct at the upper end of the tube where it blends with a fibroelastic lamina of the pharynx. The muscularis mucosae is composed of numerous closely placed bundles of smooth-muscle fibers arranged longitudinally.

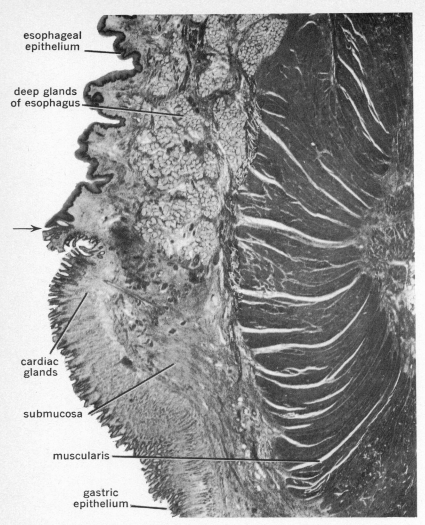

esophageal
epithelium

deep glands
of esophagus

cardiac
glands

submucosa

muscularis

gastric
epithelium

Figure 20-3 Junction of esophagus and cardiac portion of the stomach (dog) marked by an arrow. The esophagus, with deep glands, is above; the stomach, below. Photomicrograph, × 15.

The submucosa of the esophagus is thick. Its fibrous connective tissue contains many elastic networks.

Muscularis Two muscular layers are distinct in the esophagus. The upper one-third of the muscular coat is formed mainly by the skeletal variety. This is especially true of the outer longitudinal layer, which is a continuation of the inferior constrictor muscle of the pharynx. Some skeletal-muscle fibers may be found farther down the tube, but they are almost always absent in the lower one-third. A well-developed intermuscular nerve plexus containing ganglia is present.

Sphincters, i.e., high-pressure zones, are present both at the upper and lower ends of the esophagus. The upper sphincter is the cricopharyngeus muscle. There is no anatomic correlate of the lower esophageal sphincter.

Adventitia   This coat of the esophagus consists of fibrous connective tissue blending with that of the mediastinum, the partition subdividing the thorax. Where the esophagus passes through the diaphragm, it acquires a mesothelial covering for 1 or 2 cm. Many nerve fibers, notably the vagus nerves, course in the adventitia.

STOMACH

The empty stomach (ventriculus) is tubular and less of a sac than as depicted in conventional drawings in anatomy books. Its wall has great elasticity, permitting it to become distended at mealtime. Normal capacity is 1 to 1.5 liters.

Several parts of the stomach are distinguishable grossly. These are the cardiac portion, with its dilatation, the fundus; the body; and the narrow pars pylorica, consisting of the pyloric antrum and pyloric canal. The pyloric canal (or channel) connects the stomach to the duodenum. The most distal portion of the antrum is often called the "prepyloric region."

The **cardiac** portion is small and relatively unimportant histologically. The **fundus** and the main part of the stomach, called the **body,** do not differ in microscopic appearance. In histology, the term fundus is used for both parts. There are marked histologic differences between the fundus and **pylorus.**

Mucosa   The mucous membrane of the stomach is as much as 1.5 mm thick. It is folded into longitudinal ridges, called **rugae,** that disappear to a large extent during distention of the organ. The lining is beset with tiny **gastric pits,** the openings of short and relatively wide ducts of the **gastric glands.** Three to seven secreting tubules empty into each pit (Figs. 20.4 and 20.5).

The epithelium of the gastric mucosa is simple columnar, consisting of tall cells on the surface and somewhat shorter ones in the gastric pits. Their free surface displays no striated border, but a few microvilli are present. The cytoplasm is packed with the secretion antecedent, mucigen, in the form of droplets that are smaller than those in goblet cells. These **surface mucous cells** do not go through the typical filling and emptying cycle that characterizes the latter. They produce a thin mucus that coats their surface, lubricates, and possibly protects it from the digestive action of the gastric juice. The surface epithelium has noteworthy powers of regeneration. It is readily replaced by proliferation of cells in the bottom of the gastric pits.

There are three varieties of gastric glands: cardiac, principal, and pyloric. All of them open into the bottom of gastric pits (Fig. 20.6).

The **cardiac glands** resemble superficial esophageal glands and are confined to a region extending not more than 4 cm away from the opening of the esophagus; often they are not seen at all. Cells of the cardiac glands secrete mucus (Fig. 20.7A).

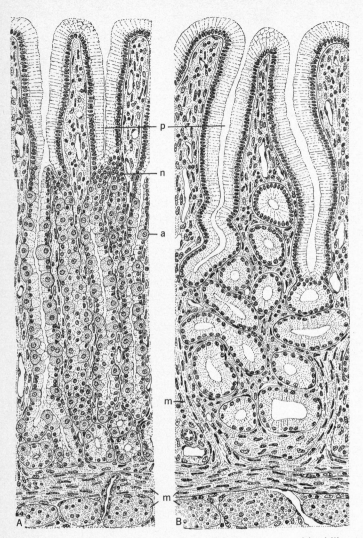

Figure 20-4 Gastric mucosa: *A*, fundus; *B*, pylorus; *a*, acidophilic parietal cell of a principal gland; *m*, muscularis mucosae, the inner layer of which sends extensions into the lamina propria; *n*, mucous neck cells; *p*, gastric pit. Compare *A* with Fig. 20-5 and *B* with Fig. 20-6. About × 150. *(JFN)*

The **principal glands**[1] of the stomach are tubular, each having a neck, or constricted portion, connecting with the bottom of a gastric pit. The body of each gland is a straight tubule ending blindly in the depth of the lamina propria upon the muscularis mucosae. The end is usually bent and may branch.

The principal glands are formed by simple columnar epithelium, with cells

[1]The principal glands of the stomach are called gastric glands by some histologists; but other types of stomach glands also are "gastric," so the term is too restrictive.

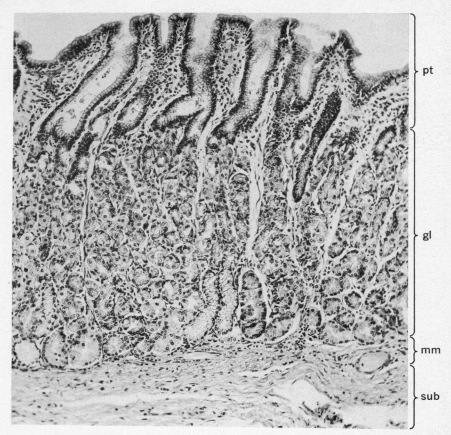

Figure 20-5 Fundus of stomach of a 17-year-old girl. The mucosa shows zones of gastric pits, *pt,* and principal glands, *gl,* but the muscularis mucosae, *mm,* is indistinct above a submucosa, *sub.* Photomicrograph, × 125.

of several kinds. Those lining the necks of the tubules are designated **mucous neck cells** and are quite difficult to see in ordinary histologic sections because they are wedged between cells of other kinds. The mucus secreted by the neck cells is similar to that produced by cardiac and pyloric glands. Droplets of mucigen in the cytoplasm are smaller than those in surface mucous cells.

Chief cells are the most numerous ones in the principal glands (Fig. 20.7*B* and *C*). They have the characteristics of other protein-synthesizing cells. The basal cytoplasm contains many lamellae of granular endoplasmic reticulum. There is a prominent golgi complex from which membrane-bounded zymogen granules move toward the free surface. Mitochondria are numerous in the basal cytoplasm. The chief cells stain with basic dyes. The zymogen granules of chief cells contain pepsinogen, the precursor of pepsin which is the main secretory product.

The cells of most striking appearance in the principal glands are the **parietal cells.** These are rather large swollen cells with one or, occasionally, two cen-

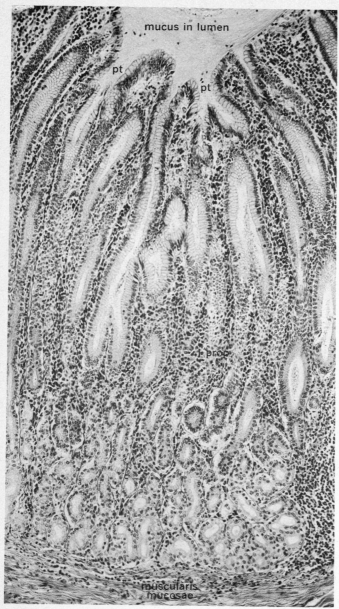

Figure 20-6 Pyloric region of human stomach. Gastric pits, *pt,* receive the long necks of branched, coiled pyloric glands, which are embedded in diffuse lymphatic tissue of the lamina propria, *l prop.* Photomicrograph, ×125.

trally located nuclei (Fig. 20.7*B* and *C*). Parietal cells are more numerous in the upper half of the tubules than in the lower half. They often appear to be crowded away from the lumen by the chief cells and look as though they are hanging onto the outer surface of each gland (Fig. 20.7*B*). Parietal cells

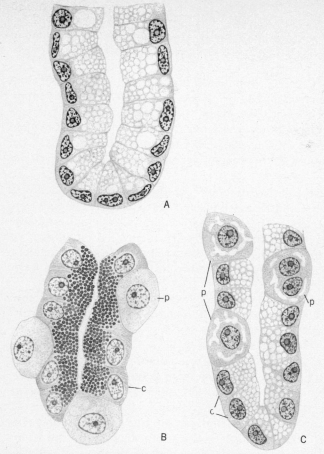

Figure 20-7 Details of cardiac and principal glands. *A,* cardiac gland showing mucin droplets in distal cytoplasm of cells. *B* and *C,* principal glands of fundus. In *B,* the chief cells, *c,* show basal striations and prominent secretion granules; in *C,* the parietal cells, *p,* have intracellular canaliculi. × 900. *(JFN)*

produce hydrochloric acid. They also produce a mucoprotein, known as the "intrinsic factor," that enhances absorption of vitamin B_{12}.

Parietal cells have a considerable amount of cytoplasm. Intracellular canaliculi can be observed with the light microscope (Fig. 20.7*C*). These are formed by invaginations of plasmolemma. Electron micrographs show many long microvilli on the borders of the canaliculi. The cytoplasm contains numerous mitochondria filled with cristae, and abundant vesicles of agranular endoplasmic reticulum. It stains strongly with acid dyes.

A fourth type of cell is found in small numbers in the principal glands. This is the **argentaffin cell**, containing silver-staining cytoplasmic granules. It is more numerous in other parts of the digestive tract. The argentaffin cells (also called enterochromaffin cells) tend to be located beneath the chief cells along the basal lamina. They are not visible in routinely stained histologic sections. Five subtypes have been identified in electron micrographs of these cells in the stomach and intestines. Just which types exist in the principal glands is still being investigated.[2]

The **pyloric glands** are confined to the antrum and are unlike the principal glands; they are more branched, and coiled (Figs. 20.4*B* and 20.6). They, too, open into gastric pits. The glands are lined with a layer of tall columnar epithelium consisting of cells with clear cytoplasm and basally placed nuclei. These cells are similar to the mucous neck cells of the principal glands. The gastrin-secreting cell (a cell of the argentaffin series) is present in the pyloric glands.

The lamina propria of the gastric mucosa is scanty in the region occupied by the glands. It is more prominent beneath the surface epithelium and between the gastric pits, as may be seen in Fig. 20.5. In addition to reticular cells and lymphocytes, the lamina propria contains a few smooth-muscle fibers. A muscularis mucosae is found just below the ends of the glands. This usually consists of two layers of smooth muscle, as shown in Fig. 20.4, and may have three layers in some places.

The tela submucosa is formed of fibrous connective tissue containing a few lipocytes. In it are the usual blood vessels, lymphatic vessels, and the submucous ganglionated autonomic plexus.

Muscularis   The muscular coat of the stomach differs from that of other tubular digestive organs. It has three layers, an inner layer, arranged obliquely, having been added to the usual circular and longitudinal layers. The circular muscle is thickened at the pylorus to form the pyloric sphincter and diminishes in size abruptly at the junction with the duodenum. No true cardiac sphincter is formed, although the inner oblique muscle is thickest at that end of the stomach. An intermuscular myenteric nerve plexus is well developed.

Serosa   A thin layer of visceral peritoneum, formed by fibrous connective tissue and mesothelium, covers the stomach and passes onto the omentum.

Function   The functions of the stomach are mechanical and chemical. Muscular movements churn its contents. **Gastric juice**, secreted by its glands, provide chemical substances that liquefy and begin digestion of the food, some of which is retained in the stomach for 3 or 4 hours. The diluted pulplike stomach contents, known as "chyme," are spurted into the intestine in small portions, beginning 15 or 20 minutes after food has been swallowed. The stomach has limited power to reject substances by initiating regurgitation.

The gastric juice secreted by gastric glands is a clear, colorless fluid containing about 0.4 to 0.5 percent hydrochloric acid and some digestive enzymes. Its production is regulated by psychic factors as well as by the stimulus of food

[2]The argentaffin cells have endocrine functions, and their secretions pass into capillaries instead of into the lumen of glands. One variety, present in the small intestine, secretes **5-hydroxytryptamine** (serotonin) which stimulates smooth-muscle contraction. Another, also present in the small intestine, secretes the hormone **enteroglucagon.** A third, located in pyloric and duodenal glands, probably secretes the hormone **gastrin.**

in the stomach and by a hormone liberated from the mucous membrane of the antrum and small intestine when the gastric contents enter the latter. The rate of secretion varies from a few to 60 ml per hour, and the total quantity may be as great as 2.5 liters per day.

Although the stomach is primarily concerned with preparation of food for absorption in the intestine, some absorption takes place in it. This is confined to a small amount of water and minute quantities of substances of low molecular weight, such as salt, sugar, and alcohol.

SMALL INTESTINE

The small intestine, a long, glandulomuscular tube extending from the pylorus to the cecum, is less distensible than the stomach. Its three subdivisions, the **duodenum**, **jejunum**, and **ileum**, merge gradually into one another and present minor structural differences. Most of the small intestine is attached by the mesentery to the posterior body wall; otherwise it is free to move about in the abdomen. Proper function is dependent upon this freedom of movement.

The small intestine differs from the stomach in the structure of its walls, especially its mucous membrane (Fig. 20.8). Instead of longitudinal rugae indented by pits, it has circular folds studded with minute projections. Glands secreting the intestinal juice are found in all parts. The structure of the small intestine is illustrated in Fig. 20.9.

Mucosa The mucous membrane of the small intestine is covered with simple columnar epithelium. The epithelium and a basal lamina rest on a highly cellular lamina propria containing many blood and lymphatic capillaries. A muscularis mucosae marks its junction with the fibrous submucous coat. The mucous membrane covers permanent transverse folds of the submucosa, the **plicae circulares**, which are not ironed out by distention of the intestine.

The absorptive surface of the small intestine is increased at least fiftyfold by minute projections, called **intestinal villi.** The villi are the most characteristic feature of the small intestine, for they are present throughout its length but are not found in any other part of the alimentary tract. These absorptive fingers of the mucous membrane diminish in number toward the lower end of the intestine but are longer there than those in the duodenum. The villi of the duodenum are leaf-shaped or tongue-shaped structures, as may be seen in Fig. 20.10. Those of the jejunum, shown in Figs. 20.9 and 20.11, are narrow. Grossly, the villi impart a velvety appearance to the intestinal lining. The intestinal villi move from side to side and are shortened by contraction of smooth-muscle fibers which are present in small numbers in their core of lamina propria. Movement of the villi enhances absorption, and shortening helps empty the contents of their lymphatic vessels into deeper channels.

The columnar epithelium of the mucosal surface covers the villi and extends down from them into cryptlike **intestinal glands.**[3] It contains five types of cell. Absorptive cells (1) are the principal ones of the villi. They are taller at the

[3]These are the "crypts of Lieberkühn."

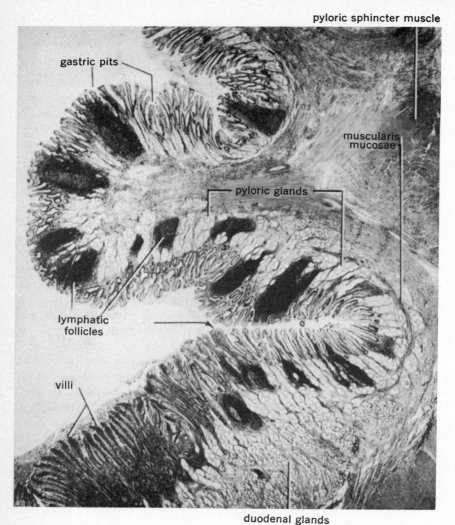

Figure 20-8 Junction of pyloric canal with the duodenum (dog) at the arrow. Photo-micrograph, × 15.

tip than toward the base. They continue into the crypts as relatively undifferentiated cells (2). Among the absorptive cells, and to a lesser extent in the necks of the crypts, are columnar goblet cells (3). Argentaffin cells (4) are found in the walls. Finally, at the bottom of the intestinal glands there is a secretory cell (5) whose precise function is unknown. Its fine structure resembles that of other exocrine-gland cells. The cell is known only by its eponym, "paneth cell" (Fig. 20.12).

Cells of the mucosal epithelium are firmly attached to one another by junctional complexes (Chap. 3). Terminal-bar structures encircle each one at its free border and strengthen the barrier between intestinal lumen and interstitial space.

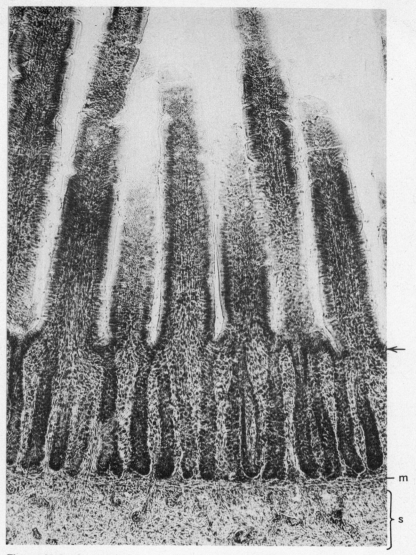

Figure 20-9 Small intestine of a kitten. Above the arrow, seven villi extend into the lumen of the intestine; below the arrow, 16 intestinal glands are embedded in the lamina propria and rest on a thin muscularis mucosae, *m;* the submucosa, *s,* is seen at the bottom of the figure. Photomicrograph, × 150.

The columnar **absorptive cells** have striated borders which may be as much as 1 or 1.5 μm thick. The border is composed of microvilli—about 3,000 on each cell. The outer component of the plasmolemma of the microvilli has minute projections, giving the surface a rough or "fuzzy" appearance in electron micrographs (Fig. 3.14). This is part of a coating of protein-polysaccharide nature containing various digestive enzymes.

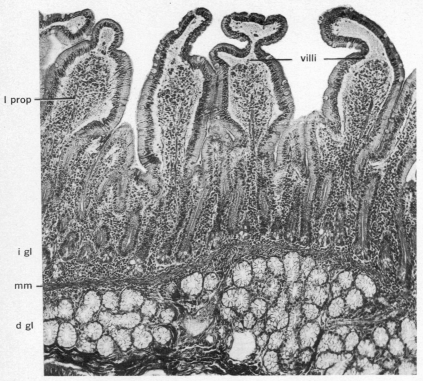

Figure 20-10 Human duodenum, showing leaf-shaped villi with cores of the lamina propria, *l prop*. Intestinal glands, *i gl*, end near the muscularis mucosae, *mm*, and duodenal glands, *d gl*, lie in the submucosa. Photomicrograph, × 125.

Each microvillus has a core of microfilaments that extends down into the terminal net of the cell. The net is formed by microfilaments running parallel to the surface and anchored into the junctional structures. Cytoplasm beneath the net contains agranular endoplasmic reticulum, pinocytotic vesicles, and the golgi complex, as well as mitochondria. The basal cytoplasm contains some ribosomes and granular endoplasmic reticulum.

Basal processes of absorptive cells rest on a basal lamina. Lateral processes display interdigitating folds (Fig. 20.13). Lateral interstitial spaces vary in width; dilatations are encountered in some places.

Mucus-secreting **goblet cells**—in essence, unicellular glands—are described in Chap. 3. There are relatively few of them in the duodenum; they become more numerous in the lower jejunum and ileum. Mucus is expelled onto the surface over the glycoprotein coating of the microvilli and helps protect it from abrasion by coarse material in the lumen.

Epithelium of the crypts is composed primarily of columnar **undifferentiated cells.** They lack striated borders. The surface epithelium of the intestinal villi is apt to be damaged and sloughed into the lumen. In the normal course of events, there is attrition, but regeneration can take place with amazing rapidity

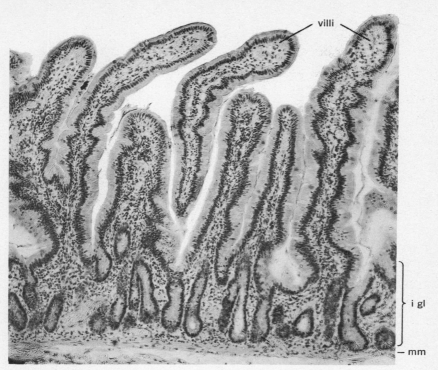

Figure 20-11　Human jejunum, showing tall villi and short intestinal glands, *i gl*. The muscularis mucosae, *mm*, is thin. Photomicrograph, × 125.

from the epithelium of the intestinal crypts. Outward migration of a cell from base to tip of a villus occurs in 36 hours. Denuded intestinal villi are usually seen in histologic sections of the small intestine. This does not indicate a normal condition but results from postmortem autodigestion of the epithelium.

Toward the bottom of the crypts there are pyramid-shaped cells with considerable amount of basal granular endoplasmic reticulum. These are the **paneth cells** (Fig. 20.12).

Argentaffin cells are more numerous in the intestine than in the stomach. Some of them secrete intestinal hormones, notably secretin and cholecystokinin, which stimulate production of pancreatic juice and also induce hepatic bile flow, duodenal-gland secretion (secretin), and gallbladder contraction (cholecystokinen).

The lamina propria of the intestinal mucosa is well defined between the intestinal glands and in the cores of the villi. It is formed by diffuse lymphatic tissue with a reticular stroma enmeshing many free cells. Lymphocytes and plasmocytes are its principal cells, although eosinophils and basophils are numerous. The lymphocyte population varies greatly. Cells escaping into the intestinal lumen are often seen in sections of the epithelium.

Throughout the intestine, the lamina propria contains solitary lymphatic follicles. The smallest are confined to the lamina propria of one villus. The larg-

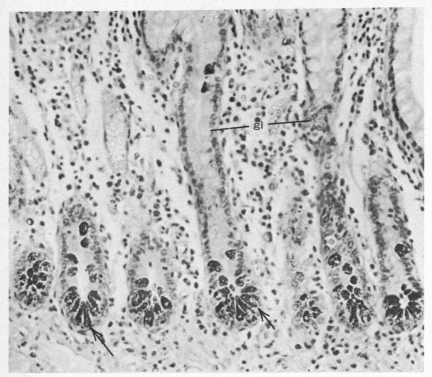

Figure 20-12 Intestinal glands, *gl*, of the human jejunum. A special method was used to stain the actively secreting paneth cells (*arrows*). Photomicrograph, × 150. *(Contributed by P. A. Laurén and T. E. Sorvari*, Stain Technology, *vol. 42, pp. 311–315, 1967.)*

est may bulge into the submucosa beneath several villi. Aggregate lymphatic follicles are found toward the lower end, especially in the ileum.[4] They somewhat resemble small tonsils and can easily be seen with the naked eye if one looks for them in the wall opposite the attachment of the mesentery. The role of lymphatic tissue in the lamina propria in antibody formation is of primary importance.

The muscularis mucosae of the small intestine consists of inner circular and outer longitudinal smooth-muscle layers. A few small bundles of muscle fibers extend into the lamina propria. The muscularis mucosae is traversed by ducts of the duodenal glands. In the duodenum, it builds the important sphincter of the bile duct.

The tela submucosa of the small intestine resembles that of the stomach but is somewhat firmer. It forms the cores of the permanent plicae circulares. A submucous nerve plexus, containing numerous small autonomic ganglia, is present. Some groups of lipocytes may be encountered. The submucosa conveys blood vessels and lymphatic vessels to and from the mucous membrane.

[4]Aggregate lymphatic follicles in the small intestine are called "Peyer's patches."

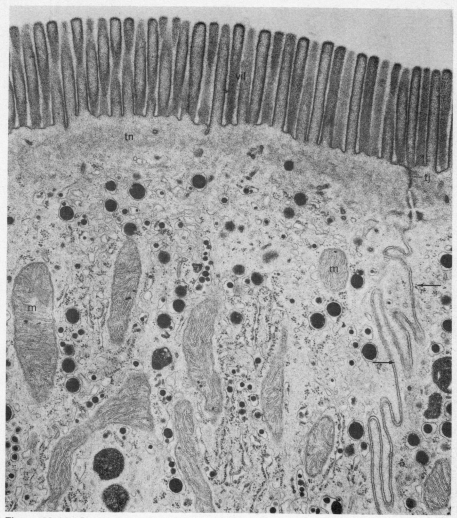

Figure 20-13 Parts of two absorptive cells on the surface of an intestinal villus (rat). Arrows mark tortuous lateral plasma membranes. Note tight junction, *tj*. Other abbreviations are: *vil*, microvilli on free border; *tn*, terminal net or web of microfilaments beneath the microvilli, *m*, mitochondria. The black bodies are membrane-bounded lipid droplets. Electron micrograph × 21,300. *(Contributed by S. L. Palay.)*

The **duodenal glands**[5] lie in the submucosa (Fig. 20.10). They are largest in the upper end, diminishing in size and number farther down. They may be absent in the lower part of the duodenum, or they may extend into the jejunum for a little way. They are made up of many small lobules, 1 mm or less in diameter, sending short ducts into some of the intestinal glands. The secretory portions are formed by branched and coiled tubules of simple columnar epithelium.

[5]Formerly called "Brunner's glands."

Their pale mucous cells have basally placed and often flattened nuclei; they resemble the pyloric glands. Secretion is primarily a thin mucus.

Muscularis   The muscular coat of the small intestine consists of two well-formed layers of smooth muscle separated by a little fibrous connective tissue. The inner layer is circular. The outer one is longitudinal. Between the two layers is the prominent **myenteric nerve plexus.**

The musculature agitates food and digestive juices, facilitating the chemical reactions and enhancing absorption of water and the products of digestion. The musculature also propels the contents by a series of nicely coordinated peristaltic movements.

Serosa   The small intestine is covered by a thin layer of fibrous connective tissue, upon which is a mesothelium. This visceral peritoneum is reflected onto the mesentery along the line of its attachment to the intestine. Most of the duodenum lacks a mesentery and has only a partial serous coat.

Digestion and Absorption   The partially liquefied contents of the stomach are admitted in small portions to the duodenum through the pylorus. In the small intestine, most of the carbohydrates, lipids, and proteins are broken down into smaller molecules by action of amylolytic, lipolytic, and proteolytic enzymes, thus facilitating their absorption by the mucosal epithelial cells.

Intestinal juice is composed of the secretions of the various glands of the digestive tract, including the pancreas and liver. It contains sloughed mucosal epithelial cells which are believed to be one source of the digestive enzymes.

Digestive processes occur not only in the intestinal lumen, but also on the surface of the striated border of the lining epithelium. There are enzymes associated with the plasmolemma and its glycoprotein coating that are capable of hydrolyzing peptides and disaccharides.

Absorption of water, electrolytes, and small molecules of the basic food substances, begins at the striated border of the epithelium. Carbohydrates are transported through it as monosaccharides, most proteins as amino acids. Only in the newborn infant can large protein molecules cross this barrier.

Dietary fat entering the small intestine is subjected to the action of pancreatic lipase. Fat digestion and absorption are complex. They involve hydrolysis to fatty acids and glycerol by the lipase, formation of micelle with bile acids, and diffusion of the fatty acids and other end products into the absorptive cells. Entrance of particles into an absorptive cell is shown in Fig. 20.14.

Another mechanism of absorption has been illustrated by using immunologic techniques. Absorption of immunoglobulin molecules from mother's milk by cells of the intestinal mucosa occurs in the newborn rat. These molecules first attach to binding sites at bases of the microvilli, stimulating pinocytosis and the subsequent intracellular transport through the endoplasmic reticulum to the interstitial spaces, as shown diagrammatically in Fig. 20.15.

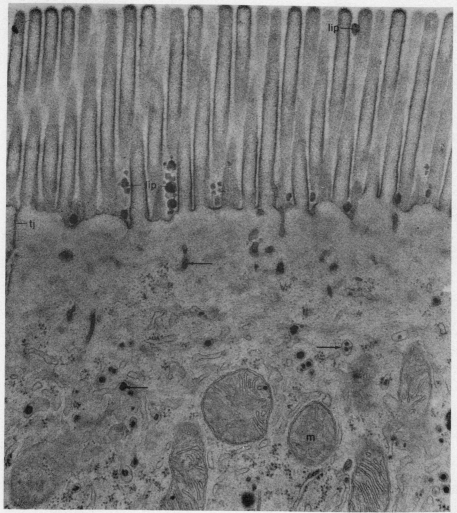

Figure 20-14 Passage of particles, *lip* (products of digestion of fat), between intestinal microvilli to be absorbed, i.e., enclosed in membranes at the plasmolemma; vesicles are marked by *arrows*. Note mitochondria, *m,* and tight junction, *tj*. Electron micrograph × 35,000. *(Contributed by S. L. Palay.)*

LARGE INTESTINE

The large intestine is a spacious sacculated tube wherein water is absorbed and the feces are formed. It may be subdivided into **cecum, colon,** and **rectum.** The **appendix** is an appendage of the cecum. The usual three tunics are present, but they differ from those of other parts of the digestive tube.

Table 20.1   Comparison of Principal Tubular Digestive Organs

	Esophagus	Stomach	Small intestine	Large intestine
Epithelium	Stratified squamous	Simple columnar	Simple columnar	Simple columnar
Villi	Absent	Absent	Present	Absent
Absorptive surface	Absent	Not marked	Marked	Present
Goblet cells	Absent	Mucus secreted, but no true goblets	Present, increasing toward lower end	Numerous
Mucosal irregularities	Longitudinal folds	Rugae; gastric pits	Plicae circulares, especially in jejunum	Ileocecal valve; anal columns
Lymphatic tissue of mucosa	Sparse	Rich	Rich; many follicles, increasing toward lower end	Rich; many follicles
Muscularis mucosae	Thick	Thin	Thin	Thin
Glands	Superficial and deep esophageal	Cardiac; principal; pyloric	Intestinal in mucosa; duodenal in submucosa	Intestinal
Muscularis	Skeletal in upper part; two layers smooth in lower	Three layers smooth	Two layers smooth	Two layers smooth, with outer longitudinal teniae; anal sphincter
Mesentery	Absent	Present (omentum)	Absent on duodenum; present elsewhere	Present on transverse colon
Digestive function	Absent	Liquefaction of food; protein digestion begins	Main digestion of proteins, carbohydrates, fats; main absorption	Absorption of water; concentration of residue

Entrance to the cecum is guarded by the **ileocecal valve**, consisting of two flaps of mucosa. Muscles of the small and large intestines are thickened there and overlap to form a sphincter. Valve and sphincter release intestinal contents into the cecum and tend to prevent flow in the reverse direction. A sharp line of

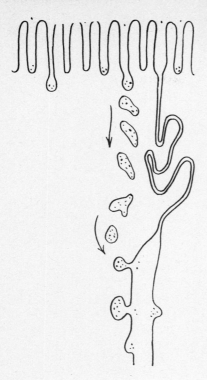

Figure 20-15 Diagram illustrating the transport of antibody (black dots) across absorptive cell in the small intestine of newborn rat. The antibodies bind to surface pits and are moved through the cell to be released into interstitial spaces. *(Redrawn from R. Rodewald,* Journal of Cell Biology, *vol. 58, pp. 89–211, 1973.) (CHP)*

transition marks the junction of the mucous membranes of small and large intestines.

The outstanding difference between mucous membrane of the small and large intestines is the absence of villi and lack of plicae circulares in the latter, giving it a smooth lining. This notable reduction in surface area does not prevent large quantities of water from being absorbed in the large intestine. The surface epithelium is simple columnar, with **absorptive cells** that have thin striated free borders. There are numerous **goblet cells**. The absorptive cells, but not the goblet cells, contain immunoglobulin A.

The intestinal glands are longer than those of the small intestine, and, as can be seen in Fig. 20.16, goblet cells are so numerous that other types of cells scarcely can be observed. **Argentaffin cells** are present. The mucus secreted by the intestinal glands and surface goblet cells lubricates and protects the mucosa. It also aids in formation of the gradually dehydrated fecal masses and facilitates progression of them toward the descending colon and rectum.

The mucosa of the rectum has intestinal glands, measuring up to 0.7 mm in length, longer than those of any other part of the intestine. However, they are not so numerous as in the colon.

The lower portion of the rectum, or anal region, is illustrated in Fig. 20.17. In it, vertical folds of the mucosa form the **anal columns**. These end about 15 or

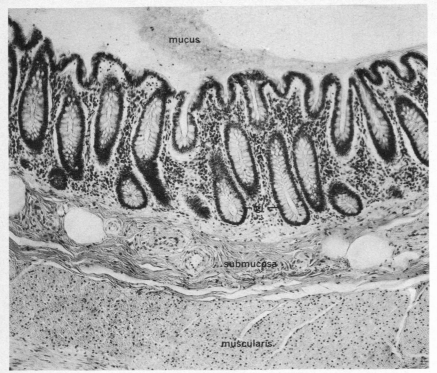

Figure 20-16 Human colon, longitudinal section. Note absence of villi and presence of intestinal glands, *gl*, filled with goblet cells. A sheet of mucus covers the surface epithelium. Photomicrograph, × 125.

20 mm from the anal orifice by uniting in crescentic folds called "anal valves." These valves enclose blind pockets, the anal sinuses or crypts. In the anal canal, the intestinal glands are no longer present, and the surface epithelium becomes noncornified stratified squamous. This transition zone extends to the anal orifice where the skin begins. Hair, sebaceous glands, and apocrine glands appear at the junction.

The lamina propria and muscularis mucosae of the large intestine are similar to those layers in the small intestine.

The submucosa presents no unusual features in the cecum and colon. That of the anal region contains sensory nerves and end organs of the baroreceptor type.

The muscularis of the human large intestine is formed by a distinct inner, circular layer and a partially deficient outer, longitudinal layer. The outer layer has been reduced to three stout bands, the **teniae coli,** arranged equidistant from one another. Contraction of these tends to throw the wall of the colon into a series of sacculations. The circular layer of muscle is thickened to form the internal anal sphincter. An external sphincter is formed by skeletal-muscle fibers.

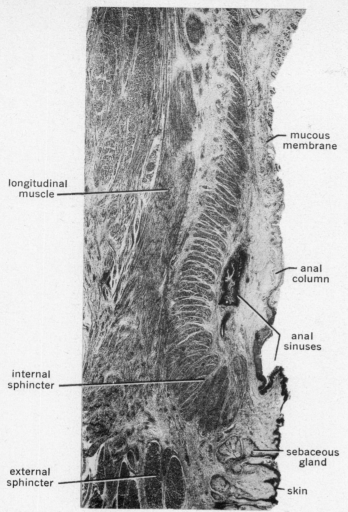

mucous
membrane

longitudinal
muscle

anal
column

anal
sinuses

internal
sphincter

sebaceous
gland

external
sphincter

skin

Figure 20-17 Anal region of the rectum of a child; longitudinal section. Photomicrograph,
× 14.

A serous coat is present in most of the colon but absent from part of the
rectum, especially the anal region. Attached to it are small pedunculated tabs of
fat covered with mesothelium. These are "appendices epiploicae."

Appendix The appendix is a blind tube 8 or 10 cm long, on the average. It
is attached to the cecum where the three teniae unite to form an outer longitudinal muscle layer. The small lumen of the appendix has an irregular, angular
form. Its mucous membrane has absorptive and goblet cells. Intestinal glands
are relatively few and are irregular in shape. They are crowded with goblet
cells.

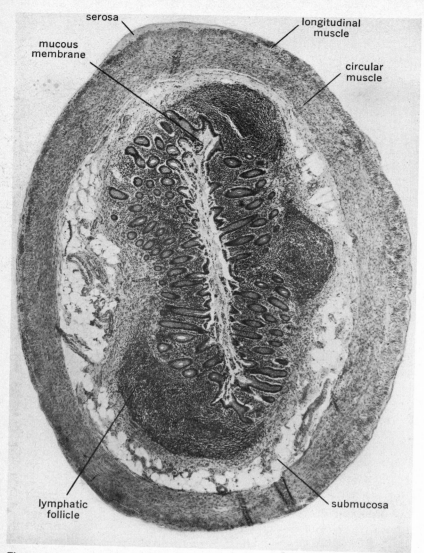

Figure 20-18 Human appendix. Photomicrograph, × 30.

The lamina propria is heavily infiltrated with lymphocytes. Lymphatic follicles, often breaking up the muscularis mucosae and penetrating the submucosa, may form a complete ring around the lumen. The submucosa contains lipocytes. Both muscular coats are complete. The serous coat is continued onto a small mesentery.

The appendix is subject to inflammation and infection and may show marked departure from normal structure, even in subjects regarded as healthy. The lumen may be partly or completely obliterated. Occasionally the mucosa is replaced by fibrous connective tissue. Figure 20.18 shows a reasonably normal appendix (see also Fig. 12.1).

BLOOD VESSELS, LYMPHATIC VESSELS, AND NERVES

The mesenteries convey arteries and nerve fibers toward the digestive tube, and veins and lymphatic vessels away from it. A general plan prevails throughout each part. Freely anastomosing arteries are found everywhere. The villi of the small intestine impose interesting differences in the vascular and lymphatic arrangements.

The connective-tissue layers of the digestive organs contain blood vessels, lymphatic vessels, and nerve plexuses. The main network of blood vessels is found in the submucosa. Branches pass out to the muscular layers and into the lamina propria of the mucous membrane. Secondary networks are formed in these locations, and capillary plexuses abound among their elements. Venous networks are similarly disposed.

Each intestinal villus is provided with an arteriole or two, which break up into capillaries. The capillaries lie close to the epithelium, where they receive absorbed materials. Venules draining the villi are usually located on the side opposite the arterioles.

Lymphatic capillaries are numerous in the lamina propria, where they collect fluid and lymphocytes. They are joined by others to form larger vessels, which build networks in the submucosa. Each villus contains one or more centrally placed lymphatic capillaries, known as "lacteals." The lacteals receive quantities of lipid droplets during digestion.

Nerves of the digestive tube are, for the most part, autonomic. They form two **enteric plexuses** between the muscle layers and in the submucosa.[6] Both these contain many small parasympathetic ganglia. Some sensory nerve fibers occur in the digestive organs, but they are relatively few compared with those of the surface of the body.

SUGGESTED READING

Brunger, O,. and J. H. Luft: Fine Structure of the Apex of Absorptive Cells from Rat Small Intestine. *Journal of Ultrastructure Research,* vol. 31, pp. 291–311, 1970.

Cardell, R. R., S. Badenhausen, and K. R. Porter: Intestinal Triglyceride Absorption in the Rat. *Journal of Cell Biology,* vol. 34, pp. 123–155, 1967.

Cheng, H., and C. P. Leblond: Origin, Differentiation and Renewal of the Four Main Epithelial Cell Types in the Mouse Small Intestine. III. Entero-endocrine Cells. *American Journal of Anatomy,* vol. 141, pp. 503–520, 1974.

Crane, R. K.: Intestinal Absorption of Sugars. *Physiological Reviews,* vol. 40, pp. 789–825, 1960.

Davenport, H. W.: Why the Stomach Does Not Digest Itself. *Scientific American,* vol. 226, no. 1, pp. 87–93, January, 1973.

[6]Often called the "plexus of Auerbach" and "plexus of Meissner."

Forsmann, W. G., L. Orci, R. Pictet, A. E. Renold, and C. Rouiller: The Endocrine Cells in the Epithelium of the Gastrointestinal Mucosa of the Rat. *Journal of Cell Biology,* vol. 40, pp. 692–715, 1969.

Friedman, M. H. F.: *Functions of the Stomach and Intestine.* University Park Press, Baltimore, 1974.

Ito, S.: The Enteric Surface Coat on Cat Intestinal Microvilli. *Journal of Cell Biology,* vol. 27, pp. 475–491, 1965.

Novikoff, P. M., and A. B. Novikoff: Peroxisomes in the Absorptive Cells of Mammalian Small Intestine. *Journal of Cell Biology,* vol. 53, pp. 532–560, 1972.

Rodewald, R.: Intestinal Transport of Antibodies in the Newborn Rat. *Journal of Cell Biology,* vol. 58, pp. 189–211, 1973.

Rubin, W., M. D. Gershon, and L. L. Ross: Electron Microscope Radioautographic Identification of Serotin-Synthesizing Cells in the Mouse Gastric Mucosa. *Journal of Cell Biology,* vol. 50, pp. 399–415, 1971.

Schafield, G. C., and A. M. Atkins: Secretory Immunoglobulin in Columnar Epithelial Cells of the Large Intestine. *Journal of Anatomy,* vol. 107, pp. 491–504, 1970.

Liver and Pancreas

Two large glands, the liver and pancreas, are associated with the alimentary tract, emptying their exocrine secretions into the duodenum. Their role in digestion supplements that of the many intrinsic gastrointestinal glands and the three pairs of salivary glands. Both the liver and pancreas have important functions besides that of contributing to the digestive juices. For a comparison of the digestive glands, see Table 21.1.

LIVER

The liver (hepar) lies in the upper right quadrant of the abdominal cavity just beneath the diaphragm. It is the largest gland of the body, weighing about 1.5 kg. It is relatively larger at birth, when it forms 5 percent of the body weight, than it is at maturity, when it accounts for approximately 2 percent.

The liver is interposed on the venous pathway between the intestines and heart, receiving blood laden with the products of absorption, except most lipids which pass first to the systemic circulation by way of the lymphatic vessels. It functions in their intermediary metabolism, altering, storing, and then releasing them to the circulation on demand. It is also concerned with metabolism of the products of erythrocyte destruction, and it secretes bile. The structure of the liver is relatively simple for an organ performing so many diverse functions.

Table 21.1 Comparison of Digestive Glands

	Parotid	Submandibular
Number of glands	Two	Two
Classification	Compound tubuloacinous	Compound tubuloacinous
Stroma	Encapsulated, lobulated	Encapsulated, lobulated
Blood vessels	Small	Small
Lymphatic vessels	Present	Present
Parenchyma		
Secretory components	Serous	Mainly serous; many demilunes
Ducts	Single main; long intercalated	Single main; short intercalated
Secretion		
Name	Saliva	Saliva
Function	Lubrication	Lubrication
Control	Neural	Neural

Hepatic Stroma   The liver is covered by a layer of dense fibrous connective tissue forming a prominent capsule (Fig. 21.1). Most of the surface is invested by mesothelium. The capsule is thickened at a hilum, known as the **hepatic portal,** and its fibrous connective tissue passes into the organ to compose the major stromal framework. The liver is lobulated by this fibrous stroma. In human beings, lobulation is incomplete because connective tissue is confined largely to the vicinity of vessels and ducts, but in some species, notably the pig, the connective tissue forms thin septa which almost completely subdivide the parenchyma into units.

The units of liver parenchyma are known as **hepatic lobules.** They are little polyhedrons of liver substance about 1 mm wide and 2 mm long, appearing roughly hexagonal in sections. In the liver of the pig, the hexagonal sections of hepatic lobules are more distinct than in human liver sections, where the amount of stroma is scanty. Human hepatic lobules are bounded at the angles by thin branches of the fibrous stroma, and the hepatic parenchyma of ad-

Sublingual	Pancreas (exocrine)	Liver (exocrine)
Two groups	One	One
Compound tubuloacinous	Compound tubuloacinous	Compound tubular
Indistinct capsule, lobulated	Encapsulated, lobulated	Heavy capsule (partial serosa); hepatic lobules
Small	Small	Hepatic artery and vein, portal vein
Present	Present	Present only in main stroma
Mainly mucous; few demilunes	Serous; marked chromophil substance and zymogen granules	Serous cells in plates
Several main; others not prominent; intercalated absent	One main, one accessory; long intercalated; centroacinous cells	Common bile duct; gallbladder; bile ductules; bile canaliculi
Saliva	Pancreatic juice	Bile
Lubrication	Carbohydrate digestion	Fat digestion
Neural	Hormonal in part	Hormonal in part

jacent lobules is coextensive along the sides of the lobules. The finest subdivisions of the hepatic stroma consist of reticular tissue which, in minute amount, separates liver cells from the sinusoids (Fig. 21.2B).

Hepatic Vessels The liver's main afferent blood vessel is the **portal vein** (Fig. 21.3). This enters the hepatic portal to break up into branches distributed through trabeculae of the hepatic stroma. The branches of the portal vein are accompanied by small hepatic arteries, bile ductules, and lymphatic vessels, as well as a few nerve fibers. The **hepatic arteries** course among the hepatic lobules in septa of the connective tissue. Branches of portal veins and hepatic arteries are sometimes designated "interlobular" veins and arteries.

In sections of liver, interlobular vessels and their accompanying **bile ductules** are easily identified in the stroma at the angles of the hepatic lobules. The group is commonly designated as a hepatic "triad," a name that is misleading because it ignores a fourth component, the important lymphatic vessels that are

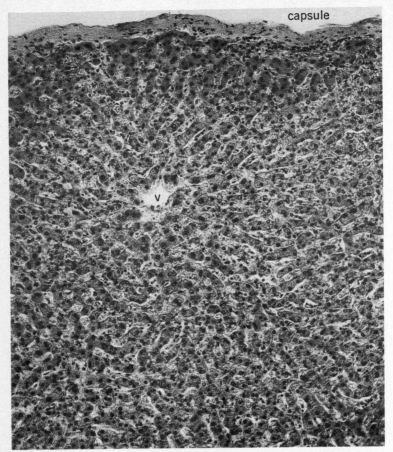

Figure 21-1 Human liver with fibrous-connective-tissue capsule; one central venule is shown, *v;* radiating from it are hepatic-cell cords and hepatic sinusoids. Photomicrograph, × 150.

always associated with the other vessels, although often difficult to see. A triad at a place where branching of the venule and ductule occurs is illustrated in Fig. 21.4.

Innumerable short branches spring from the interlobular portal venules as they course between the hepatic lobules. Similarly, branches of lesser prominence arise from the interlobular hepatic arterioles. Almost immediately, these terminal branches open into a myriad of **hepatic sinusoids** in the parenchyma of the liver. The hepatic sinusoids, like those of the bone marrow and spleen, are wide fenestrated channels wherein blood can move slowly. Their walls are composed of thin cells and appear to have no basal laminae.

There is a **perisinusoidal space**[1] between the sinusoids and the parenchymal

[1]This is called the "space of Disse."

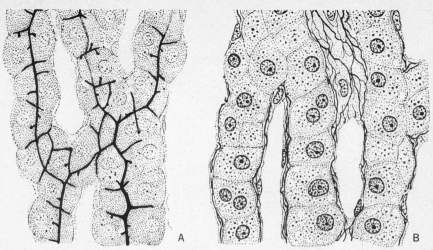

Figure 21-2 Hepatic cell cords. Bile canaliculi are blackened with silver in *A*. Reticular fibers around hepatic cells are stained by the silver carbonate method in *B*. × 900. *(JFN)*

hepatic cells (Fig. 21.5). The lining cells of the sinusoids, and gaps between them, permit fluid to pass from the sinusoidal lumen into the perisinusoidal space.

The sinusoids anastomose and converge toward the center of the hepatic lobule, where they come together to enter a **central venule** in the core of the lobule (Fig. 21.6).

Arterial blood entering a hepatic lobule at its periphery contains more oxygen, and portal venous blood more metabolic substances than blood leaving the lobule by the central venule. Thus there is a gradient across the lobule, resulting in a structural zonation of the hepatic parenchyma.

The cells lining the hepatic sinusoids resemble those of thin endothelium. They have dark ovoid or irregularly shaped nuclei, but the cytoplasm usually cannot be seen with the light microscope. These cells can give rise to macrophages and even hemocytoblasts. Many **macrophages** are found in the walls of the sinusoids, often protruding from the walls, as illustrated in Fig. 21.5.[2] These phagocytes remove and digest cellular detritus and other foreign material from the blood while it moves slowly through the hepatic sinusoids. They can become free macrophages. The number of macrophages in the liver is greater than in any other organ, with the possible exception of the bone marrow.

Hemocytoblasts are not found in the normal adult liver, but **hemopoiesis** is a normal hepatic function during part of prenatal life, and under certain abnormal conditions it can recur in the adult.

The central venules of the hepatic lobules join one another to form tributaries of the **hepatic veins.** These tributaries are designated "sublobular" veins

[2]The eponym for hepatic macrophages is "Kupffer cells."

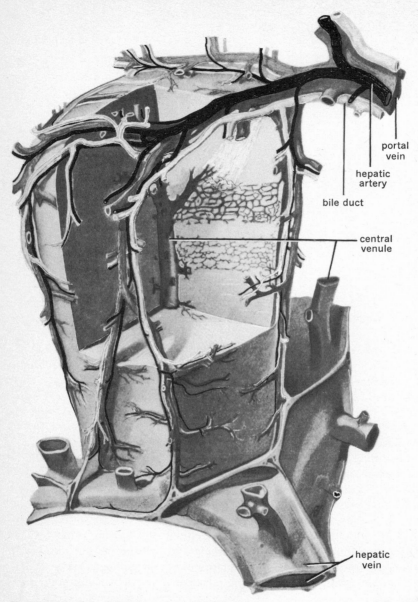

portal
vein

hepatic
artery

bile duct

central
venule

hepatic
vein

Figure 21-3 Reconstruction of a liver lobule of a pig, showing relation of blood vessels and bile ducts to liver parenchyma. *(Modified from H. Braus.)*

after they have left the lobules. The central venules are not surrounded by fibrous connective tissue, but the larger sublobular venules and veins are. They enter the stromal trabeculae, where they course unaccompanied by other blood vessels or ducts. The sublobular veins ultimately become the hepatic veins draining into the inferior vena cava, and thence to the heart.

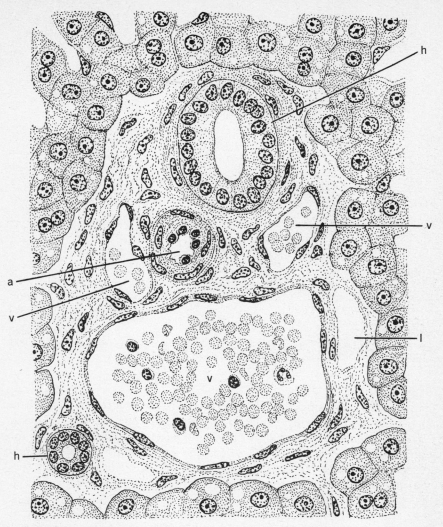

Figure 21-4 Hepatic vessels and ducts in interlobular connective tissue: *a*, hepatic arteriole; *h*, bile ductules; *l*, lymphatic vessel; *v*, portal venules containing blood. × 900. *(JFN)*

Numerous **lymphatic vessels** course through the capsular and stromal connective tissue of the liver (Fig. 21.4). Fluid from the hepatic blood plasma, enriched by the contributions from hepatic cells, passes through the walls of the sinusoids and enters the perisinusoidal spaces. This is a tissue fluid of high protein content. Upon reaching the interlobular stroma, it is collected by lymphatic capillaries, to be conveyed by larger lymphatic vessels to the systemic circulation. A large volume of lymph, rich in proteins, leaves the liver. It may amount to 30 to 50 percent of the lymph formed in the body.

Hepatic Parenchyma　The hepatic lobule is composed of many irregularly

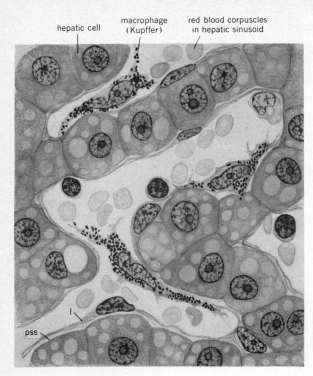

hepatic cell   macrophage   red blood corpuscles
                (Kupffer)   in hepatic sinusoid

pss

l

Figure 21-5 Hepatic sinusoids, showing macrophages. Thickness of lining cells, *l,* and width of perisinusoidal spaces, *pss,* are exaggerated, × 900. *(JFN)*

branching and anastomosing plates of hepatic cells, **hepatocytes,** organized in radial manner around the central venule. The plates are one cell thick in many places. The arrangement of the plates provides a parenchymal spongework for the hepatic sinusoids (Figs. 21.2 and 21.5). The polyhedral hepatocytes, as a rule, present two surfaces to the perisinusoidal spaces, while their other surfaces are in close apposition to one another except at **bile canaliculi** (Fig. 21.2*A*).

Each hepatic cell has one or, occasionally, two nuclei, each containing at least one distinct nucleolus, but scanty chromatin. The cytoplasm is somewhat basophilic and has a granular appearance under the light microscope. Special staining methods show varying amounts of glycogen particles and lipid droplets, depending on the functional state of the cell and its location in the hepatic lobule (Fig. 21.7).

Glycogen is stored first in cells at the periphery of the lobule, the process extending gradually toward the center, where glycogen is seldom seen. Similarly, conversion of glycogen to glucose proceeds along the hepatic lobular gradient. Lipids, when stored in the liver, tend to be deposited first in hepatocytes adjacent to central venules.

The fine structure of hepatocytes is illustrated in Figs. 21.8 and 21.9. The cytoplasm contains both types of endoplasmic reticulum. The granular form is

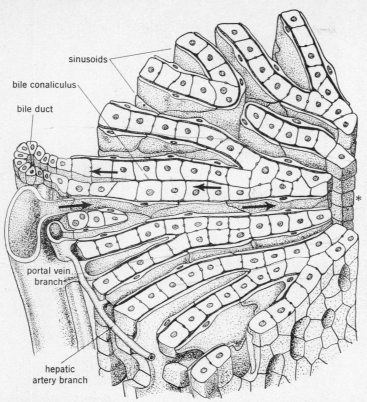

sinusoids

bile conaliculus

bile duct

portal vein
branch

hepatic
artery branch

Figure 21-6 Diagram illustrating radial arrangement of plates of hepatocytes in relation to hepatic sinusoids. Arrows indicate direction of blood flow from a branch of the portal vein, and bile flow from canaliculi to tributary of the bile-duct system. Asterisk (*) indicates position of central venule. *(Modified from A. W. Ham,* Histology, *6th ed., J. B. Lippincott Company, Philadelphia, 1969.) (CHP)*

represented by groups of flat cisternae; the agranular form, by anastomosing tubular structures. Free ribosomes and polysomes are present. The golgi complex appears in several locations as groups of lamellae with dilated ends. Mitochondria are numerous and vary regionally in complexity of their structure. Lysosomes and microbodies are encountered, usually near the bile canaliculi. Glycogen granules, often in clumps, appear among the vesicles of agranular endoplasmic reticulum.

The free borders of hepatocytes have microvilli. Those projecting into the lumen of bile canaliculi are short; those in the perisinusoidal spaces are long (Fig. 21.9).

Liver Function   The liver is the main metabolic center of the body. Glucose absorbed by the intestinal mucosa is transported to the liver in the blood by the portal venous system. There the parenchymal cells polymerize it into glycogen by a process known as glycogenesis. Glycogen is formed also

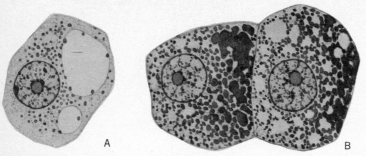

Figure 21-7 Hepatocytes. *A.* Lipid-filled spaces and dark granules of bile pigment. *B.* Glycogen in clumps of granules, *gl. (JFN)*

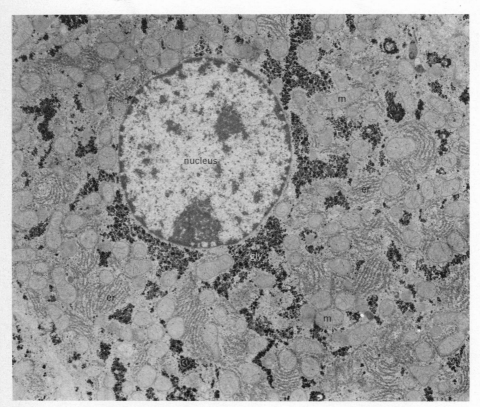

Figure 21-8 Part of a hepatocyte from a fasted rat, taken from the midportion of a lobule. Numerous mitochondria, *m,* clumps of glycogen granules, *gly,* and parallel arrays of granular endoplasmic reticulum, *er,* are seen. Electron micrograph, × 6,000. *(Contributed by R. R. Cardell, Jr.)*

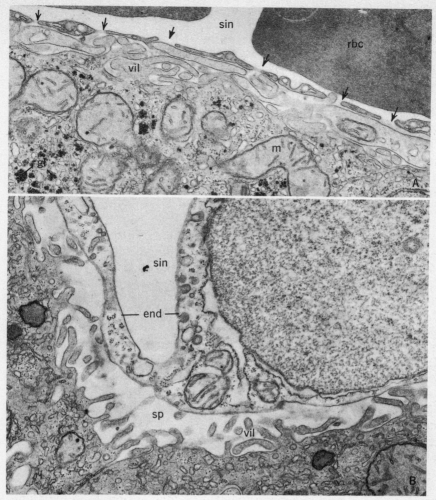

Figure 21-9 Hepatic sinusoids, *sin*, and perisinusoidal spaces, *sp;* the latter contain microvilli, *vil*, of adjacent hepatocytes. The space in *A* is collapsed; that in *B* is open. Marked discontinuity of the endothelial cells, *end*, is seen at arrows in *A*. The hepatocytes contain mitochondria, *m*, glycogen, *gl*, and other organelles and inclusions. *A*, from the normal liver of a hamster; *B*, from that of a rat that had been fasted for 24 hours. Electron micrographs: *A*, × 17,600; *B*, × 19,600. *(Contributed by A. L. Jones.)*

during protein and lipid metabolism. Glycogenolysis is the process by which the hepatic cells change their glycogen to glucose, through phosphorylation, and release it into the perisinusoidal spaces. A balance between glycogenesis and glycogenolysis is maintained through hormonal regulation.

Lipids are synthesized by hepatocytes from carbohydrate, protein, and other precursor substances. They are combined with protein molecules to form lipoproteins which are either stored in the cells or released into the perisinusoidal spaces. Synthesis of cholesterol also occurs in the liver.

Plasma proteins, such as albumins, fibrinogen, and prothrombin, are synthesized by hepatocytes. Urea is formed in the process of deaminization. Toxic substances reaching the liver are degraded by hepatocytes to forms that can be excreted by the kidneys. Storage functions of the liver have been mentioned: mainly glycogen and lipids, but also vitamins and heparin, are stored in hepatic cells.

Production of bile represents both secretion and excretion. Bile pigments come from the hemoglobin of destroyed erythrocytes and bile acids from cholesterol. Lecithin is also secreted in bile.

Intrahepatic Duct System   Most of the substances synthesized by the hepatocytes are passed into the sinusoids. Bile is secreted into bile canaliculi, which are tiny tubules lying in the plates between adjacent hepatocytes (Fig. 21.2A). These canaliculi have no wall of their own but utilize small parts of the plasma membranes of cells as a wall; short microvilli project into the lumen of the bile canaliculus. The bile canaliculi course toward the periphery of the hepatic lobule between rows of hepatocytes, as shown in Fig. 21.6, and empty into **interlobular bile ductules,** whose epithelial cells are directly continuous with the hepatocytes at the periphery of the lobule.

Bile ductules are small tubes of nonsecretory low columnar epithelium, into which the bile canaliculi empty. At their junction with hepatocytes, the ductules are formed by cells that are a little smaller than the hepatocytes with which they are continuous.[3] The ductules are surrounded by fibrous connective tissue of the interlobular trabeculae. As they join one another to form larger ductules, their epithelial cells become taller. Bile ductules thus form larger **intrahepatic bile ducts.**

BILE DUCTS AND GALLBLADDER

Union of intrahepatic bile ducts ultimately forms left and right **hepatic ducts** in the hepatic portal. These two come together as they emerge from the hilum, and a duct from the gallbladder, known as the **cystic duct,** is received. The large intrahepatic and extrahepatic ducts are lined with tall simple columnar epithelium with a basal lamina, beneath which is a lamina propria of connective tissue containing a few lymphocytes but no smooth-muscle fibers.

A **common bile duct** is formed by the union of hepatic ducts and cystic duct. This passes to the duodenum, running obliquely through the wall of that organ to open into its lumen. The wall of the common bile duct contains very few smooth-muscle cells, but near the duodenum a thick smooth-muscle layer is present. This forms a sphincter. As the common bile duct passes through the wall of the duodenum, it is joined by the pancreatic duct, and a slight expansion of the lumen, known as the **ampulla,**[4] is formed. This opens into the duodenum

---

[3]This part of the passage is sometimes called the "canal of Hering."
[4]Also known as the "ampulla of Vater."

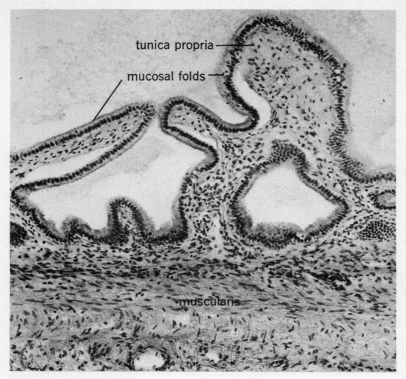

tunica propria

mucosal folds

muscularis

Figure 21-10 Gallbladder (cat). Photomicrograph, × 150.

on an elevation, the **duodenal papilla.**[5] The smooth-muscle **sphincter** of the bile duct is formed around the duct just before it unites with the pancreatic duct. This sphincter remains closed most of the time, but relaxes when food is ingested and allows bile to flow into the duodenum. Humoral and neural mechanisms are involved in this process.

The **gallbladder** (visica fellae) is a small elongated sac that receives, stores, and concentrates bile during intervals between meals when the sphincter of the bile duct is closed. Its structure resembles that of the tubular digestive organs. The mucosa of the gallbladder consists of a layer of tall simple columnar epithelium with a basal lamina on connective tissue (Fig. 21.10). The epithelial cells have a striated border that is not always distinct under the light microscope. Electron micrographs show microvilli on the surface. No glands are present in the lamina propria, and there is no muscularis mucosae, but the mucous membrane adjoins a thin layer of irregularly arranged smooth-muscle bundles. The gallbladder has a thick perimuscular layer of connective tissue containing blood vessels, small nerves, and lymphatic vessels. A serous layer is found on the free surface of the organ.

[5]Called the "papilla of Vater."

The lining of the gallbladder is extensively folded, and some of the folds remain intact even when the organ is distended. So complex are some of the folds that sections through them may give an erroneous impression that glands are present in the lamina propria (Fig. 21.10). The neck of the gallbladder tapers into the cystic duct, where the folds are especially prominent and have an arrangement known as the spiral fold.[6] A few small tubuloacinous mucous glands are present at the neck of the gallbladder and in the cystic duct.

The gallbladder empties during digestion of a fatty meal by contraction of its musculature. The concentrated bile is evacuated through the cystic duct, bile duct, and opened sphincter into the duodenum where it aids in digestion of the fat. The mechanism of emptying can be activated in the denervated gallbladder by the hormone cholecystokinin, formed in the duodenal mucosa.

PANCREAS

The pancreas is an elongated gland lying behind the stomach on the posterior abdominal wall, embraced on the right by the duodenum. It is a duplex organ. One portion is a tubuloacinous exocrine gland; the other is endocrine, consisting of many pancreatic islands embedded in the exocrine gland (Fig. 21.11).

Pancreatic Stroma   The pancreas is surrounded by loose fibrous connective tissue forming a thin and indefinite capsule. Septa carry blood vessels, lymphatics, and nerves[7] into the gland and subdivide it into numerous lobules. The septa are quite thin and send fine wisps of areolar tissue into the lobules, but the acini are separated from one another by only a little reticular tissue.

Exocrine Parenchyma   The acini of the pancreas are serous and resemble those of the parotid gland. Their pyramidal cells have a characteristic two-toned appearance when stained with hematoxylin and eosin or similar dyes. They are basophilic and longitudinally striated at the base. Apically, they are lighter in color, and zymogen granules can be seen in the cytoplasm when appropriate techniques are used. The basal cytoplasmic striations are formed by well-developed, longitudinally oriented mitochondria and parallel arrays of granular endoplasmic reticulum. Free ribosomes are present. The golgi complex is distinct. The prominence of these organelles in the pancreatic acinous cells is correlated with vigorous synthesis of the pancreatic enzymes.

The pancreas daily produces 1 liter or more of alkaline secretion containing enzymes that split proteins, fat, and starch into simpler compounds for absorption, e.g., trypsin, lipase, and amylase. Pancreatic secretion accumulates during fasting and is released into the intestine in response to the hormones secretin and cholecystokinin which are liberated from the duodenal mucosa by gastric

---

[6]Formerly described as the "valve of Heister."
[7]Sensory end organs of the lamellated type are often encountered in sections of the pancreas. These lie in the capsule and septa.

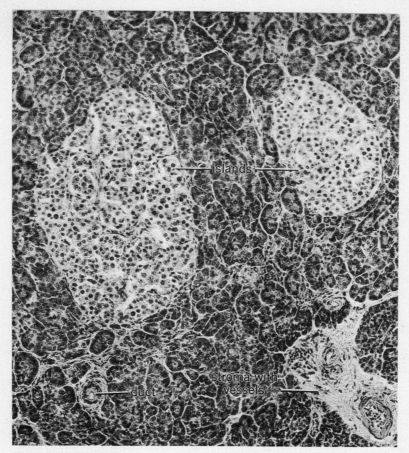

Figure 21-11   Human pancreas showing two islands. Compare the exocrine portion with the parotid gland (Fig. 19-18). Photomicrograph, × 150.

hydrochloric acid, and bile acids and fat, respectively, at the beginning of intestinal digestion.

The acini contain a few centrally placed low columnar or squamous cells protruding into their lumen. These are the **centroacinous cells** (Fig. 21.12). They represent the beginning of the pancreatic duct system. To a varying extent, each acinus folds around its intercalated duct, often bulging to one side like a boxing glove over the hand and wrist.

Intercalated ducts have low epithelium, are long and branched, and enter interlobular ducts directly. No secretory ducts are present in the pancreas. All excretory ducts are lined with tall simple columnar epithelium and are surrounded by fibrous connective tissue.

The main pancreatic duct and an accessory pancreatic duct have thick

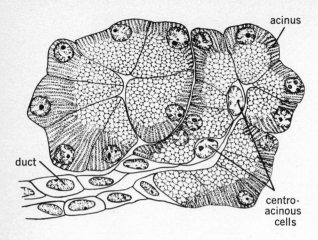

acinus

duct

centro-
acinous
cells

Figure 21-12 Centroacinous cells in the pancreas of a guinea pig. *(Redrawn from Bensley.)* *(MWS)*

coats of dense fibrous connective tissue. Their epithelium contains goblet cells, and a few tiny mucous glands may be encountered in their walls.

The endocrine portions of the pancreas are described in Chap. 24.

SUGGESTED READING

Burkel, W. E.: The Fine Structure of the Terminal Branches of the Hepatic Arterial System of the Rat. *Anatomical Record,* vol. 167, pp. 329–349, 1970.

Cardell, R. R., Jr.: Action of Metabolic Hormones on the Fine Structure of Liver Cells. II. Effects of Hypophysectomy and Chronic Administration of Somatotropin. *American Journal of Anatomy,* vol. 139, pp. 49–79, 1974.

Elias, H., and J. C. Sherrick: *Morphology of the Liver.* Academic Press, Inc., New York, 1969.

Fawcett, D. W.: Observation on the Cytology and Electron Microscopy of Hepatic Cells. *Journal of the National Cancer Institute,* vol. 15, pp. 1475–1502, 1955.

Greenway, C. V., and R. D. Stark: Hepatic Vascular Bed. *Physiological Reviews,* vol. 51, pp. 23–65, 1971.

Jamieson, J. D., and G. E. Palade: Condensing Vacuole Conversion and Zymogen Granule Discharge in Pancreatic Exocrine Cells: Metabolic Studies. *Journal of Cell Biology,* vol. 48, pp. 503–522, 1971.

Matter, A., L. Orci, and C. Rouiller: A Study on the Permeability Barriers between Disse's Space and the Bile Canaliculus. *Journal of Ultrastructure Research,* Suppl. 11, pp. 1–71, October, 1969.

Novickoff, A., and E. Essner: The Liver Cell. *American Journal of Medicine,* vol. 29, pp. 102–131, 1960.

Wisse, E.: An Electron Microscopic Study of the Fenestrated Endothelial Lining of Rat Liver Sinusoids. *Journal of Ultrastructure Research,* vol. 31, pp. 125–150, 1970.

Respiratory System

The respiratory system is composed of the lungs and passages carrying air to and from them. The lungs are elastic, permitting them to expand and collapse with movements of the ribs and diaphragm, but the air passages are constructed in such a way that they remain open and in free communication with the exterior. The lungs are protected in several ways from accidental admission of food and foreign bodies. The lining of the airway is kept warm by blood vessels, moist by serous secretions, and sticky by mucus. One portion of the airway, the larynx, has become specialized for vocalization. The olfactory organ lies in the upper end of the airway.

NASAL CAVITY AND NASOPHARYNX

The nasal cavities have bony and cartilaginous walls (Fig. 19.1). They can be divided into three regions on the basis of structural differences. The epithelium of each region is securely attached to the subjacent bone and cartilage by a lamina propria, containing few elastic fibers and numerous small glands.

Vestibular Region The stratified squamous epithelium of the vestibule resembles that of skin but is lightly cornified. This part of the nasal cavity is a transition zone; toward the nostrils, the epithelium is thick and has large hairs, or "vibrissae," as well as sebaceous glands, the hair and glands diminishing in number and size toward the respiratory region.

Respiratory Region   The main part of the nasal cavity is lined by a mucous membrane varying in thickness from several millimeters over the inferior turbinate bone to less than a millimeter elsewhere. It has pseudostratified epithelium made up of ciliated columnar cells, with many interspersed goblet cells secreting mucus. The epithelium rests on a basal lamina.

The lamina propria is formed by fibrous connective tissue, containing many lymphocytes, plasmocytes, eosinophils, and other cells. Rich vascularity is the main feature. It contains an extensive capillary bed and many wide, thin-walled, anastomosing venules, especially prominent on the inferior turbinate bones, where they form pseudoerectile bodies. Engorgement of the venous channels in the mucous membrane can occlude the airways of the nose. The vascular plexus of the lamina propria forms a radiator that warms the air as it passes through the respiratory region of the nose. Figure 22.1 illustrates the structure of this mucous membrane.

The thick lamina propria is filled with small tubuloacinous glands emptying onto the epithelium by numerous ducts. These have mixed serous and mucous acini, as do most glands of this type throughout the respiratory tract. The deep layer of the lamina propria blends with the perichondrium or periosteum.

Cilia of the respiratory epithelium move the nasal secretions toward the nasopharynx. The intrinsic glands and one large extrinsic gland, the lacrimal (Fig. 17.14), supply serous fluid that moistens the epithelium and the air passing over it. Foreign particles, bacteria, and pollen grains are picked out of the air by a film of mucus lying on the epithelial surface.

Olfactory Region   The upper part of the nasal cavity is lined by a special neuroepithelium. This pseudostratified epithelium, about 60 μm thick, contains no goblet cells. It consists of short basal and tall "sustentacular" cells surrounding cell bodies of the **olfactory neurons.** The sustentacular cells have striated free borders but lack cilia. Each olfactory nerve cell has a slender body with an ovoid nucleus in the deep portion of the epithelium. Neurofibrils and, in electron micrographs, microtubules can be demonstrated in the cytoplasm. The dendritic process ends at the epithelial surface in a little swelling, or olfactory vesicle, from which spring six or eight motile olfactory cilia, each about 2 μm long (Fig. 22.2). The cilia have basal bodies in the vesicle. The axon extends through the lamina propria and unites with others to form olfactory nerve filaments that pass through the cribriform plate of the ethmoid bone to enter the olfactory bulbs of the brain.

The lamina propria of the olfactory mucous membrane contains small tubuloacinous **olfactory glands**. These are serous glands, opening by many rather wide ducts onto the olfactory epithelium. Their thin, lipid-containing secretion provides a solvent for airborne scents.

Olfaction plays a relatively unimportant role in human beings, in contrast to that in many other species. On the other hand, the sense of smell is absent in

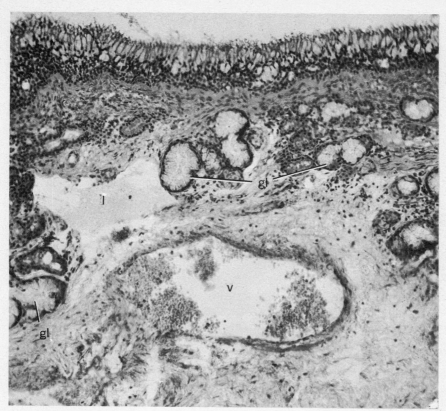

Figure 22-1 Nasal mucous membrane from human inferior turbinate bone. Note the lymphatic vessel, *l*, venule, *v*, and mixed mucous and serous glands, *gl*. The surface epithelium is pseudostratified and contains many goblet cells. Compare with the tracheal mucosa in Fig. 22-6. Photomicrograph, × 150.

some (dolphins). Human beings are sometimes rendered anosmic by injury or disease, without leaving them with serious handicaps.

Appendixes of the Nasal Cavity The maxillary, frontal, sphenoid, and ethmoid bones contain cavities lined by thin mucous membranes, continuous with the respiratory mucous membrane of the nose. Tiny apertures of these **paranasal sinuses** permit no significant circulation of air into them from the nasal passages. Their epithelium is pseudostratified but thinner than that of the nasal cavity. Cilia of the epithelial cells move secretions toward the apertures. A few small mucous glands are found in the lamina propria of the maxillary mucous membrane. Elsewhere the lamina propria is meager and indistinguishable from the periosteum.

Besides the paranasal sinuses, the **nasolacrimal duct** opens into the nasal cavity on either side. This is a tube lined with pseudostratified epithelium and surrounded by a lamina propria containing a venous plexus. Its dilated upper end, the **lacrimal sac**, receives two small lacrimal canaliculi carrying the secre-

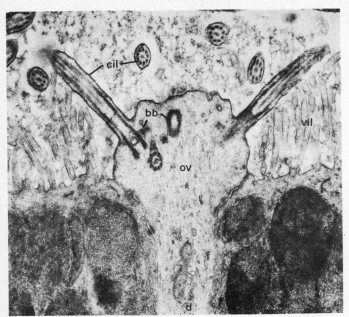

Figure 22-2   Olfactory epithelium (frog). The dendrite of an olfactory neuron here terminates in an enlargement, or olfactory vesicle, *ov*, from which spring cilia, *cil*. Two cilia are cut longitudinally and several others in cross section. The vesicle contains basal bodies, *bb*, of the cilia; also other organelles. On either side of the dendrite, *d,* are epithelial cells with long microvilli, *vil*, on their surface. Electron micrograph, × 23,500. *(Contributed by T. S. Reese.)*

tion that has bathed the cornea and conjunctiva of the eye. The lacrimal sac has an epithelium similar to that of the nasolacrimal duct, but the lacrimal canaliculi are lined with stratified squamous epithelium. The lacrimal gland was considered in Chap. 17.

Nasopharynx   The nasal cavities open into the nasopharynx. Laterally, the **auditory tube**[1] opens from the middle ear. The structure of the nasopharyngeal lining is similar to that of the nasal respiratory mucous membrane. A thick lamina propria contains many lymphocytes; dense lymphatic tissue forms pharyngeal and tubal tonsils. Glands are of the tubuloacinous mixed type in contrast to the purely mucous glands of the oral pharynx.

There is no sharp line of demarcation between nasal and oral pharynx, nor is the laryngeal pharynx clearly bounded. Stratified squamous epithelium of the oral pharynx continues down to the upper end of the larynx, covering a plate of elastic cartilage and forming the **epiglottis** (Fig. 22.3). The opening of the larynx, known as the **glottis**, is closed reflexly when food is swallowed and when foreign bodies or noxious fumes enter the nose and nasopharynx. It is closed automatically during tensing of the abdomen in straining and can be

[1]Commonly called "Eustachian tube."

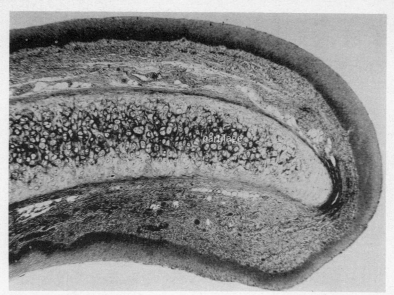

cartilage

Figure 22-3 Human epiglottis; longitudinal section; dorsal surface above. Photomicrograph, × 50

closed voluntarily. Closure is accomplished by sphincter muscles, rather than by any trapdoor action of the epiglottis.

LARYNX

The larynx can be studied advantageously by gross dissection. It has a cartilaginous skeleton to which are attached a number of small skeletal muscles, serving as part of the speech mechanism. The mucous membrane of the larynx is mainly of the respiratory type. Cilia move surface secretions toward the pharynx. The lamina propria contains a few mixed glands, many elastic fibers, and some lymphatic tissue with an occasional lymphatic follicle. A submucosa is present. With aging, the cartilagenous skeleton of the larynx undergoes partial ossification.

Part of the larynx is shown in Fig. 22.4. Its mucous membrane has two sets of prominent folds: the **ventricular** and **vocal folds,** or false and true vocal cords, above and below a space called the **laryngeal ventricle.** The vocal folds contain the **vocal ligaments** of elastic fibers to which skeletal-muscle fibers of the thyroarytenoid muscles are attached. Contraction of muscles relaxes the vocal ligaments, changes the shape of the laryngeal ventricle, and thus makes is possible to produce different sounds. Muscles of the larynx are supplied by the inferior laryngeal nerve. The superior laryngeal nerve is sensory.

The epithelium becomes stratified squamous over the vocal folds in consequence of their active movement. The epithelium at the junction of the

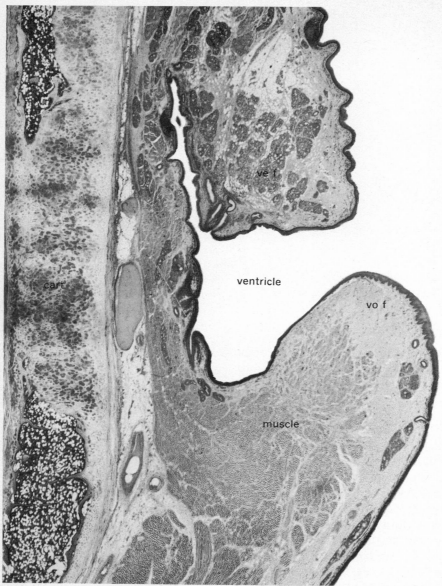

Figure 22-4 Human larynx; frontal section through the partly ossified thyroid cartilage, *cart,* on the left and the laryngeal ventricle with ventricular folds, *ve f,* and vocal folds, *vo f,* at the upper and lower right. Note the stratified squamous epithelium with papillae of lamina propria on the lip of the vocal fold. Photomicrograph, × 13.

two types of fold is ciliated stratified columnar. Glands are present in the ventricular folds.

TRACHEA AND BRONCHI

The trachea is a fibrocartilaginous tube about 10 to 12 cm long extending from the larynx to its bifurcation into the bronchi. One can distinguish a mucous membrane, a submucous layer containing glands, a fibrous and cartilaginous layer, and an adventitia of loose fibrous connective tissue continuous with the fascia of the neck and mediastinum.

Cartilage forms the skeleton of the trachea and gives it some rigidity. There are 16 to 20 hyaline **tracheal cartilages** forming incomplete, and occasionally branching, C-shaped rings deficient dorsally toward the esophagus. Dense fibrous connective tissue completes this coat by bridging the gaps in the rings and becoming continuous with the perichondrium on both sides of the cartilages. It forms a dense lamina at the open ends of the cartilages, where it extends from one cartilage ring to the next. A layer of smooth muscle, the **tracheal muscle,** lies in front of the fibrous membrane connecting the ends of the tracheal rings. These structures are shown in Fig. 22.5. Tracheal cartilages, unlike those of the larynx, do not ossify with aging, but the collagenous fibers in them do increase in number.

The mucous membrane of the trachea, shown in Fig. 22.6, is lined with pseudostratified epithelium, most columnar cells of which have cilia beating toward the mouth. Goblet cells are numerous. The epithelium rests on a well-defined basal lamina. The lamina propria is formed by reticular and elastic fibers and contains numerous lymphocytes. A distinct elastic layer is present between it and the submucosa.

The submucosa of the trachea is composed of fibrous connective tissue containing the larger vessels and the **tracheal glands.** The latter are tubuloacinous mixed glands with many ducts piercing the lamina propria and opening onto the epithelium.

The trachea bifurcates to form two smaller tubes of similar structure. These are the **primary bronchi**. The right bronchus has six or eight cartilagenous rings; the left, nine to twelve. Each primary bronchus enters the hilum of the lung and immediately begins a series of branchings that culminate in the smallest air passages and the lung alveoli.

Within the lung, the main branches of the pulmonary tree are the **intrapulmonary bronchi.** They are tubes of dense fibrous connective tissue in which are embedded rings or plates of hyaline cartilage of odd and irregular shape, often appearing as crescents or ovoid masses in sections. The smooth muscle of an intrapulmonary bronchus is arranged in long spirals, coursing clockwise and counterclockwise down the wall of the tube.

The mucous membrane of the intrapulmonary bronchus in histologic sections appears to be thrown into projections or ridges (Fig. 22.7) because of constriction of the tubes by the smooth muscle and diffuse elastic fibers in the wall.

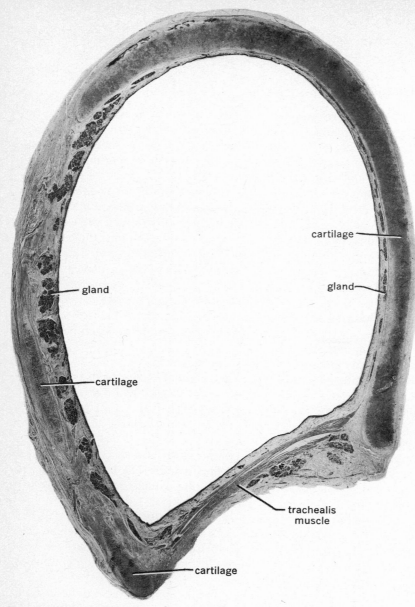

Figure 22-5 Human trachea, sectioned through a cartilage on the right and through parts of the intercartilaginous membrane on the left. Tracheal glands are few and compressed on the right; they are more prominent on the left. Note the tracheal muscle below. Photomicrograph, × 6.

Otherwise, the mucous membrane has much the same structure as that of the trachea and primary bronchi. As a bronchus branches and becomes smaller, the muscle bands come to lie closer to the epithelium. Glands are found external to the muscle.

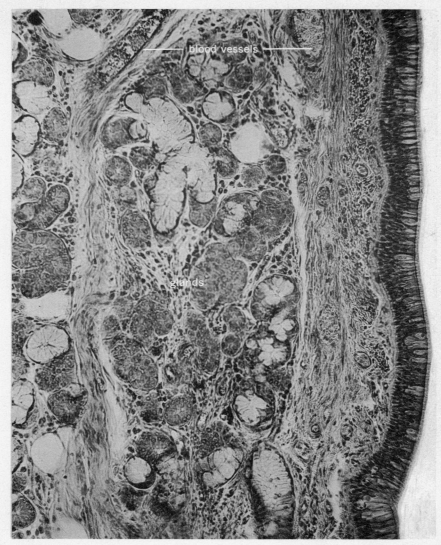

Figure 22-6   Human tracheal mucous membrane showing ciliated pseudostratified epithelium and mixed glands. Compare with Fig. 22-1. Photomicrograph, × 150.

The tracheal and bronchial musculature has a double innervation, from vagus and sympathetic nerves. Small ganglia may be encountered occasionally.

LUNGS

The lung (pulmo) is the vital organ for exchanging oxygen and carbon dioxide. Essentially, it is an airway that, after some 23 successive subdivisions, ends in about 300 million minute alveoli. These terminal functional elements have a

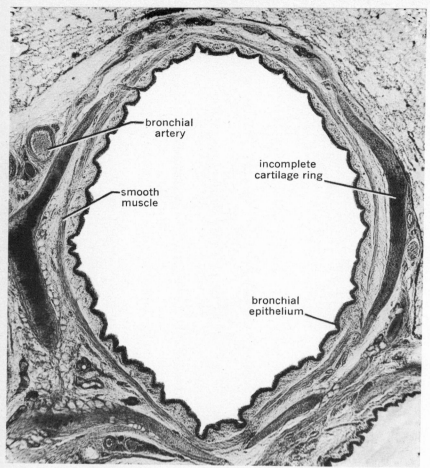

Figure 22-7 Small bronchus in a human lung. Photomicrograph, × 40.

total surface of nearly 600,000 cm². The two lungs occupy most of the thorax, which alternatively expands and contracts under neural control of intercostal and diaphragmatic muscles.

Histologic sections present an appearance that may be puzzling unless it is recognized that the lung is much like a large gland in which the acini have become expanded into minute balloons. The ducts are the bronchi which, with their many subdivisions, conduct air instead of fluid secretion.

The similarity between lung and gland structure is especially striking in the fetus and newborn infant before the first breath has been drawn. Prior to inspiration, portions of the lung resemble an extraordinarily vascular exocrine gland, as will be seen in Fig. 22.8. The alveoli are only partially expanded and are lined with low simple columnar epithelium that flattens out when the lung is first expanded with air.

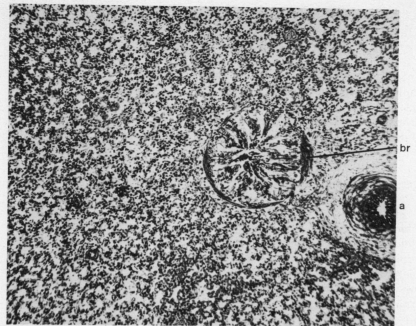

Figure 22-8 Unexpanded lung of a newborn guinea pig before taking a breath. A bronchiole, *br,* and an arteriole, *a,* are seen on the right. Note that magnification is equal to that of Figs. 22-9 and 22-10. Photomicrograph, × 150.

Just as a gland is surrounded by a capsule and subdivided by trabeculae of fibrous connective tissue, so the lung is provided with a similar connective-tissue stroma. The lung capsule is the visceral pleura, covered with mesothelium.

Intrapulmonary Bronchi There are ten bronchopulmonary segments in the right lung and eight in the left. Main branches of the primary bronchi pass into each lobe of the lungs from the hilum accompanied by blood vessels, lymphatic vessels, and nerves. The trabeculae of fibrous connective tissue, in which these structures course, are rich in elastic fibers. The secondary bronchi divide into tertiary bronchi, and smaller and smaller subdivisions are formed through 50 or more generations, as it were. A bronchus of small size is shown in Fig. 22.7.

As airways diminish in size, bronchial epithelium is reduced in thickness until it becomes a ciliated simple columnar lining containing a few goblet cells. The cilia increase in number, and goblet cells disappear in the smallest bronchi. The lamina propria, containing lymphocytes, is a thin layer of connective tissue in which reticular and elastic fibers predominate.

Just beneath the mucosa of the bronchus, there is a layer of smooth muscle. This is not a complete coat but consists of diagonal spirals of muscle running both to the left and to the right and becoming relatively greater in amount as the bronchus decreases in size. As this muscle contracts, it not only constricts the bronchus but shortens it. It plays an important part in adjusting the length of the bronchus to contraction and expansion of the lung during breathing.

The cartilaginous C-shaped rings of the main bronchi give way to irregular and incompletely encircling plates of cartilage in the lesser bronchi. In the larger bronchial branches, no posterior deficit, like that in the trachea and primary bronchi, is produced by the cartilages. The cartilaginous plates disappear altogether in the smallest bronchi, which are only about 1 mm in diameter.

The bronchial glands are mixed, as in the trachea. They lie outside the smooth muscle and are found in the smallest bronchi, sometimes extending a little farther peripherally along the respiratory tree than do the cartilaginous plates.

Bronchioles   When the air passages become less than 1 mm in diameter, they are called bronchioles. These little conducting tubes are lined with simple columnar epithelium, many cells distally becoming nonciliated. The bronchiolar epithelium lacks goblet cells, and there are no glands beneath it; mucus is not present in the lumen of these small passages. Bronchioles have no cartilages, but there is a relatively great amount of smooth muscle which, upon contraction, can constrict and shorten them. The surrounding stroma is continuous with that of adjacent pulmonary alveoli and contains abundant elastic fibers. Bronchioles are illustrated in Figs. 22.9 and 22.10.

Respiratory Bronchioles   Terminal bronchioles are lined with low simple columnar epithelium, mostly lacking cilia. They have diagonal bands of smooth muscle forming an incomplete layer in their walls. This fenestration leaves regions in which the walls of these small tubes are unusually thin, such tubes being designated respiratory bronchioles. Each terminal bronchiole divides into two or more respiratory bronchioles, as a rule. The thin wall of the latter passages become bubbled out into air sacs between the crisscrossing bands of smooth muscle. These air sacs are exactly like the terminal lung alveoli. A respiratory bronchiole will be seen in Fig. 22.10.

Alveolar Ducts   As the respiratory bronchioles are followed peripherally, each one branches into several incompletely circumscribed alveolar ducts. These are seen in Figs. 22.10 and 22.11. Each alveolar duct may have several branches. The walls of these channels are even more extensively ballooned out into air sacs than those of the respiratory bronchioles. Their interlacing diagonal bands of smooth muscle appear in sections as little knots of tissue.

Alveoli   The terminal subdivisions of the respiratory tract are the alveoli, or air sacs, the first of which are encountered as outpocketings of the respiratory bronchioles. Most alveoli occur in clusters opening from the alveolar ducts (Fig. 22.10). Small apertures in alveolar walls provide a few intercommunications between alveoli.

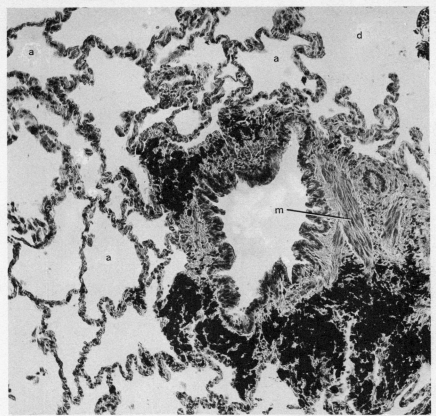

Figure 22-9 Bronchiole in a lung of a city dweller. Note the extensive deposition of carbon pigment in the peribronchial lymphatic tissue. Smooth muscle, *m*, is prominent. Numerous alveoli, *a*, and one alveolar duct, *d*, are shown. Distorted boundaries of the alveoli resulted from postmortem fixation of a piece of lung by immersion in formaldehyde solution. Photomicrograph, × 150.

In studying the alveoli in histologic sections of pieces of lung that collapsed when it was removed from the body, one must bear in mind that the walls appear to be somewhat folded, owing to the presence of elastic fibers in the surrounding stroma. In the lung during life, the alveoli are larger and have smoother, more even contours than in fixed preparations. The amount of elastic tissue in alveolar walls can be appreciated only by employing special elastic-tissue stains, after which the fibers appear as in Fig. 22.12.

The structure of the **interalveolar walls** is not easy to interpret from ordinary histologic sections. One can observe that these partitions are thin and that their principal component is an extensive capillary network, supported by some delicate stroma, rich in elastic fibers. Most of the cells seen in the interalveolar walls are endothelial cells of the capillaries. There are a few connective-tissue cells, such as fibrocytes and macrophages.

The structure of the walls has been clarified by electron microscopy.

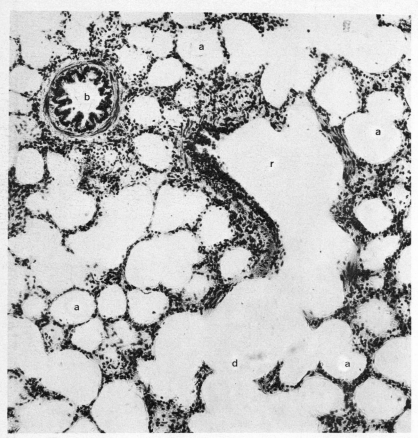

Figure 22-10 Lung of a human infant: small bronchiole, *b;* respiratory bronchiole, *r;* alveolar duct, *d;* alveoli, *a.* Note the ring of smooth muscle in the bronchiole and patches of smooth muscle in the alveolar ducts. Photomicrograph, × 150

Simple squamous epithelium on each side forms a complete lining; adjoining cells show tight junctions. Beneath this is a basal lamina and varying numbers of collagenous and elastic fibrils. In the middle are capillaries made up of non-fenestrated endothelium whose cells overlap. The endothelium has a basal lamina, frequently fused with that of the alveolar epithelium (Fig. 22.13).

The **air-blood barrier,** consisting of one-half of the interalveolar wall, is reduced in some places to the following elements: (1) a fluid film containing phospholipids; (2) the very thin alveolar epithelium; (3) basal lamina of the epithelium and that of the capillary endothelium, often fused; and (4) the non-fenestrated endothelium of the capillaries. Both epithelium and endothelium exhibit numerous pinocytotic vesicles, indicative of active movement of substances in solution across the barrier. The passage of gases probably occurs passively by simple diffusion.

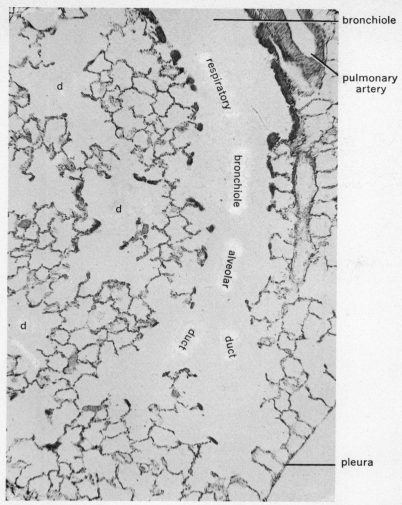

Figure 22-11 Lung of a cat showing continuity of bronchiole, respiratory bronchiole, branching alveolar duct, and many alveoli. The alveoli are the smallest openings. Other alveolar ducts, *d*, are present. Photomicrograph, × 50.

Three types of cell can be identified on the alveolar side. In addition to the thin epithelial **lining cells,** there are secretory great alveolar cells and alveolar macrophages.

The fine structure of the **great alveolar cells** is noteworthy (Fig. 22.14). Short microvilli occur on their free surface. Their cytoplasm contains agranular endoplasmic reticulum, well-developed golgi complex, lysosomes, and prominent multivesicular bodies that are sometimes seen in the process of extruding their contents into the alveolar cavity. The secretion of these cells contains

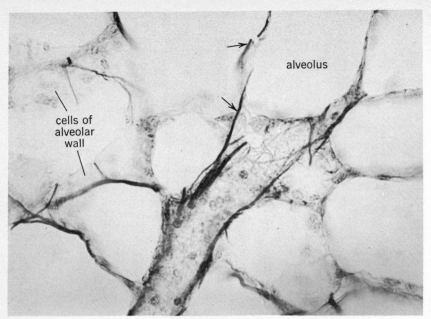

Figure 22-12 Expanded lung; thick section stained for elastic fibers (*arrow*) in the finest subdivisions of the pulmonary stroma. Photomicrograph, about × 450.

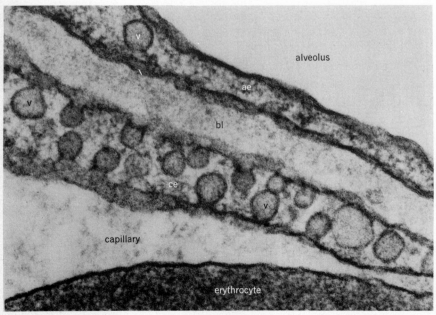

Figure 22-13 A section through the alveolar wall; capillary below, alveolus above. The capillary endothelium, *ce,* is separated from the alveolar epithelium, *ae,* by conjoined basal laminae, *bl;* note pinocytotic vesicles, *v.* Part of an erythrocyte is seen in the capillary. Electron micrograph, × 120,000. *(Contributed by E. R. Weibel.)*

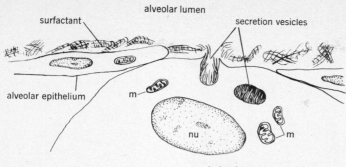

surfactant

alveolar lumen

secretion vesicles

alveolar epithelium

m

nu

m

m

great alveolar cell

Figure 22-14 Great alveolar cell in alveolar wall. Inclusion bodies are releasing their contents into alveolar lumen. Mitochondria, *m;* nucleus, *nu. (Modified from R. J. King.) (CHP)*

phospholipids and becomes part of a fluid coating of the alveoli, to which the name "surfactant" has been applied. Surfactant has a detergent property that tends to prevent cohesion of alveolar walls.

Alveolar macrophages are found in the interalveolar wall and occur as free cells in the alveolar lumen. Particulate matter that was not removed from the inspired air by mucus of the epithelial surface of trachea, bronchi, and bronchioles is phagocytized by these cells. Carbon particles are commonly seen in the macrophages of city dwellers and usually accumulate in the peribronchial lymphatic tissue, as seen in Fig. 22.9. Blood erythrocytes that enter lung alveoli in a certain type of heart disease are phagocytized; the swollen macrophages, filled with products of digestion of hemoglobin, may be seen in the sputum, being designated "heart-failure cells."

Blood Vessels, Lymphatic Vessels, and Nerves Blood of diminished oxygen content is brought to the lungs by the **pulmonary arteries** for aeration. Branches accompany the bronchial tree. The smallest pulmonary arterioles convey blood to the alveolar plexuses beginning at the level of alveolar ducts. **Pulmonary veins** take oxygenated blood back to the heart. Their tributaries do not accompany the bronchial tree, but course independently in the pulmonary stroma (Fig. 22.15).

Another system of arteries enters the lungs. These are the **bronchial arteries.** They arise from the aorta and supply the bronchi and the pleura with oxygenated blood. The blood carried by them may return by way of bronchial veins or may join that of the pulmonary veins.

Lymphatic vessels of the lung form two plexuses. Those coursing through the pleura form a superficial plexus. A deep plexus follows the course of the bronchial tree. There are a few communications between these two plexuses. Lymph nodes occur in the root of the lung. The afferent lymphatic vessels of these nodes come from both lymphatic plexuses. The efferent vessels from the lymph nodes enter the mediastinum.

There are no lymph capillaries in the walls of lung alveoli, but lymphatic

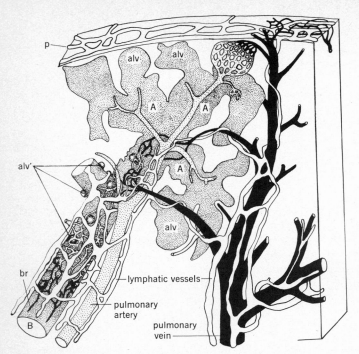

Figure 22-15 Schematic drawing of a primary pulmonary lobule (gray) in relation to blood and lymphatic vessels. Abbreviations: *A*, atria; *B*, bronchiole; *alv,* alveoli; *alv',* small alveolar buds in wall of respiratory bronchiole; *p*, pleura. The pulmonary artery and its branches are stippled; pulmonary veins and tributaries are black; bronchial artery on the respiratory bronchiole, *br*; lymphatic vessels are white. *(Redrawn from W. S. Miller.) (CHP)*

vessels do course in the stroma around the bronchioles. Tissue fluid in the delicate stroma between the alveolar epithelium and capillary endothelium diffuses into the trabecular lymphatic vessels.

Nerves course along the bronchial tree from the pulmonary plexus in the root of the lung. They are concerned mainly with motor innervation of the blood vessels and the bronchial musculature, but sensory nerve fibers also are present.

PLEURA

The lungs occupy closed pleural cavities in the chest which are lined with a serous membrane consisting of mesothelium resting on a basal lamina and a layer of fibrous connective tissue. The lungs are covered by an extension of this membrane known as the visceral pleura. That lining the cavities composes the parietal pleura. Should a pleural cavity become opened to the air, the lung of that side will collapse immediately. This condition is known as "pneumothorax."

Little **interstitial tissue** is seen in routinely prepared sections through the renal cortex, but there is an appreciable amount in the medulla. There, in addition to the usual connective-tissue elements, some elongated cells are closely applied to renal tubules. These cells have cytoplasmic microfilaments and lipid inclusions; their function has not been ascertained. The renal interstitial space contains water and solutes that are passing from renal tubules to the capillaries.

Lobulation is clearly indicated on the surface of the kidney at birth, but the lobes soon become fused, and are infrequently observed in the adult. The only regular indications of lobulation in the adult kidney are the projections of renal medullary substance into the renal sinus. Each projection forms a conical **renal papilla**, clasped by a minor calyx, into the lumen of which urine is emptied from openings of 10 to 20 papillary ducts.

Renal papillae are the apices of **renal pyramids**. Vertical sections through the pyramids have a striated appearance when viewed with the naked eye. The papillae and pyramids compose the medulla of the kidney. The base of each pyramid is parallel to the surface of the kidney, but it has a ragged border because stripes of its medullary substance extend into the cortex of the kidney, forming the **medullary rays**, seen in Fig. 23.3.

Each renal pyramid is completely surrounded by cortex, which reaches inward to the renal sinus, forming **renal columns** between adjacent pyramids. They are not actually columns, but regions of cortical substance surrounding the cones of medullary tissue. Portions of the cortical parenchyma between medullary rays compose the **cortical labyrinth** (Fig. 23.3).

Medullary rays and renal pyramids contain the straight portions of renal tubules and ducts, whereas the renal columns and the cortical labyrinth contain the convoluted tubules and renal corpuscles.

The Nephron The unit of renal structure corresponding to the secretory portion of a gland lobule is called a **nephron**. It consists of glomerular and tubular portions. The tubular portion of the nephron is further subdivided into proximal and distal segments, formed by simple columnar epithelium; these are joined by a thin middle segment, composed of simple squamous epithelium. The parts of three nephrons are illustrated diagrammatically in Fig. 23.4. There are more than 1 million nephrons in each human kidney.

The **glomerular capsule**[2] is a little sac of simple squamous epithelium, invaginated by a tuft of capillaries forming a glomerulus. The capsule and its glomerulus together form a small body about 0.2 mm in diameter, called the **renal corpuscle**.[3] A full complement of corpuscles is present in each kidney at birth, and none is added thereafter. In the fetus, the capsule has a wall formed by simple columnar epithelium, but after birth, when the kidney takes over the excretory function of the placenta, the capsular epithelium becomes flattened. It is possible to see the squamous lining of the capsule, but its reflection onto

[2]Commonly called "Bowman's capsule."
[3]Formerly designated "Malpighian corpuscle."

capsule

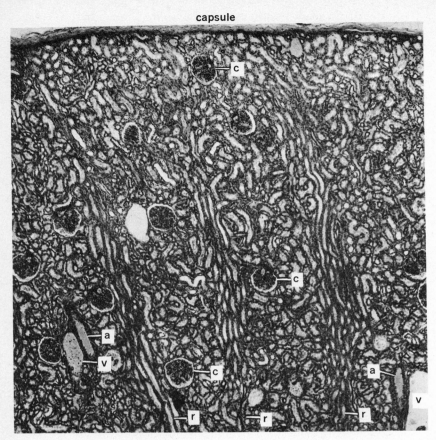

Figure 23-3 Human kidney: section through the labyrinth of the cortex and parts of three medullary rays, *r;* a number of renal corpuscles, *c*, interlobular arteries, *a*, and veins, *v*, can be seen. Photomicrograph, × 40.

the capillaries of the glomerulus is difficult to observe (Figs. 23.5 and 23.6). This part is spoken of as the visceral layer of the capsule. It is the renal filtration site where fluid from the blood, with solutes up to about 65,000 molecular weight, enters the capsular space.

The visceral layer of the capsule consists of thin epithelial cells with many basal processes, or feet, giving the cells the name **podocyte.** The processes, or "pedicles," of these cells are covered with a glycoprotein surface coat and rest on a prominent basal lamina. Gaps of 250 Å or more between the pedicles are bridged by extremely thin diaphragms of electron-dense material. On the other side of the basal lamina the capillary endothelium is fenestrated, with gaps of 500 Å or more between the cells. Figure 23.7 is a low-magnification electron micrograph of a glomerular lobule. It and Fig. 23.8 show these features.

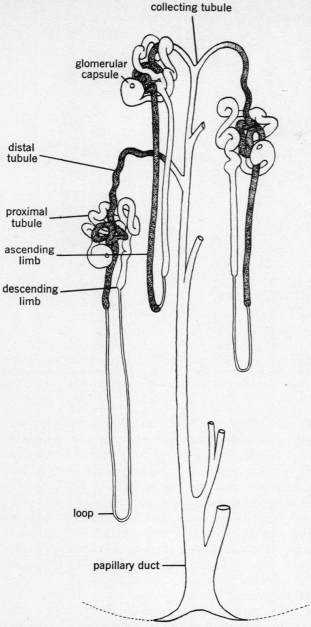

collecting tubule

glomerular
capsule

distal
tubule

proximal
tubule

ascending
limb

descending
limb

loop

papillary duct

Figure 23-4   Diagram of three nephrons, their collecting tubules and ducts. Distal tubules are stippled; other parts of the nephron are unshaded. *(Redrawn after G. C. Huber.)(MWS)*

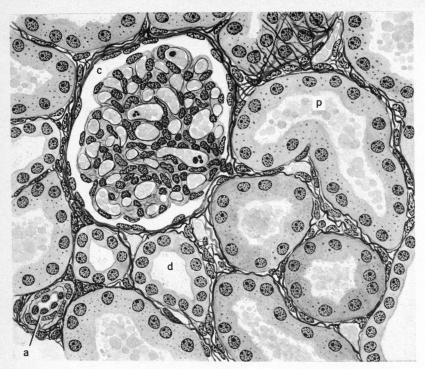

Figure 23-5 Renal corpuscle and tubules of a human kidney. The glomerulus is sectioned near its vascular pole; *a*, arteriole; *c*, exaggerated capsular space; *d*, distal convoluted tubule; *p*, proximal convoluted tubule. Reticular fibers of the renal stroma are stained. × 300. *(JFN)*

Each renal corpuscle has a vascular pole, where an afferent arteriole enters and an efferent arteriole leaves the glomerulus, and a tubular pole, where the lumen of the capsule becomes confluent with that of the proximal tubule. The confluence can be seen in Fig. 23.6. Not more than one in ten sections of a renal corpuscle cut 10 μm thick will show the tubular pole.

The **renal tubule** begins at a glomerular capsule, pursues a tortuous course through the cortical labyrinth near its corpuscle, and then enters an adjacent medullary ray to form a long straight-sided loop in the medulla. Returning to the site of its corpuscle in the cortical labyrinth, it engages in another, smaller series of convolutions before joining a collecting tubule. Three parts of the renal tubule are distinguishable on the basis of its course, namely, the proximal convoluted tubule, the distal convoluted tubule, and the loop, as shown in Fig. 23.4. The collecting tubule also is part of the functional nephron because urine concentration occurs in it as it passes through the medulla.

The **proximal convoluted tubule** composes nearly half the length of the entire nephron. Because of its great tortuosity in the neighborhood of the glomerular capsule from which it arises, a section through the cortical labyrinth

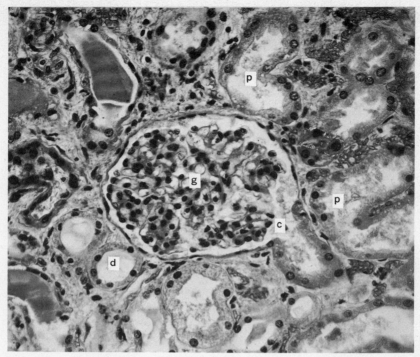

Figure 23-6 Renal corpuscle and tubules of a human kidney. The glomerulus is sectioned through its tubular pole, *c*, where the glomerular capsule joins a proximal convoluted tubule; *d*, distal convoluted tubule; *g*, glomerulus; *p*, proximal convoluted tubule. Photomicrograph, × 300.

always traverses it many times. The straight portion of the proximal tubule, spoken of as its medullary segment, passes into a medullary ray to begin the descending limb of the loop.

The proximal convoluted tubule is the thickest part of the nephron. Its columnar epithelium consists of wide cells with a high brush border on the free surface (Fig. 23.9). The brush border is formed by tall, closely packed microvilli. Pinocytotic vesicles are numerous at the base of the villi (Fig. 23.10). Junctional complexes, including tight junctions, are encountered at places where cells adjoin.

The epithelium stands on a distinct basal lamina separating its cells from the fenestrated endothelium of capillaries. The basal border of the epithelial cells is deeply folded, and many elongated mitochondria are present therein. Intercellular boundaries are indistinct under the light microscope, but electron micrographs reveal extensive interdigitating folds. About four-fifths of the glomerular filtrate is reabsorbed in the proximal convoluted tubule, passing from it into the interstitial spaces and thence to the capillaries.

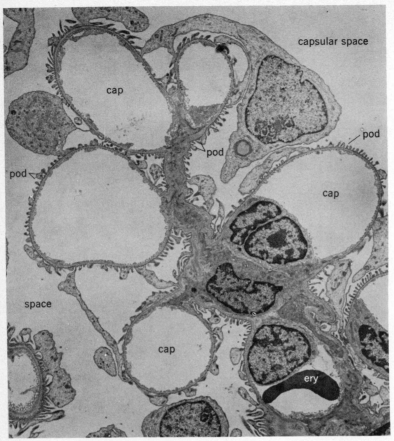

Figure 23-7 A lobule of a glomerulus (rat) showing capillaries, *cap*, distended by the perfusion fluid; one contains an erythrocyte, *ery*. Processes of podocytes, *pod*, are seen between capillaries and capsular space, *space*. Electron micrograph × 4,650. *(Contributed by H. Latta, Journal of Ultrastructure Research, vol. 45, pp. 149–167, 1973. Reproduced with permission of the publishers.)*

The **thin segment** of the **loop**[4] usually passes downward for a variable distance from the medullary segment of the proximal tubule. When it is associated with a renal corpuscle located in the outer part of the cortex, it is short. Nephrons with corpuscles lying near the base of a pyramid have long, thin segments which may extend almost to the apex of the pyramid, bend sharply there, and then return for some distance as the ascending limb of the loop. Cross sections of thin segments can be seen in Fig. 23.11

[4]This is known as "Henle's loop."

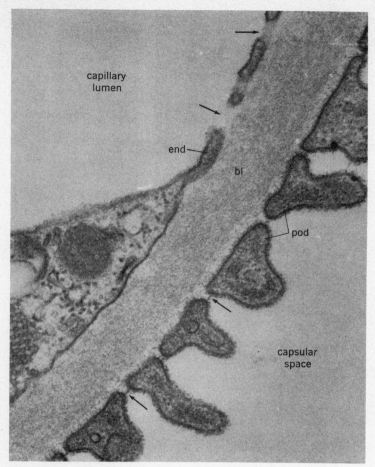

Figure 23-8 Relation of glomerular capillary to glomerular capsular space. The capillary endothelium, *end*, is fenestrated *(left arrows)*. Processes of podocytes, *pod*, are connected by electron-dense membranes *(right arrows)*. The basal lamina, *bl*, between the endothelium and podocytes has a filamentous appearance; its mesial substance is darker than its outer borders. Electron micrograph × 75,000. *(Contributed by H. Latta, Journal of Ultrastructure Research, vol. 32, pp. 526–544, 1970. Reproduced with permission of the publishers.)*

The thin segment is formed by simple squamous epithelium, consisting of cells appreciably thicker than those of the fenestrated endothelium lining adjacent capillaries. Although the tubular epithelium may be reduced in thickness gradually as the descending segment is formed, the fine structure of its cells changes abruptly. The cells lose the brush border and basal cytoplasmic striations. Surface microvilli become few and short.

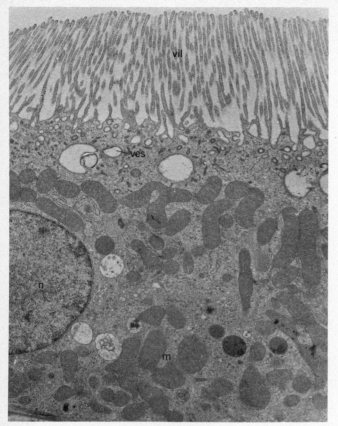

Figure 23-9 Proximal convoluted tubule. Part of one cell with a brush border composed of microvilli, *vil.* Note pinocytotic vesicles, *ves;* invaginations at the base of microvilli; mitochondria, *m;* and nucleus, *n.* Electron micrograph, × 12,000. *(Contributed by W. H. Johnston and H. Latta.)*

The **thick segment** of the ascending limb of the loop (Fig. 23.12) has low columnar epithelial cells with marked interdigitations and tight junctions. The cytoplasm contains numerous mitochondria. This segment extends as far as the macula densa, after which it becomes the distal convoluted tubule. The thick ascending limb is known also as the "diluting segment of the distal nephron."

The upper part of the thick segment of the loop makes contact with the juxtaglomerular portion of the afferent and efferent arterioles at the vascular pole of the capsule. The epithelial cells of the tubule there become taller, forming a **macula densa** (Fig. 23.15).

The distal convoluted tubule displays some structural differences in its

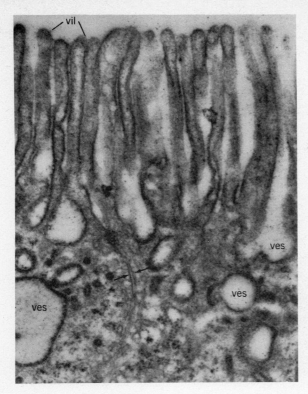

Figure 23-10 Parts of two cells of a proximal convoluted tubule with a deep brush border composed of long microvilli, *vil*. The cell boundaries are marked by arrows. Prominent vesicles, *ves*, are in continuity with spaces between microvilli. Electron micrograph, × 25,000. *(Contributed by D. Pease.)*

early and late course. The first part of the distal tubule is formed by low simple columnar epithelium, the cells of which are smaller and narrower than those of the proximal tubule. Their nuclei are close together, and their intercellular boundaries are slightly more distinct in routinely stained sections than those of the proximal-tubule cells. The cytoplasm usually appears lighter.

The cells of distal tubules display basal processes packed with mitochondria (Fig. 23.13). Their lateral borders also show extensive folds, increasing the cellular surface area considerably. The free border has only short microvilli. These become more numerous near the terminal end of the tubule, and pinocytotic vesicles appear there. The seond or late part of the distal convoluted tubule is structurally similar to the collecting tubule.

Because the convoluted portion of the distal tubule is considerably shorter than that of the proximal tubule, sections divide it into fewer pieces. The lumen is wider than that of the proximal tubule. One or two pieces usually are seen near the vascular pole of the renal corpuscle (Figs. 23.5 and 23.6).

The first part of the **collecting tubule** consists of a short arched segment passing directly from the cortical labyrinth into a medullary ray. There it

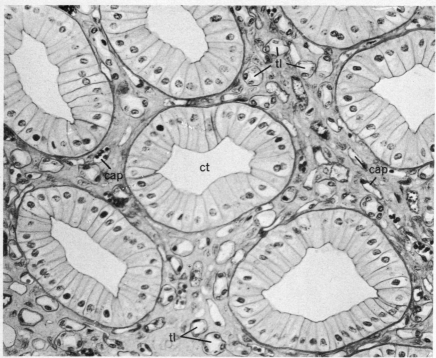

Figure 23-11 Inner zone of the medulla of a rabbit kidney sectioned across a renal papilla and stained with iron hematoxylin. Large ducts are collecting tubules, *ct;* small ducts are thin limbs of nephron loops, *tl,* and blood capillaries, *cap;* some of the latter are identified by dark-stained erythrocytes inside. Photomicrograph, × 600.

becomes a straight collecting tubule, descending into the pyramid among the straight portions of the nephrons. As it approaches the renal papillae, it is joined by other collecting tubules and increases in diameter from about 40 to 200 μm. The largest collecting tubules join **papillary ducts** which open into minor calyces on the apex of the renal papillae.

Collecting tubules are formed by low simple columnar epithelium (Fig. 23.13). Cell boundaries and basal laminae are distinct. The cells increase in height in the larger tubules and become tall as they reach the papillary ducts. The term "distal nephron" is used to designate the several segments begin-ning with the thick ascending (diluting) portion of the loop.

Renal Blood Vessels Approximately 1,300 ml of blood flow through the two kidneys of an adult person each minute. This amounts to nearly one-fourth of the total cardiac output. The **renal artery** forms branches in the renal sinus, and these give rise to **interlobar arteries** passing into the kidney through the

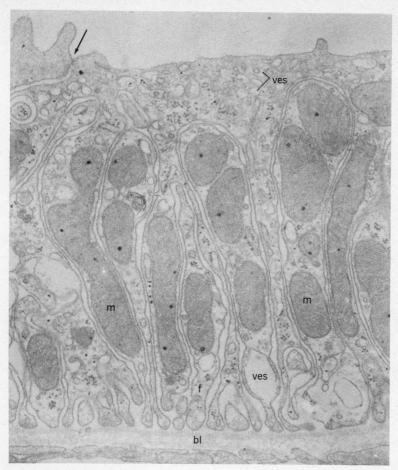

Figure 23-12 Thick segment of the descending limb of the nephron loop. Part of a cell showing marked foldings, *f*, of the plasmolemma, and many mitochondria, *m*. Note the vesicles, *ves*, beneath the free surface and in the basal folds. An arrow indicates tight junction with an adjacent cell. The basal lamina, *bl*, is prominent. Electron micrograph, × 28,500. *(Contributed by H. Latta.)*

renal columns of cortical substance surrounding the renal papillae. Each interlobar artery runs straight toward the surface of the kidney but ends abruptly in a spray of terminal branches at the level of the bases of the renal pyramids. Its terminal branches curve away from the parent stem and course parallel to the surface of the kidney as **arcuate arteries**. The arcuate branches of one interlobar artery do not anastomose with those of another interlobar artery.

The arcuate arteries give rise to many branches that come off at right

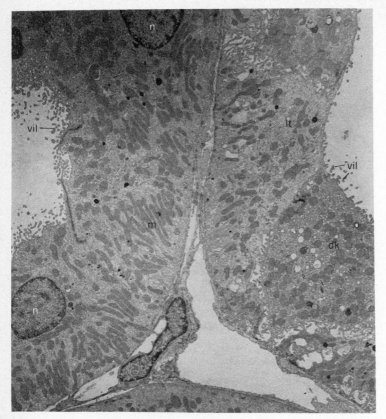

Figure 23-13 Portions of distal convoluted tubule (left) and collecting tubule (right), the latter containing light, *lt,* and dark, *dk,* cells. Note the short microvilli, *vil,* and numerous long mitochondria, *m,* in the distal tubule. Nuclei, *n,* are seen in the distal tubule. Electron micrograph, × 5,000. *(Contributed by W. H. Johnston and H. Latta.)*

angles and pass straight toward the surface of the kidney in the substance of the cortical labyrinth, one between each two medullary rays, as a rule. These branches of the arcuate arteries are called **interlobular arteries**. They should not be confused with the larger interlobar arteries.

Each interlobular artery, like the trunk of a tree, gives off numerous lateral branches, the **afferent glomerular arterioles**. Interlobular arteries are so numerous in the cortex that their afferent glomerular arterioles need not course far before entering the vascular pole of a renal corpuscle (Fig. 23.14).

At the vascular pole of each corpuscle, the afferent glomerular arteriole divides into four or five branches, each dividing again to form a series of anastomosing capillary loops in the glomerulus. These capillaries then recombine

1

2

3

4

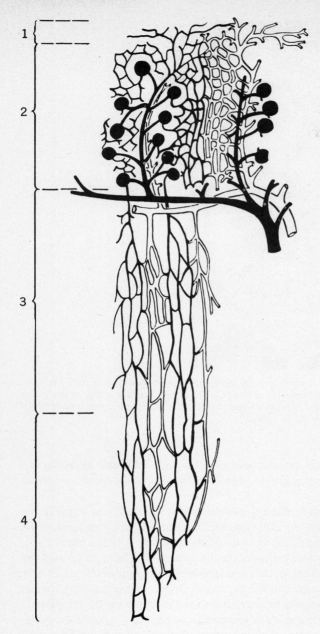

Figure 23-14 Diagram of the kidney cortex and medulla. Arteries and capillaries on arterial side are black; veins and capillaries on venous side are white; *1,* fibrous capsule; *2,* cortex; *3,* outer zone of medulla; *4,* inner zone of medulla. *(Redrawn from A. A. Maximow and W. Bloom.) (MWS)*

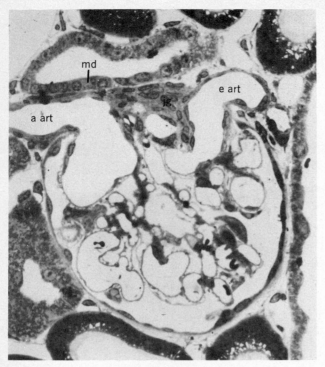

Figure 23-15 Juxtaglomerular complex in a rat kidney. A mass of juxtaglomerular cells, *jg,* lies at the hilum of the glomerulus between afferent, *a art,* and efferent, *e art,* arterioles. The mass of cells is also adjacent to the macula densa, *md,* of the distal convoluted tubule. Photomicrograph, ×600. *(Contributed by H. Latta.)*

and leave the vascular pole as another arteriole, the **efferent glomular arteriole**—not a venule, as one might expect. This vessel has a smaller caliber than the afferent arteriole.

The walls of afferent and efferent glomerular arterioles, just outside the glomerular capsule adjacent to the macula densa, assume an endocrine glandular appearance. The epithelioid cells of their media contain membrane-bounded secretion granules and a distinct golgi complex. These cells and the adjacent macula densa constitute the **juxtaglomerular complex** (Fig. 23.15), which is believed to be the source of the hormone, renin. The latter functions in the elaboration of angiotensin and in secretion of aldosterone by the suprarenal cortex. The juxtaglomerular complex is thought to be part of a feedback mechanism in autoregulation of the rate of glomerular filtration, renal blood flow, and systemic blood pressure.

As soon as the efferent arteriole leaves the glomerulus, it breaks up into another series of capillaries, forming a network around tubular portions of the nephron in the renal labyrinth and medullary rays. A reticular stroma supports this capillary bed.

The renal pyramids are supplied by capillary networks arising from the efferent arterioles of glomeruli nearest the medulla. The capillary bed around tubular loops in the medulla is less torturous than that around the convoluted tubules in the cortical labyrinth. All parts of the renal tubule are supplied by blood, at reduced pressure, that has already traversed the filtration units of the kidney, i.e., the renal glomeruli.

The interlobular, arcuate, and interlobar arteries are accompanied by veins bearing the same names. Tributaries of the interlobular veins are venules draining the capillary bed of the cortex. Straight venules collect blood from the capillaries of the medulla and are tributaries of the arcuate veins (Fig. 23.14). Thus it is probable that blood traversing some of the glomeruli nearest the medulla does not reach the capillaries of either proximal or distal convoluted tubules.

Renal Function   Urine formation involves glomerular filtration from the blood, reabsorption of water and some solutes from the filtrate, and selective secretion by tubular epithelial cells. The daily turnover of water and essential electrolytes is indicated in Table 23.1.

The process begins in the renal corpuscle. Renal arteries are large, short, direct branches of the abdominal aorta, conveying blood to the kidney. Even after traversing their many branches, the blood reaches the renal glomerulus with a capillary pressure sufficiently high to maintain the process of ultrafiltration at a rate of approximately 125 ml per minute in the two kidneys. This process takes place at the blood-capsular barrier consisting of fenestrated capillary endothelium, basal lamina, and capsular epithelium formed by podocytes. The elements involved are illustrated in Fig. 23.16. Water and solutes of molecular weights less than about 65,000 pass across the barrier. The capillary blood retains its cells, platelets, chylomicrons, plasma proteins, and other large molecules, with enough water to flush them into the efferent arterioles.

Table 23.1 Daily Turnover of Water and Principal Essential Electrolytes in Adult Human Beings

Substance	Amount filtered,* mEq/day	Amount excreted,* mEq/day	Amount reabsorbed,* mEq/day	Proportion reabsorbed, %
H_2O	180	1.5	178.5	99.2
Na^+	25,000	150.0	24,850.0	99.4
HCO_3^-	4,500	2.0	4,498.0	99.9
Cl^-	18,000	150.0	17,850.0	99.2

*Water is given in liters per day.

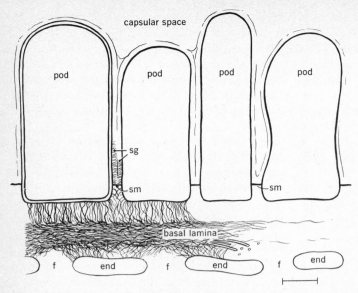

Figure 23-16 Diagrammatic representation of the elements involved in glomerular filtration. The filtration pathway involves capillary endothelium, *end*, and its fenestrations, *f;* trilayered basal lamina; surface glycocalyx, *sg,* of the podocyte processes, *pod,* and their silt membranes, *sm:* and capsular space. The marker indicates 1000 Å. *(Modified from H. Latta.)*

The glomerular filtrate enters the proximal convoluted tubule, and there the process of reabsorption, essential for maintenance of homeostasis, begins. Glucose and sodium ions are transported actively through the tubular epithelial cells (not between cells), all the former and about 80 percent of the latter being conserved. Water and chloride ions are transported passively across the tubular wall into the interstitial spaces. A small amount of urea is reabsorbed, but most of it and other nitrogenous metabolic waste products do not leave the tubule.

The process of reabsorption continues in the descending limb of the tubular loop. There, more of the water leaves, and the fluid in the lumen becomes more concentrated. Toward the bottom of the loop in the renal medulla, salt concentration increases, both within the tubule and outside it in the interstitial spaces. Thus, a salinity gradient is established through which the loop of the nephron passes, making possible the movement of water into the interstitial spaces while keeping metabolic waste products inside the lumen.

The hypertonic state of the renal interstitial substance is believed to be produced by a sodium-pumping action of epithelial cells in the ascending limb of the loop. However, water is not lost from that part of the nephron, so there is a gradual shifting from hypertonicity to hypotonicity toward the distal convoluted tubule.

Water passes out of the nephron again in the distal convoluted and collecting tubules. Its transport through the epithelial cells is controlled by the antidiuretic hormone, vasopressin, which is produced and secreted by cells of the hypothalamus and released in the neurohypophysis. The final step in urine formation, then, occurs in collecting tubules in the medulla where water passes into the interstitial space while salts are retained in the lumen.

A number of substances of high molecular weight, that cannot enter the renal capsule but must be eliminated from the body, find their way into the urine. Tubular secretion supplements the processes of ultrafiltration and reabsorption. These substances include certain drugs, excess hormones, and some vitamins.

One should not think of the kidneys as simply waste-removing organs. They are regulatory organs that actively conserve water and essential solutes to maintain the constancy of the internal environment, i.e., homeostasis.

The kidneys are vital organs, but an individual can thrive with only one. Knowledge of renal function and structure, technical advances in vascular surgery, and an appreciation of the role of the immune system have greatly advanced the conquest of renal diseases. Successful employment of peritoneal dialysis, use of the "artificial kidney," and perfection of kidney transplantation from one person to another are among the great accomplishments in medical science during the last two decades.

RENAL DUCTS

The duct of the kidney is the **ureter** with its expanded proximal end, the **renal pelvis**. The **calyces** clasping the papillae are extensions of the renal pelvis. The ureters terminate by passing diagonally through the wall of the urinary bladder. The walls of the several parts of the renal duct are of similar structure, consisting of three tunics, the mucosa, muscularis, and adventitia.

The mucous membrane is lined with transitional epithelium, several cells thick. The lamina propria, beneath this, merges directly with the fibrous connective tissue among the bundles of smooth muscle of the middle coat. It contains no glands, and there is no submucosa. In the ureter, the mucous membrane is thrown into longitudinal folds, imparting a stellate appearance to its lining in cross sections (Fig. 23.17).

The muscular coat consists of inner longitudinal and outer circular layers—just the opposite of the arrangement of the muscularis of the digestive organs. Near the bladder, an accessory outer longitudinal layer is added to the wall. In the calyces, the circular muscle is thick. Both layers are well developed in the renal pelvis, but the longitudinal layer consists only of scattered bundles throughout most of the ureter. The muscularis of the renal calyces and pelvis undergoes peristaltic contractions squeezing the urine on into the ureters. The well-developed longitudinal layer at the lower end of the ureter tends to maintain the integrity of the ureteral orifice in the bladder.

The adventitia of the ureter consists of fibrous connective tissue containing blood vessels, lymphatics, and nerves. A considerable quantity of adipose tissue is found around it in the renal sinus.

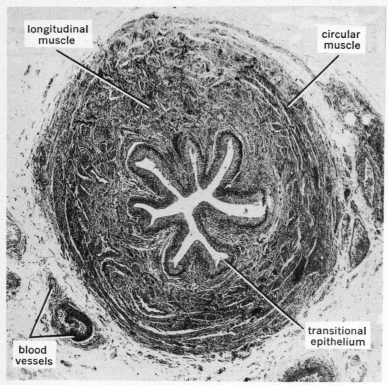

Figure 23-17   Human ureter. Photomicrograph, × 40.

URINARY BLADDER

Although the urinary bladder (vesica urinaria) has a structure much like that of the ureter, its wall is thicker, mainly because of an increase in smooth muscle (Fig. 23.18). Its appearance varies with the degree of distention of the bladder.

The mucous membrane of the empty bladder is thrown into heavy folds, and its transitional epithelium may be six or eight cells thick. When greatly distended, the bladder has only two or three layers of cells in its epithelium, and the surface cells are flattened (Fig. 3.10). The lamina propria is loose and contains many elastic fibers and small blood vessels. It, too, is capable of accommodation to changing conditions in the bladder.

The muscularis has three layers. The muscle fibers of the inner and outer layers run parallel to each other. The middle layer is thickest, and its fibers run at right angles to those of the inner and outer layers. Much loose fibrous connective tissue separating the muscle bundles permits them to shift during filling and emptying. An internal **urinary sphincter** muscle is present at the place where the urethra begins.

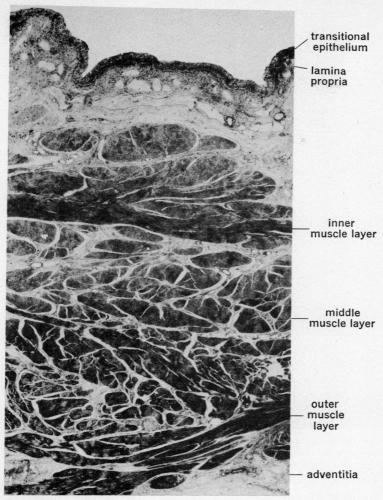

transitional epithelium

lamina propria

inner muscle layer

middle muscle layer

outer muscle layer

adventitia

Figure 23-18 Human urinary bladder: contracted state. Photomicrograph, × 20.

The adventitia, or outer coat of the bladder, contains the largest blood vessels, lymphatic vessels, and nerves. Part of the bladder is covered by mesothelium of the peritoneum.

URETHRA

The urethra is a duct connecting the lower end of the bladder with the exterior. It is much shorter in the female than in the male, measuring only about 3 or 4 cm in length. The female urethra presents a structure of no great complexity. It is illustrated in Fig. 23.19.

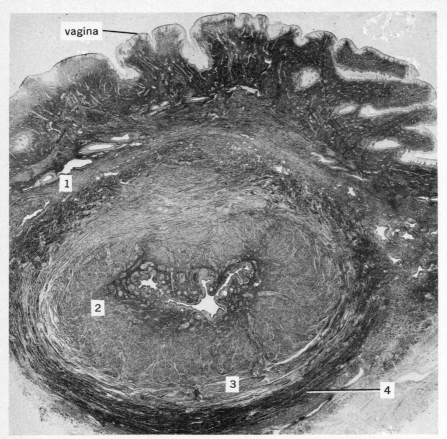

Figure 23-19 Human female urethra (below) and anterior wall of the vagina (above), sectioned at the level of the urogenital diaphragm; connective-tissue stain. The adventitia of the vagina and urethra join at *1;* the inner longitudinal and outer circular smooth-muscle layers are shown at *2* and *3;* the sphincter of skeletal muscle is seen, darkly stained, at *4*. Photomicrograph, × 10.

The mucous membrane, like that of other large ducts reaching the body surface, has an epithelium that changes to stratified squamous near its orifice. Stratified or pseudostratified columnar epithelium may be present just before the stratified squamous epithelium begins. Elsewhere the epithelium is the same transitional type as that of the bladder.

The mucous membrane of the female urethra is folded longitudinally, and there is an especially prominent fold posteriorly. A few small urethral glands of the tubuloacinous type secrete mucus. Some of them empty into little epithelial pockets. All the glands of the female urethra are homologous with those of the prostate in the male. The lamina propria of the female urethra resembles that of the bladder, with which it is continuous. It does not form a true corpus spongiosum, as does that of the male urethra.

The muscularis of the urethra is formed by prominent inner longitudinal and outer circular layers, separated by a venous plexus. The circular muscle forms an internal sphincter at the junction of the urethra with the bladder. An external sphincter of skeletal muscle is present at the lower end of the urethra, as shown in Fig. 23.19.

The adventitia contains blood vessels, lymphatics, and nerves coursing in fibrous connective tissue, continuous with that of the surrounding perineum.

The structure of the male urethra differs considerably from that of the female, because it is incorporated into the penis. Its glands have undergone extensive development, and on occasion it serves as a genital passage. Consequently it is described in Chap. 25.

SUGGESTED READING

Barajas, L.: The Ultrastructure of the Juxtaglomerular Apparatus as Disclosed by Three-dimensional Reconstructions from Serial Sections. *Journal of Ultrastructural Research*, vol. 33, pp. 116–147, 1970.

Brenner, B. M. (chairman): Symposium on Renal Handling of Sodium. *Federation Proceedings*, vol. 33, pp. 13–36, 1974.

Hamburger, J., G. Richet, and J. P. Grünfeld: *Structure and Function of the Kidney*. W. B. Saunders Company, Philadelphia, 1971.

Latta, H.: The Glomerular Capillary Wall. *Journal of Ultrastructure Research*, vol. 32, pp. 526–544, 1970.

McGiff, J. C., K. Crowshaw, and H. D. Itskovitz: Prostaglandins and Renal Function. *Federation Proceedings*, vol. 33, pp. 39–47, 1974.

Osvaldo, L., and H. Latta: The Thin Limb of the Loop of Henle. *Journal of Ultrastructure Research*, vol. 15, pp. 144–168, 1966.

Parker, M. V., H. G. Swann, and J. G. Sinclair: The Functional Morphology of the Kidney. *Texas Reports on Biology and Medicine*, vol. 20, pp. 425–445, 1962.

Pease, D. C.: Fine Structure of the Kidney as Seen by Electron Microscopy. *Journal of Histochemistry and Cytochemistry*, vol. 3, pp. 295–308, 1955.

Pitts, R. F.: *Physiology of the Kidney; An Introductory Text*. Year Book Medical Publishers, Chicago, 1968.

Valtin, H.: *Renal Function: Mechanisms Preserving Fluid and Solute Balance in Health*. Little, Brown and Company, Boston, 1973.

Wearn, J. T., and A. N. Richards: Observations on the Composition of Glomerular Urine, with Particular Reference to the Problem of Reabsorption in the Renal Tubules. *American Journal of Physiology*, vol. 71, pp. 209–227, 1924.

Endocrine System

Regulation of body functions is effected by the nervous and endocrine systems, both of which respond to changes in the external and internal environments, pervading nearly all tissues to transmit appropriate messages from one region to another. The nervous system carries messages with great speed. Transmission in the endocrine system is relatively slow, because transmitting substances depend on circulation through the blood rather than being sped along nerve fibers.

HORMONES

Cells of the endocrine system secrete chemical substances which, as a rule, pass directly into the surrounding interstitial spaces and capillaries. The substances, called **hormones**, are the factors that convey information to specific sites of action.

Hormones are present in the blood in varying amounts and are accessible to any and all tissues as they circulate, but in most cases they influence some specific "target" organ and do not affect all indiscriminately. Thus an endocrine organ may be related to some other endocrine or nonendocrine organ for which it serves as a regulator. The amount of circulating hormone can be controlled by feedback influences from the target organs as well as by stimuli from the environment through the nervous system.

There are three main categories of hormone. One is secreted by gland cells in response to a chemical stimulus (e.g., from another hormone); another is secreted by gland cells in response to nerve impulses (e.g., in the suprarenal medulla); the third is secreted by nerve cells (e.g., in the hypothalamus).

Several types of activity are regulated by hormones. Stimulation or inhibition of smooth-muscle contraction, control of metabolic functions, and regulation of growth and development are examples. The responses to some hormones are relatively quick. Others, however, such as the growth hormone, exert prolonged or continuous control over many tissues.

CYCLIC NUCLEOTIDES AND PROSTAGLANDINS

Mediation of hormonal stimulation is effected in the specific receptor sites by certain nucleotides. One of these, adenosine 3',5'-monophosphate, is known as **cyclic AMP**. Another, present in lesser amounts, is guanosine 3',5'-monophosphate, or **cyclic GMP**. These two components appear to interact antithetically in regulating such events as glycogen synthesis—glycogen breakdown. These nucleotides are not hormones, but have been called "second messengers."

Other mediators of hormonal action are fatty-acid substances, known as **prostaglandins.**[1] These appear to be derived from phospholipids in the plasma membranes of cells. The richest source of them is the seminal vesicles. Specific prostaglandins have been found in many human tissues.

Prostaglandins also may be considered as true hormones, for they circulate in the blood to specific action sites. Some have been found to stimulate contraction of smooth muscle of the gravid uterus, for example. They are involved in energy transfer by affecting the concentration of cyclic AMP at the cell.

NONSPECIFIC ENDOCRINE ORGANS

Organs of the endocrine system are formed by or derived from epithelium. The classical endocrine or "ductless" glands are sources of many of the better-known hormones, but they are not the only organs of the endocrine system in which hormones are formed. Table 24.1 lists a number of organs and the hormones they are known to secrete. Some have been mentioned in preceding chapters, and others will be discussed in later ones. Primary emphasis in the present chapter is given to the hypothalamus, hypophysis, pancreas, parathyroid glands, pineal gland, suprarenal glands, and thyroid gland. The testes and

---

[1]These substances are found in semen and were once thought to be secreted by the prostate gland; hence, the name prostaglandin.

Table 24.1 Organs of the Endocrine System and Their Secretions

Organ	Hormone	Function
Brain (hypothalamus)	(a) Releasing factors (RF)	Stimulate release of hormones of anterior hypophysis
	(b) Inhibiting factor (IF)	Inhibits, e.g., secretion of prolactin by anterior hyphophysis
	(c) Oxytocin	Stimulates contraction of uterine muscle, milk ejection
	(d) Vasopressin (ADH)	Stimulates reabsorption of water by renal tubules
Duodenum	(a) Secretin	Stimulates exocrine pancreatic secretion
	(b) Cholecystokinin	Stimulates release of bile
	(c) Enterogastrone	Inhibits gastric secretion
Hypophysis (anterior lobe)	(a) Growth hormone (GSH)	Stimulates bodily growth
	(b) Adrenocorticotropic hormone (ACTH)	Stimulates secretion of suprarenal glucocortical hormones
	(c) Thyroid-stimulating hormone (TSH)	Stimulates secretion of thyroid hormones
	(d) Follicle-stimulating hormone (FSH)	Stimulates ovarian follicle development, testicular tubule development
	(e) Lutenizing hormone (LH) (ICSH)	Stimulates ovulation, corpus luteum development, estrogen and progesterone secretion, testosterone secretion
	(f) Melanocyte-stimulating hormone (MSH)	Stimulates melanocyte expansion
	(g) Prolactin	Stimulates and maintains milk secretion
Hypophysis (posterior lobe)	Storage site for: (a) oxytocin; (b) vasopressin	See Brain, above
Kidney	(a) Renin	Stimulates suprarenal cortex (aldosterone)
	(b) Erythropoietin	Stimulates erythropoiesis in bone marrow
Ovary	(a) Estrogens	Stimulate development of female secondary sexual characteristics, stimulate periodic hypertrophy of endometrinum, inhibit secretion of FSH
	(b) Progesterone	Stimulates development of female secondary sexual characteristics, stimulates uterine glandular development, maintains endometrium, inhibits LH and FSH
	(c) Relaxin	Stimulates relaxation of pelvic ligaments.

Pancreas (islands)	(a) Insulin	Stimulates reduction of blood-glucose level, stimulates carbohydrate storage by cells
	(b) Glucagon	Stimulates conversion of liver glycogen to glucose (raising blood-sugar level)
Parathyroid gland	Parathormone	Regulates metabolism of calcium and phosphorus
Pineal gland	"Melatonin"	Regulates other endocrine regulators
Placenta	(a) Gonadotropic hormones	Mimic adenohypophyseal hormones
	(b) Relaxin	Stimulates relaxation of pelvic ligaments
Stomach	(a) Gastrin	Stimulates exocrine pancreatic secretion
	(b) Enteroglucagon	See Pancreas above
Suprarenal cortex	(a) Glucocorticoid hormones	Stimulate glycogen formation, maintenance of normal blood-sugar levels
	(b) Mineralocorticoid hormones	Regulate sodium-potassium metabolism
	(c) Adrenosterone	Stimulates secondary sexual characteristics
Suprarenal medulla	(a) Epinephrine	Augments actions of sympathetic nervous system; increases blood-sugar levels
	(b) Norepinephrine	Stimulates vasoconstriction
Testis	Testosterone	Stimulates development of male secondary sexual characteristics
Thymus	Thymosin	Stimulates formation of lymphocytes in lymphatic tissue
Thyroid gland	(a) Thyroxine, triiodothyronine	Stimulate oxydative metabolism
	(b) Calcitonin	Inhibits excessive blood-calcium rise

ovaries are described in Chaps. 25 and 26. Some nonspecific endocrine organs are the thymus, gastrointestinal mucosa, kidneys, skin, and the fetal placenta.

Thymic epithelial cells secrete **thymosin** (Chap. 13), a hormone that stimulates formation of lymphocytes in lymphatic tissues. Production of it appears to be regulated by a hormone from the adenohypophysis.

Several hormones are formed in the mucosa of the gastrointestinal tract (Chap. 20). The enterochromaffin (argentaffin) cells, of which as many as five varieties have been identified by electron microscopy and histochemical techniques, appear to secrete them. **Gastrin** and **secretin**, stimulating secretion of the exocrine pancreas; **enteroglucagon,** stimulating conversion of liver glycogen to glucose; **cholecystokinin,** stimulating release of bile; and **enterogastrone**, inhibiting gastric secretion, have been identified as the main gastrointestinal hormones. The enterochromaffin cells are thought also to synthesize certain catecholamines.

The kidneys are the site of formation of hormones. **Renin,** secreted by the juxtaglomerular cells (Chap. 23), acts on a substrate in the blood to form **angiotensin** which stimulates the suprarenal cortex to increase production of the hormone, aldosterone. **Erythropoietin** is another hormone of renal origin (or perhaps stored in the kidneys). Its function is the initiation and regulation of erythropoiesis in the bone marrow.

Vitamin D is synthesized by cells of the epidermis when stimulated by ultraviolet light. A product of it, affecting specific target organs through circulation in the blood, may be considered a hormone.

Hormones are formed in the reproductive organs, both male and female. In addition, the fetal part of the placenta is a site of hormone synthesis (Chap. 26).

HYPOTHALAMUS

That neurons can secrete should not be surprising because they are modified epithelial cell derivatives. Most of them produce neurohumoral transmitter substances that are released at synapses from the presynaptic microvesicles in the endings of axonal telodendria (Chap. 14). The transmitter substances are not hormones, for they act locally and do not circulate in the blood stream. Some neurons, however, do secrete hormones. They are found particularly in the hypothalamus.

The hypothalamus composes the ventral portion of the diencephalon. It forms the floor and lateral walls of the third brain ventricle. Its components are the optic chiasm, mamillary bodies, tuber cinereum, funnel-shaped infundibulum, and the neurohypophysis (Fig. 24.1). Several groups of neurons in the hypothalamus compose the neuroendocrine nuclei. Synaptic connections by other neurons of the brain put them in touch with impulses from the environment.

The hypothalamic relationship to the hypophysis is close, not only anatomically, but also functionally. The hormones of the former can pass into the

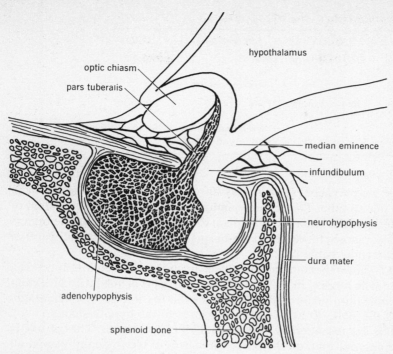

Figure 24-1 The hypothalamus and hypophysis, and their relation to the skull. *(CHP)*

latter where they are either stored (neurohypophysis) or directly affect secretion of other endocrine cells (adenohypophysis). The principal hormones stored in the neural lobe of the hypophysis are secreted by nerve cells in the supraoptic and paraventricular nuclei of the hypothalamus and transported through the axons.

Other hormones of the hypothalamus are known as **releasing factors** and **inhibiting factors.** They are secreted by collections of small nerve cells of the hypothalamus and transported through their axons to a network of capillaries and venules at the base of the hypothalamus composing the hypophysioportal system into which the secretions pass. A separate releasing or inhibiting factor has been found for each of the seven principal hormones secreted by the adenohypophysis. Figure 24.1 diagrammatically illustrates relations of the hypothalamus to the hypophysis.

HYPOPHYSIS

The hypophysis, commonly called the "pituitary gland," used to be considered the "master endocrine gland," but it is now evident that it has fallen to a position of servant to the brain. It is actually two endocrine organs of very different

Table 24.2   Components of the Hypophysis

Division	Origin	Subdivisions	Lobes
Adenohypophysis	Oral ectoderm	Pars distalis Pars tuberalis Pars intermedia	Anterior
Neurohypophysis	Diencephalon	Pars nervosa Stalk Median eminence and infundibulum	Posterior

functions. The **neurohypophysis** arises as an evagination of the diencephalic portion of the neural tube. The **adenohypophysis** comes from a diverticulum of the oral ectoderm of the embryo.[2] The main divisions are two separate organs in some animals, but are fused in human beings. Classifications of the parts of the gland are listed in Table 24.2.

Figure 24.2 shows the human hypophysis in midsagittal section. It lies in a bony fossa, the **sella turcica,** in the base of the skull. This is lined with an extension of the cranial dura mater that also bridges the fossa to form a diaphragm through which the stalk of the hypophysis passes to the hypothalamus.

The gland is encapsulated by an extension of the pia mater. The capsule is thicker on the anterior than on the posterior aspect of the hypophysis, and no trabeculae of size pass from the capsule into the gland. The stroma is confined to the portions of the gland derived from the oral ectoderm, especially the adenohypophysis (anterior lobe). It consists mainly of reticular connective tissue and contains an extensive system of sinusoidal capillaries. The neurohypophysis, like other parts of the central nervous system, has invading collagenous fibers only along blood vessels.

The blood vessels of the hypophysis bear an important relation to functions of the gland. These vessels arise from superior hypophyseal branches of the internal carotid arteries, and anastomose over the median eminence at the base of the stalk of the hypophysis. There they form a plexus from which a number of venules course down the stalk to the sinusoids of the adenohypophysis, forming the **hypophyseoportal system** (Fig. 24.3). Secretory neurons of the hypothalamus discharge their hormones into these vessels. Veins leaving the hypophysis drain into the cranial cavernous sinus. The neurophypophysis has a blood supply (the inferior hypophyseal branches) separate from that of the adenohypophysis.

A remnant of the lumen of the embryonic oral diverticulum may be found in the human hypophysis. It is represented by the occasional epithelial cleft or follicle in the pars intermedia (Fig. 24.4). No vestige of the ventricular cavity

---

[2]This is known as "Rathke's pouch." A small group of cells constituting the **pharyngeal hypophysis** is consistently encountered in the roof of the nasopharynx beneath the posterior vomerosphenoidal articulation. It may be a remnant of the oral diverticulum.

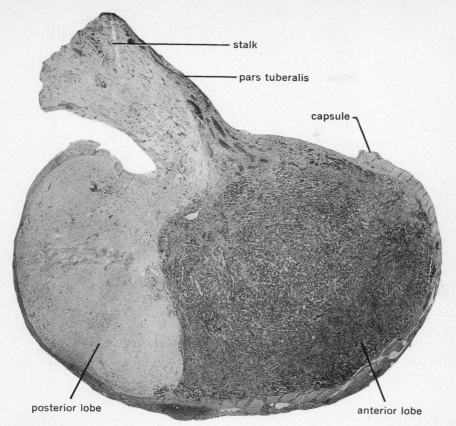

Figure 24-2 Human hypophysis, midsagittal section to show its general topography. Photomicrograph, × 12.

remains in the human hypophysis, though it may be seen in some other species, notably the cat.

Neurohypophysis This term is used for the **posterior lobe** of the hypophysis plus the **median eminence** and the **infundibulum**. It consists of cells called **pituicytes**, nerve fibers with their terminal dilatations, and fenestrated capillaries. The prominent **hypothalamohypophyseal tract** arises in supraoptic and paraventricular nuclei, the cells of which produce neurosecretions that pass down the tract fibers to end in close relation to the fenestrated capillaries (Fig. 24.5).

Electron microscopy reveals many neurosecretory granules in the nerve terminals but none in interstitial spaces.[3] The pituicytes are nonsecretory and

[3]Masses of secretory material seen under the light microscope are called "Herring bodies."

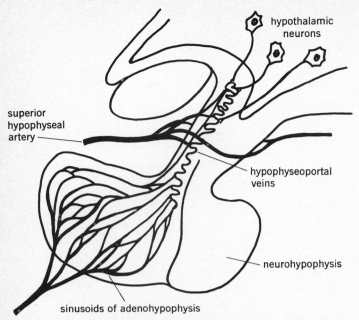

Figure 24-3 Diagrammatic representation of the hypophyseoportal system, consisting of tortuous vessels in the stalk that connect the superior hypophyseal artery with sinusoids of the adenohypophysis. Axons of hypothalamic neurons convey releasing factors to the tortuous vessels. *(Modified from R. Guillemin and R. Burgus,* Scientific American, *vol. 229, November, 1972.) (CHP)*

are comparable with neuroglia cells of the brain. Thus, there appears to be no endocrine secretion by the neurohypophysis, in the true sense. Instead, the organ should be considered as only a storage site for hypothalamic hormones.

Neurosecretory granules differ in weight. The lighter ones contain the hormone **oxytocin**, the heavier ones **vasopressin**—also called antidiuretic hormone (ADH). The granules give up their hormones at their contacts with the fenestrated capillaries. Oxytocin can stimulate contraction of smooth muscles of the gravid uterus. It also stimulates contraction of myoepithelial cells of the mammary glands (milk ejection). The antidiuretic hormone, vasopressin, increases water resorption in distal renal tubules, thus helping control water balance (Chap. 23).

Adenohypophysis The **pars distalis**, or **anterior lobe**, is the largest subdivision of the hypophysis (Fig. 24.2). Its parenchyma consists of clusters and cords of epithelioid secreting cells (Fig. 24.4). The cells lie in close proximity to adjacent sinusoids, walls of which are fenestrated. Thin basal laminae and very little reticular connective tissue intervene.

Only three types of cell can be recognized in sections routinely stained with such dyes as hematoxylin and eosin (Fig. 24.6). These have been desig-

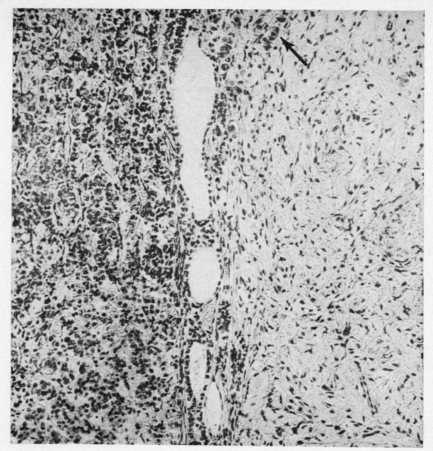

Figure 24-4 Human hypophysis, showing colloid-filled follicles of the pars intermedia in the middle, the pars distalis on the left, and the neurohypophysis on the right. Small basophilis (*arrow*) invade the pars nervosa. Photomicrograph, × 150.

nated "chromophobe," "acidophil," and "basophil" cells. However, electron microscopic and various modern histochemical methods have led to recognition of seven types of cell in the adenohypophysis, one specifically for each of its hormones. Table 24.3 lists the hormones of the anterior lobe and the cells producing them; secretion in all cases is controlled by hypothalamic hormones as well as by chemical feedback from target organs.

The **growth hormone** (GH), also known as somatotropin (STH), has no specific target organ, but stimulates growth of tissues in general. Its cell of origin (GH cell) has been identified among acidophils. Excessive amounts of this hormone in young individuals cause acceleration of body growth leading to "gigantism," and, in the adult, "acromegaly" (thickening of bones). Deficiency

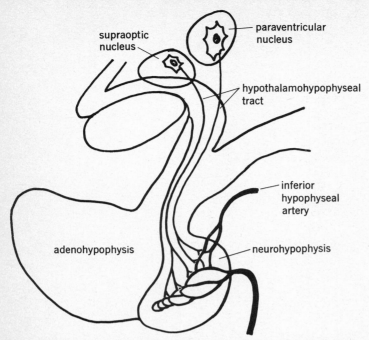

Figure 24-5 Diagrammatic representation of the hypothalamohypophyseal tract, over which the hormones from supraoptic and paraventricular nuclei pass to capillaries in the neurohypophysis. *(Modified from R. Guillemin and R. Burgus,* Scientific American, *vol. 229, November, 1972.) (CHP)*

of the hormone leads to cessation of growth of cartilage cells and, consequently, cessation of growth in length of bones, with "dwarfism" resulting.

Prolactin stimulates and maintains lactation. It also maintains the corpus luteum of the ovary, in some species (e.g., rat) permitting continued secretion of progesterone. Its cell of origin (PS cell) may be found among the acidophils.

Table 24.3 Hormones of the Anterior Lobe of the Human Hypophysis

Name of hormone	Names of cell	Hypothalamic factor
Growth stimulating	GH cell (alpha)	GRF
Adrenocorticotropin	ACTH cell (gamma)	CRF
Thyrotropin	TSH cell (theta)	TRF
Follicle stimulating	FSH-LH cell (delta)*	FSH-RF
Leutinizing		LH-RF
Melanocyte stimulating	MSH cell (zeta)	MSH-IF
Prolactin	PS cell (episilon-eta)	P-IF

*Subtypes of the delta cell have been observed in electron micrographs.

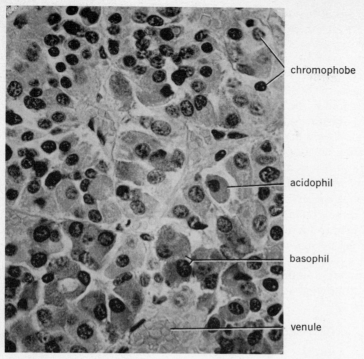

chromophobe

acidophil

basophil

venule

Figure 24-6   Human adenohypophysis. Photomicrograph, × 600.

Thyrotropin (TSH) stimulates the thyroid gland to produce thyroid hormones. Its secretion is reciprocally controlled by the thyroid hormones. Its cell of origin (TSH cell) is thought to be among the basophils (theta basophils).

Adrenocorticotropin (ACTH), or corticotropin, primarily stimulates the suprarenal cortex to produce hydrocortisone. It maintains the size of the suprarenal gland. The hormones of the suprarenal cortex, in turn, control output of adrenocorticotropin. The cell of origin (ACTH cell) appears to be among chromophobes or basophils.

The two gonadotropic hormones of the anterior lobe appear to be formed by cells with basophil characteristics, and specific ones are believed to exist for the **follicle-stimulating** hormone (FSH) and **luteinizing** hormone (LH). The former brings about maturation of ovarian follicles in the female and stimulates development of seminiferous tubules and differentiation of sperm in the male. The luteinizing hormone (LH) in the female not only stimulates formation of the corpus luteum, but also stimulates estrogen secretion and causes ovulation. In the male, it stimulates development of testicular interstitial cells and their secretion of testosterone. For this reason it is sometimes called "interstitial-cell-stimulating hormone" (ICSH). Further discussion of these anterior-lobe hormones is found in later chapters.

The **pars tuberalis** of the adenohypophysis is a small portion derived from the oral diverticulum. It extends onto the hypophyseal stalk (Fig. 24.2), forming a collar of cellular tissue. The cells tend to form alveolar clusters. Their function is unknown.

The **pars intermedia** lies between anterior and posterior lobes of the hypophysis. Remnants of the lumen of the oral diverticulum are represented by follicles, often elongated in the plane of separation between the lobes, containing a little colloidal substance (Fig. 24.4). Some of the cells in this region are basophilic and may be seen invading the substance of the neurohypophysis. A **melanocyte-stimulating** hormone (MSH) is produced by certain basophils (zeta basophils). Its cells of origin are found in the intermediate lobe of animals in which that structure is present. Its function in human beings is unclear.

Since the adenohypophysis regulates the activities of many other endocrine glands, its removal leads to atrophic changes in these organs. Tumors of the pars distalis lead to increased activity with hypertrophy of the other endocrine glands. In the normal course of events, the latter organs exert inhibitory effects on the hypophysis and hypothalamus, preventing overproduction of the trophic hormones, and their releasing factors. This feedback mechanism is illustrated in the following schema.

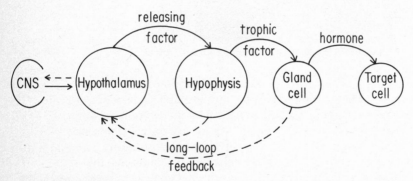

PINEAL GLAND

The mammalian pineal gland is a neuroendocrine organ, secretions of which regulate other endocrine regulating organs. It is an unpaired bud of highly cellular tissue, weighing only about 0.1 g, attached to the brain behind the roof of the third ventricle and in front of the midbrain. It is encapsulated by fibrous connective tissue continuous with the dura mater.

The principal cells of the pineal gland are designated **pinealocytes**. They form irregular cords among which capillaries course. Their fine structure resembles that of other endocrine secreting cells, varying with the state of activity of the gland (Fig. 24.7). A second type of cell, more numerous than the pinealocytes, is known as an "interstitial" cell; it is similar to the astrocyte of nervous tissue. Finally, a few nerve cells have been found in the pineal gland of human beings and in some other species.

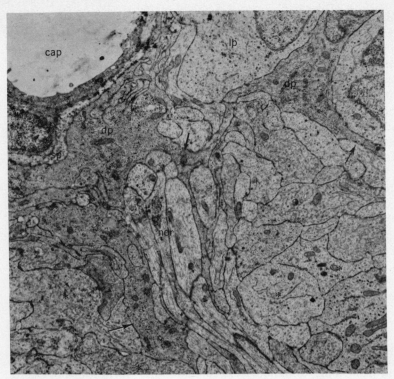

Figure 24-7 Medulla of pineal gland (mouse). Two dark pinealocytes, *dp*, have irregularly shaped processes marked by arrows; one lies adjacent to a capillary, *cap*, from the wall of which it is separated by perivascular space, *sp*. Light pinealocytes, *lp*, at the upper right have many processes, some sections of which are marked by asterisks (*). Terminal sympathetic noradrenergic nerve fibers, *ner*, are seen in the center of the picture. Electron micrograph, × 9,000. *(Contributed by H. J. Romijn.)*

The pineal gland arises embryologically from neuroepithelium, but in the mature condition it has no direct connection with the brain. It is an end organ of the autonomic nervous system. Nerve fibers—both myelinated and unmyelinated—enter the gland. The unmyelinated fibers are postganglionic neurons from the superior cervical sympathetic ganglia. The myelinated ones are believed to be preganglionic parasympathetic (from the brain stem) that synapse with the intraglandular nerve cells. Terminals of nerve fibers ramify among pinealocytes in the interstitial spaces. Thus it appears that the pineal gland, like most visceral organs, has a double innervation by sympathetic and parasympathetic neurons.

The principal hormone of the pineal gland is generally considered to be **melatonin.** It is synthesized by the pinealocytes in response to nerve impulses, and secreted into the capillaries of the gland. The amount of secretory activity varies with daylight and darkness. Afferent nerve impulses from the retinae reach the superior cervical sympathetic ganglia, from which postganglionic nerve fibers transmit them to the pineal gland. By this neural pathway, the exact course of which is unknown, the photoperiod regulates secretion of melatonin. Thus the gland serves as the "master clock" for circadian rhythms regulating some biologic activities.

Evolution of the pineal gland has been traced to an active unpaired photoreceptor organ in primitive animals. Certain lower forms today have such organs. The gland of mammals continues to be influenced by environmental lighting, though no trace of a "median eye" remains.

Melatonin, so called because it was found to contract larval frog melanocytes, modifies activities of other endocrine organs. In excessive amounts, as from certain pineal neoplasms, it affects male and female reproductive systems, delaying onset of puberty, for example. Recent data suggest that an as yet unidentified polypeptide may be the true pineal hormone.

One of the characteristic histologic features of human pineal glands, especially those from elderly subjects, is the presence of laminated concretions of mineral salts. These small bodies, seen in Fig. 24.8, are called **corpora arenacea,** and were quite erroneously spoken of as "brain sand" by earlier writers. It is doubtful that they bear any significant relationship to function of the gland.

SUPRARENAL GLANDS

The two suprarenal glands, commonly called "adrenals," form triangular caps for the rostral ends of the kidneys, from which they are separated by fibrous connective tissue. Each weighs 5 or 6 g and is in reality a duplex organ, consisting of coretex and medulla. The two parts of the gland produce different secretions, the one upon stimulation by hormones from the adenohypophysis, the other by nerve impulses from the spinal cord. Figure 24.9 illustrates the appearance of a section of a human suprarenal gland.

Early in development each suprarenal gland consists of two components that become combined during the fetal period. The cortex arises in the fifth week from cells of the peritoneum. This early mesodermal cellular accumulation forms an inner zone of the cortex, the so-called "fetal cortex," while another migration of smaller, more basophilic, cells encapsulates it during the early part of the sixth week and becomes the outer permanent cortex.

The fetal suprarenal gland attains a size at 2 months of gestation that is out of proportion to that of the fetal kidneys. At birth the glands are relatively about twenty times their adult size. The fetal cortex undergoes involution postnatally, and the glands lose one-third of their birth weight in the first 2 weeks.

The suprarenal medulla is derived from chromaffin cells migrating from neural-crest primodia of the celiac plexus. These cells begin invasion of the cortical mass in the seventh week of gestation.

The adult human suprarenal gland has a fibrous connective-tissue capsule from which trabeculae pass into its substance. The hilum of the gland is made

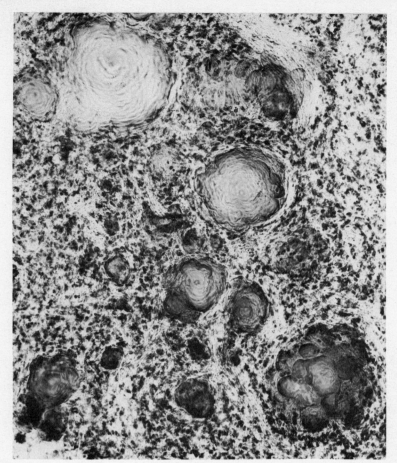

Figure 24-8 Human pineal gland. Note the lobulated and lamellated corpora arenacea. Photomicrograph, × 150.

prominant by emergence of a single suprarenal vein with an abundance of smooth muscle arranged longitudinally in its wall (Fig. 24.9). Arteries from several sources enter the gland through the capsule and trabeculae. Most of them supply the cortex, but some pass directly through it to the medulla. No veins accompany the cortical arteries.

Some reticular connective tissue surrounds the smallest blood vessels. The cortical arterioles soon branch into sinusoids that pursue rather straight courses through the cortex parallel to the cords of epithelioid secretory cells. Reticular connective tissue likewise surrounds capillaries and venules of the medulla. Cortical sinusoids become continuous with capillaries of the medulla.

More blood flows through the suprarenal gland than through any other comparable amount of tissue of the body, a point that cannot be appreciated by

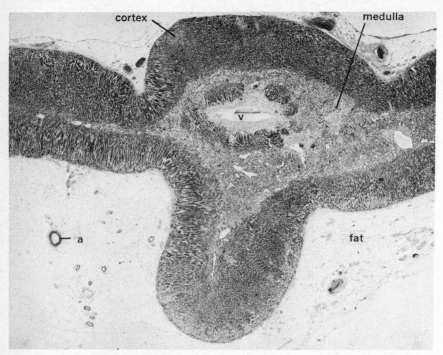

Figure 24-9 Human suprarenal gland, showing its division into cortex, the darker peripheral region, and medulla, the lighter central area. The suprarenal vein, *v*, is sectioned near the hilum, and cortical tissue indents the gland here to form an incomplete dark ring. Longitudinal smooth-muscle bundles lie inside this ring. A branch of one suprarenal artery, *a*, appears in the surrounding tissue. Photomicrograph, × 13.

studying ordinary histologic sections in which the capillaries and sinsusoids are empty and collapsed.

Lymphatic capillaries occur in trabeculae of the cortex and in the capsule. They are absent in the medulla.

Nerve fibers in small bundles pass from the capsule through the suprarenal cortex to the medulla. A few of them supply smooth-muscle cells of blood vessels, but most of the nerve fibers course freely among the medullary secretory cells upon which their terminal telodendria end synaptically. Fibers so doing are preganglionic sympathetic neurons from the spinal cord, reaching the suprarenal gland over splanchnic nerves.

Suprarenal Cortex　The fundamental plan of the cortex is an arrangement of parallel cords of cells looped at the periphery and branched and anastomosed at their medullary ends. The sinusoids, arising beneath the capsule, pass toward the medulla among the cords. When the cords branch, they do likewise. All the blood enters the suprarenal cortex at the periphery and leaves the cortex at its

deep border. Consequently, there is a gradient in respect to diffusion of substances, and it is not surprising to find a marked change in the appearance of
cells from the exterior toward the interior of the cortex.

   Three zones can be distinguished in the adult suprarenal cortex. The outermost is called the **zona glomerulosa.** This narrow zone is formed by columnar
cells (Fig. 24.10), and is not always very distinct in the human suprarenal gland.
Adjacent to it, the cords become straight, forming the **zona fasciculata.** There

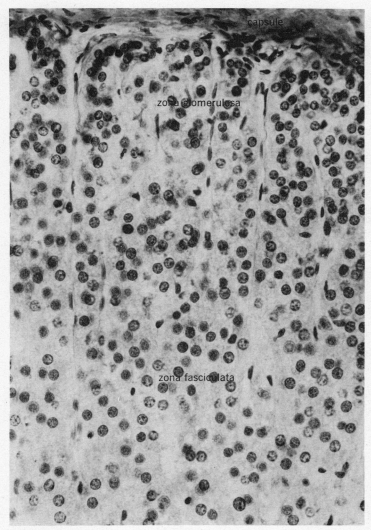

Figure 24-10 Human suparenal cortex, ("outer region") showing capsule, zona glomerulosa, and zona fasciculata.Photomicrograph, × 600.

the cells are polyhedral, and the cords tend to be two cells thick. This is the widest zone. Its cords become continuous with the branching and anastomosing cords of cells in the narrow **zona reticularis,** or innermost zone of the cortex next to the medulla (Fig. 24.11). The anastomosing cords of this zone are usually one cell wide.

The cortical cells are separated from the sinusoids by a perisinusoidal space, similar to that found in the liver. The endothelial lining of the sinusoids is the fenestrated type.

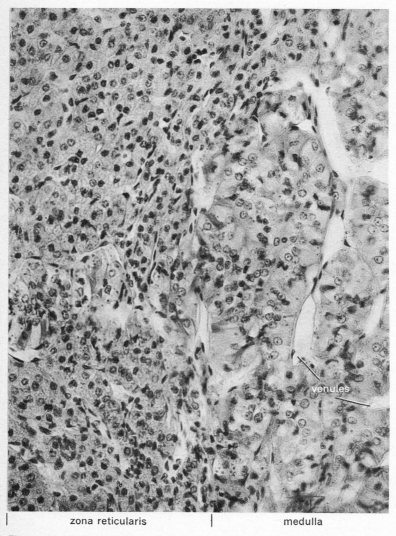

zona reticularis | medulla

Figure 24-11 Human suprarenal gland. Junction of the zona reticularis of the cortex (left) with the medulla (right). Photomicrograph, × 300.

Cortical-cell cytoplasm is characterized by the presence of massed vesicles of agranular endoplasmic reticulum. The cells of the zona glomerulosa are more basophilic than in other layers. Lipid droplets in those of the zona fasciculata impart a yellow color to the cortex of the fresh unstained gland. Both light and dark cells are seen in the zona reticularis. The dark ones are thought to be degenerating, for their nuclei are dark and their cytoplasm contains lipofuscin.

Many steroid substances with hormonal properties have been isolated from the suprarenal cortex. Three of these corticosteroids appear to be naturally secreted. They are **hydrocortisone** (cortisol), **corticosterone,** and **aldosterone**. The first two are secreted by cells of the zona fasciculata and zone reticularis, while the last-named hormone is a product of cells of the zona glomerulosa.

Aldosterone is called a "mineralocorticoid" hormone because it regulates electrolyte and water balance, acting on the distal tubule of the nephron in regulation of sodium metabolism. Hydrocortisone and corticosterone are called "glucocorticoids" because they control carbohydrate balance. They are concerned with glucogenesis in the liver, and also help mobilize free fatty acids from adipose tissue.

Other hormones secreted by the suprarenal cortex, particularly in the zona reticularis, are **androgenic corticoids** with minimal effects in normal individuals.

Stimulation of secretion in the suprarenal cortex is effected by the hypophyseal adrenocorticotropic hormone (ACTH) and its hypothalamic releasing factor (CRF). The glucocorticoid hormones, in turn, exert a negative feedback action on the hypothalamohypophyseal complex, regulating the output of ACTH.

The suprarenal cortex is essential for life. When the glands are removed or destroyed by disease, the individual loses ability to regulate water balance and mineral metabolism; water and sodium chloride are lost through renal excretion, and the blood potassium level rises excessively.

The role of the suprarenal cortex in resistance to stress is noteworthy. In the absence of the glands, animals become sensitive to emergency situations, such as exposure to cold or to conditions that cause a decrease in blood sugar or a fall in blood pressure. Administration of cortical hormones restores their resistance. Stress situations in normal animals result in hypertrophy of the suprarenal cortex in compensation for the increased demand upon the glands for more hormones. Normally the thickness of the cortex and amount of lipid in the zona fasciculata vary to some extent with bodily activity, with the seasons, and with pregnancy.

Suprarenal Medulla   This is a neuroendocrine organ. The histologic appearance of it differs from that of the cortex. Its cells are arranged in irregular anastomosing cords in close association with nerve endings as well as with capillaries and venules. Cells around some venules resemble simple columnar epithelium (Fig. 24.11). The secretory cells of the human gland contain granules, some clear and others with electron-dense material in them. The two hormones of the medulla are produced by the same cell. Fixing fluids containing chromic acid impart a brown color to the cytoplasm of the secretory cells. This is called the "chromaffin reaction." The brown-staining granules are precursors of the two medullary hormones.

The capillaries and venules of the medulla receive blood from the cortical sinusoids as well as from arterioles that penetrate the cortex to reach the medulla. Venules drain into the single suprarenal vein that leaves the gland through the hilum.

Nerve cells are encountered occasionally in the medulla. Nerve fibers are both myelinated and unmyelinated. The former may be preganglionic parasympathetics to the intrinsic neurons. The unmyelinated fibers are postganglionic sympathetic neurons. The medullary gland cells thus receive a double innervation.

Two catecholamines are secreted by cells of the suprarenal medulla. One of these is **epinephrine**. The other is **norepinephrine**, which occurs also in other organs, such as the heart, but especially is found at synaptic endings of neurons throughout the body. Production of epinephrine by the medulla is about five times that of norepinephrine. The medullary catecholamines are secreted directly into venules as well as capillaries. Control of their secretion is neural rather than hypophyseal. The cardivascular system is one of the main sites of action of medullary catacholamines; the mechanism by which they act is a complex one.

Paraganglia   Some neural-crest cells of the embryo migrate to various positions along the posterior wall of the abdomen. They tend to form small groups, more prominent in infancy than in the adult. These **paraganglia** are associated with some of the sympathetic ganglia, especially around major branches of the abdominal aorta. They contain epithelioid cells in clusters and cords that are closely applied to capillaries and bear some resemblance to suprarenal medullary tissue. The cells contain granules exhibiting the chromaffin reaction and rich in norepinephrine. Figure 24.12 illustrates the microscopic appearance of one of these paraganglia.

THYROID GLAND

The largest endocrine gland is the thyroid, that of an adult person weighing 20 to 30 g. It lies in the neck, embracing the upper end of the trachea and lower portion of the larynx. The gland consists of lateral lobes, one on either side of a connecting isthmus. In about one-third of all individuals, a median pyramidal lobe lies in front of the larynx.

The thyroid gland is encapsulated by fibrous connective tissue of the deep cervical fascia. Trabeculae pass from the capsule into its substance, subdividing it into lobules and carrying blood vessels, lymphatic vessels, and nerves into it (Fig. 24.13). The finer subdivisions of the thyroid stroma consist of loose fibrous and reticular connective tissue supporting a rich capillary bed (Fig. 24.15).

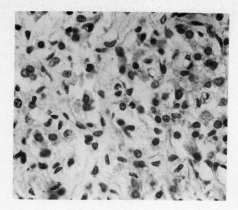

Figure 24-12 Human paraganglion ("organ of Zuckerkandl"). Photomicrograph, × 300.

The thyroid parenchyma consists of epithelial **follicles** and a few interfollicular cells. The follicles vary in size from small clumps of cells with hardly any lumen to globoid structures 100 to 200 μm in diameter. The adult human follicular epithelium under normal conditions is cuboidal (Fig. 24.14), but height of the cells varies with status of glandular activity; the cells become squamous during hypoactivity and tall columnar when the gland is hyperactive.

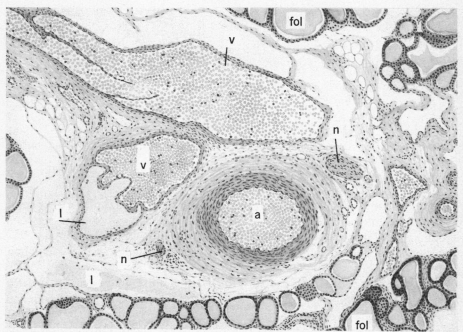

Figure 24-13 Stroma of the thyroid gland containing a small artery, *a*, veins, *v*, and lymphatic vessels, *l*, as well as nerves, *n*. Note the valve in a vein. The parenchyma is represented by a few follicles, *fol*. ×75. *(JFN)*

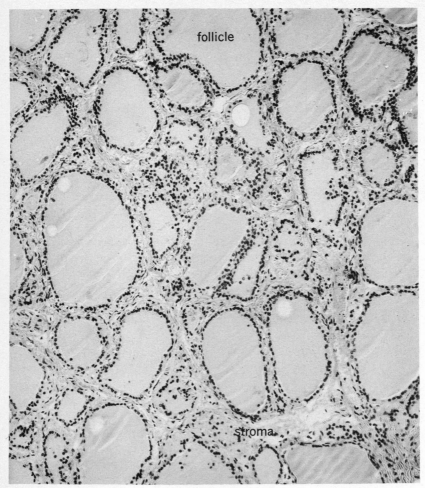

Figure 24-14 Human thyroid gland. Follicles are filled with colloid during life, and the few vacuoles seen here are artifacts. Photomicrograph, × 150.

Thyroid follicles contain a slightly gelatinous substance, known as **colloid.** The usual histologic preparation shows artificial shrinkage spaces between epithelium and the colloid, but in the specimen of Fig. 24.14 contact was preserved. The colloid is usually acidophilic. Occasionally, a few detached epithelial cells or lymphocytes are seen in it.

The follicular epithelium rests on a thin basal lamina. The follicular surface of the cells shows microvilli and often pinocytotic vesicles. Among organelles of the cytoplasm are mitochondria and lysosomes. Prominence of the golgi complex varies with secretory activity of the thyroid gland. Lateral borders of cells present junctional structures.

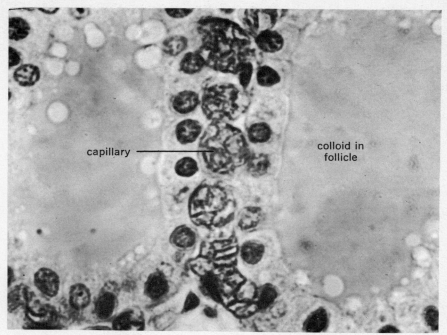

Figure 24-15   Thyroid of a rat, showing a row of blood-filled capillaries between the walls of adjacent follicles. Photomicrograph, × 1,200.

A second type of cell is present in the thyroid parenchyma. It occurs in the follicular epithelium or between it and the basal lamina. Groups of these cells are sometimes encountered between follicles, and so the name **parafollicular cell** has been applied to them. They appear as clear cells in routine preparations, but when their numerous secretory granules are stained by silver methods, as in Fig. 24.16, they are darker than the principle follicular cells.

Nearly one-fifth of the body iodine is contained in the thyroid gland. This is an essential component of the principle thyroid hormone. **Thyroglobulin** of the follicular colloid is the storage form of the hormone secreted by the epithelial cells. **Thyroxine** (tetraiodothyronine) and **triiodothyronine** are the principal components constituting thyroid hormone. They are secreted into the colloid where they remain in bound form until they are withdrawn and actively transported to extrafollicular capillaries. The thyroid gland is sensitive to deficiency of iodine, an optimum amount of which must be present to maintain normal production of thyroid hormone and normal glandular structure.

The thyroid hormone regulates, i.e., stimulates, the rate of cellular oxidation in practically all tissues of the body. Another quite different hormone, **thyrocalcitonin**, is produced by the parafollicular cells. It functions in regulation of blood-calcium level, inhibiting an excessive rise. The hormone has been synthesized and is in clinical use.

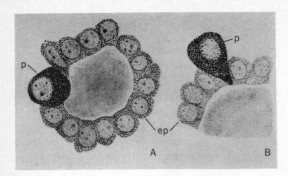

Figure 24-16 Thyroid of a young dog. *A.* A parafollicular cell, *p,* with dark granules in the cytoplasm is seen among principal cells of the follicular epithelium, *ep. B.* A parafollicular cell partly withdrawn from the epithelium. × 900. *(JFN)*

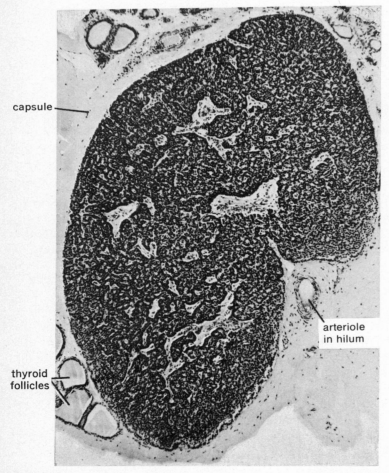

Figure 24-17 Human parathyroid gland showing general histologic features. Note capsule and hilum; trabeculae are the light regions in the gland. Parenchymal cell cords can be discerned. Photomicrograph, about × 75.

Thyroid gland function is directly controlled by thyrotropin (TSH), one of the hormones secreted by the adenohypophysis. Thyrotropin, in turn, is regulated by a hypothalamic hormone, thyrotropin-releasing factor (TRF), the first releasing factor to be synthesized. A negative feedback relationship exists between thyroid gland and hypophysis, and probably also hypothalamus.

Hypothyroidism, with attendant deficiency of thyroid hormone, results in marked decrease in metabolic rate and extensive changes in connective tissue leading to puffy appearance of the skin, known as "myxedema." Administration of thyroid hormone can remedy this condition. When thyroid deficiency develops in early life, growth is inhibited, and the resulting dwarfism associated with a myxedematous condition and impaired intellectual development is known as "cretinism." Hyperthyroidism is associated with increase in the metabolic rate. The follicles are depleted of colloid, the epithelial cells are tall, and the epithelium is often folded. In one form of hyperthyoidism, known as "exophthalmic goiter," the gland may be somewhat enlarged, the individual is readily fatigued, loses weight, and exhibits a characteristic protrusion of the eyeballs. Simple enlargement of the thyroid gland is known as "goiter," a condition related to iodine deficiency.

PARATHYROID GLANDS

The parathyroid glands are small bodies, measuring approximately 3 by 6 mm, located on the posterior surface of the lateral lobes of the thyroid gland close to the anastomosing superior and inferior thyroid arteries. Usually there are four glands, but sometimes only two can be found, and occasionally one to several accessory or aberrant glands may be present. The typical appearance of a parathyroid gland is illustrated at low magnification in Fig. 24.17.

A thin fibrous connective-tissue capsule surrounds each gland and separates it from the thyroid. This gives rise to small trabeculae that convey the blood vessels of the gland. The stroma generally is inconspicuous, the finer subdivisions of it being formed by reticular fibers around capillaries. A variable amount of adipose tissue may be found in the trabeculae.

The parathyroid parenchyma consists of cords of epitheloid cells closely associated with the capillaries. Only the basal laminae and a few reticular fibers intervene. Occasionally small colloid-filled follicles occur among the cell cords, but these are not the same as thyroid follicles, for they contain little iodine.

The parenchymal cells of the parathyroid glands are of a single type in young individuals, but at some time before puberty another, the **acidophil cell,**[4] makes its appearance. The **principal cells** (chief cells) of the glands have characteristics similar to those of some other epithelioid endocrine cells. They do not display a clear polarization toward surrounding capillaries, and their secretory organelles are less well formed than in some other endocrine organs. The

[4]Most writers retain the name oxyphil cells. Oxyphil is synonymous with acidophil, and was widely used 50 years ago, e.g., "oxyphil leucocyte" for blood eosinophil. Acidophil cells are not found in parathyroid glands of most mammals.

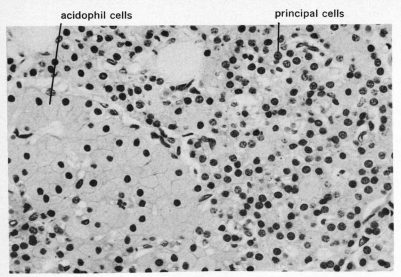

acidophil cells   principal cells

Figure 24-18 Human parathyroid gland showing a group of pale-staining acidophil cells among cords of principal cells. Photomicrograph, × 300.

principal cells exhibit some variability in staining, and one can find a few that appear to be intermediate between principal and acidophil cells. The acidophil cells tend to occur in clumps (Fig. 24.18) and are considered to be nonsecretory. Their fine structure differs markedly from that of the principal cells. The cytoplasm of acidophil cells is packed with mitochondria, contains few if any secretory granules, and has a poorly defined golgi complex.

Parathormone, the parathyroid hormone, is secreted by the principal cells. Its essential function is maintenance of blood-calcium at a level of approximately 10 mg per 100 ml of blood. Reciprocally, the blood calcium level controls secretions of the hormone. Parathormone also regulates the concentration of inorganic phosphorus in the blood.

The parathyroid glands are essential for maintenance of life, and their removal leads to a condition known as "parathyroid tetany." Administration of parathormone or elevating the blood calcium level can compensate for parathyroid insufficiency. Hyperparathyroidism, which may result from tumors or parathyroid glands, leads to mobilization and removal of calcium and phosphorus from bones. Excessive intake of calcium or of vitamin D can suppress activity of the parathyroid glands, leading to atrophic changes in the glands.

The action of parathormone is the opposite of that of thyrocalcitonin from the parafollicular cells of the thyroid gland. Parathormone (and vitamin D) can raise the serum calcium level, while thyrocalcitonin can dampen a tendency for it to exceed normal levels. The one regulates the other by a double feedback mechanism. Growth hormone from the hypophysis may also have a role in maintaining normal levels of serum calcium.

PANCREATIC ISLANDS

The pancreas is described in Chap. 21. It is principally an exocrine gland with a well-formed duct system. During its early development, however, groups of cells arise from the duct primordia and become the endocrine components of the pancreas; these are the pancreatic islands.[5] There are about 1 million of these minute ductless glands, each 0.5 mm or less in diameter, totalling only about 1 g in weight.

The pancreatic islands are distributed throughout the organ, although they are slightly more numerous in the tail of the gland than in its main portion. They are composed of irregularly arranged cords of epitheliod cells polarized toward fenestrated capillaries coursing adjacent to the cords. Reticular connective tissue within the islands is sparce, but each island is separated from the surrounding exocrine pancreatic acini by a delicate layer of it.

The pancreatic islands can be recognized easily in routinely stained sections by their pale appearance (Fig. 21.11). Special staining methods and electron micrographs reveal cytoplasmic granules that differ in three principal types of cell composing the cords. The three types are designated **alpha, beta,** and **delta** (Fig. 24.19).[6] Beta cells are the most numerous ones in the human pancreatic islands. The fewer alpha cells tend to be arranged peripherally. Delta cells appear to represent an altered form of alpha cell.

The secretory granules of beta cells are distinctly different from those of alpha cells. Both contain electron-dense material, but in the beta cells it takes the form of irregularly shaped crystalloid bodies, while it appears as round masses in the alpha cells.

Insulin is secreted by the beta cells. The crystalloid bodies may represent a storage form of this hormone. Insulin stimulates glucose uptake by cells and promotes conversion of glucose to glycogen. Removal of the pancreas or destruction of the beta cells results in "diabetes mellitus," a condition in which the blood sugar level exceeds the capacity of the kidney to absorb it, so that sugar appears in the urine, which in turn is copious.

Another hormone of the pancreatic islands is **glucagon,** a product of the alpha cells. Its action is reciprocal to that of insulin, for it causes reduction of liver glycogen and elevation of the blood-sugar level.

Control of insulin secretion is exerted by the level of glucose in the blood. Furthermore, a rise in amino-acid level increases the output of insulin. Glucagon and gastrointestinal hormones can increase insulin secretions. The role of cyclic AMP was noted earlier.

---

[5]They are commonly called "islands of Langerhans" after the man who discovered them a century ago.

[6]A fourth type, known as C cell, is found in some animals. Its cytoplasm is agranular.

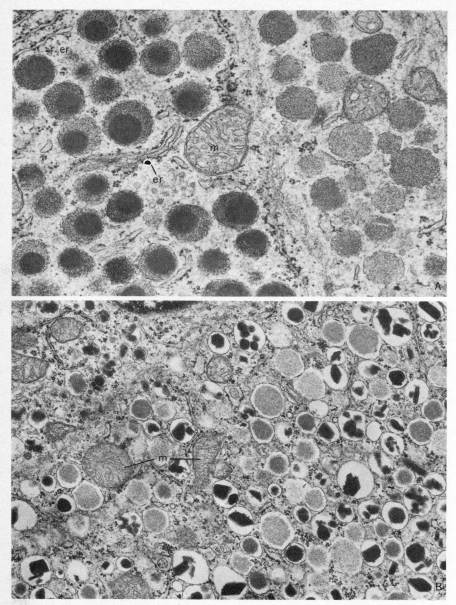

Figure 24-19 Human pancreatic island cells. *A.* Alpha cell on left and delta cell on right; the former has granules containing round electron-dense inclusions. *B.* Beta cell granules contain crystalloid inclusions. Note mitochondria, *m,* and granular endoplasmic reticulum, *er.* Electron micrographs, *A,* about × 25,000; *B,* about × 15,000. *(Contributed by A. A. Like and L. Orci, Diabetes, Suppl. 2, vol. 21, pp. 511–534, 1972.)*

SUGGESTED READING

Axelrod, J.: The Pineal Gland: A Neurochemical Transducer. *Science,* vol. 184, pp. 1341–1348, 1974.

Brownstein, M. J., M. Palkovits, J. M. Saavedra, R. M. Bassiri, and R. D. Utiger: Thyrotropin-Releasing Hormone in Specific Nuclei of Rat Brain. *Science,* vol. 185, pp. 267–269, 1974.

Canadian Association of Anatomists Symposium: Functional Morphology of the Hypothalamus. *Canadian Journal of Neurobiological Sciences,* vol. 1, pp. 23–84, 1974.

David, G. F. X., and G. D. S. Wright: The Ultrastructure of the Pineal Ganglion in the Ferret. *Journal of Anatomy,* vol. 115, pp. 79–97, 1973.

Ezrin, C., J. O. Godden, R. Volpé, and R. Wilson: *Systematic Endocrinology.* Medical Department, Harper & Row, Publishers, Incorporated, New York, 1973.

Gabbay, K. H., J. Korff, and E. E. Schneeberger: Vesicular Binesis: Glucose Effect on Insulin Secretory Vesicles. *Science,* vol. 187, pp. 177–179, 1975.

Guillemin, R., and R. Burgus: The Hormones of the Hypothalamus. *Scientific American,* vol. 227, no. 5, pp. 24–33, November, 1972.

Harris, G. W.: *Neural Control of the Pituitary Gland.* Edward Arnold (Publishers) Ltd., London, 1955.

Like, A. A.: The Ultrastructure of the Secretory Cells of the Islets of Langerhans in Man. *Laboratory Investigation,* vol. 16, pp. 937–951, 1967.

Locke, W., and A. V. Schlally, (eds.): *The Hypothalamus and Pituitary in Health and Disease.* Charles C Thomas, Publisher, Springfield, Ill., 1972.

Pastan, J.: Cyclic AMP. *Scientific American,* vol. 227, no. 2, pp. 97–105, August, 1972.

Pike, J. E.: Prostaglandins. *Scientific American,* vol. 225, no. 5, pp. 84–92, November, 1971.

Pitt-Rivers, R. V., and W. R. Trotter (eds.): *The Thyroid Gland,* vol. 1. Butterworth, London, 1964.

Roediger, W. E. W.: A Comparative Study of the Normal Human Neonatal and the Canine Thyroid C Cell. *Journal of Anatomy,* vol. 115, pp. 225–276, 1973.

Sutherland, E. W., G. A. Robison, and R. W. Butcher: Some Aspects of the Biological Role of Adenosine 3′,5′-monophosphate (Cyclic AMP). *Circulation,* vol. 37, pp. 279-306, 1968.

Werner, S. C., and S. H. Ingbar (eds.): *The Thyroid: A Fundamental and Clinical Text,* 3d ed., pt. I, pp. 1–158. Medical Department, Harper & Row, Publishers, Incorporated, New York, 1971.

Weymouth, R. J., and H. R. Seibel: An Electron Microscopic Study of the Parathyroid Glands in Man. Evidence of Secretory Material. *Acta Endocrinologicia (Kobenhavn),* vol. 61, pp. 334–342, 1969.

Chapter 25

Male Reproductive Organs

The main organs of reproduction in the male are the gonads, or testes, which have a twofold function, namely the production of the sex cells and male sex hormones. Three glands, the seminal vesicles, prostate, and bulbourethral glands, provide a fluid vehicle for the sex cells. A system of ducts, the epididymis, spermatic ducts, and urethra, transports the mixture of sex cells and exocrine secretion, constituting the semen. The penis provides the means of introducing the semen into the female reproductive system. The components of this system are shown by diagram in Fig. 25.1.

Marked differences in structure and function of the male reproductive organs are encountered at the various stages in development. Gonadal secretion of hormones begins early in the fetal period (6 weeks). Development of testes from cells in the interior of the primordial gonad was determined genetically, and thereafter the hormones of the fetal testes regulate growth and development of internal and external genital organs. For that matter, practically all systems, including the brain, are affected by the presence of optimal amounts of hormones of the fetal testes.

After gonadal differentiation has occurred (seventh week), a testicular hormone, called "testis inducer," stimulates the formation of male genital ducts and external genitalia. The embryonal müllerian system (the primordium of rine tube, uterus, and upper vagina) is caused to undergo atrophy, while the

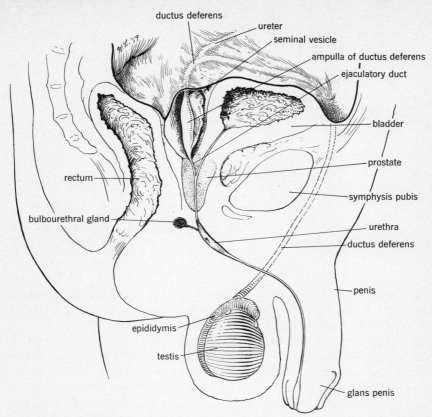

Figure 25-1 Diagram of the male reproductive system to show the relations of the various organs to each other *(WEL)*

wolffian ducts go on to form epididymis, ductus deferens, and seminal vesicle. Testosterone from the fetal testes appears to be necessary for development of the penis and for fusion of the lateral components of the scrotum.

Regulation of fetal hormones appears to be placental, for, at least in some animals, maternal gonadotropins do not traverse the placental barrier. Chorionic gonadotropin secretion begins early in pregnancy and is available before the fetal hypophysis begins to function. The stage is set for sexual function before birth, but, thereafter, there appears to be little gonadal activity until puberty.

TESTES

The **testis** is essential for maintenance of the species but is not a vital organ. It only makes hormones and spermatozoa. Its structure, illustrated diagrammatically in Fig. 25.2, is that of a compound tubular gland with about 250 lobules.

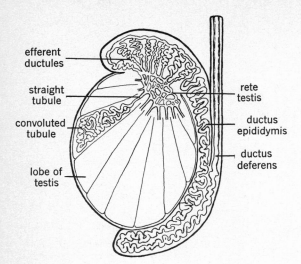

efferent
ductules

straight
tubule

convoluted
tubule

lobe of
testis

rete
testis

ductus
epididymis

ductus
deferens

Figure 25-2 Diagram of the relation between the testis, epididymis, and ductus deferens. *(MWS)*

It has a heavy capsule of dense fibrous connective tissue, called the **tunica albuginea** (Fig. 25.3). The testis lies in a mesothelium-lined sac that developed as an evagination of the peritoneum into the scrotum.

At the hilum, called the **mediastinum testis,** the connective tissue is thickened. Septa pass through the testis from hilum to capsule and incompletely subdivide the organ into lobules. Within each lobule, the connective tissue forms an abundant stroma around the **convoluted seminiferous tubules**, carrying blood vessels, lymphatics, and nerves and containing the endocrine interstitial cells.

A lobule of the testis contains one to three extensively convoluted seminiferous tubules, each of which may be as long as 70 cm—well over a half mile of tubules in each testis. Each convoluted seminiferous tubule forms a loop, the two ends joining a **straight tubule** in the mediastinum testis. The convoluted loops occasionally anastomose and may give off branches.

The straight tubules are short ducts connecting the seminiferous tubules with a network of thin, irregular channels in the mediastinum testis, called the **rete testis.** About a dozen **efferent ductules** connect the rete testis with the head of the epididymis.

The efferent ductules and the **ductus epididymis** are other types of convoluted tubes in the head of the epididymis. Toward the lower pole of the testis, the ductus epididymis becomes less tortuous and ultimately joins the **ductus deferens.** The latter is the excretory duct of the testis; it enters the spermatic cord and passes with it into the abdomen.

Prepubertal Seminiferous Tubules   The appearance of the seminiferous tubules is different before and after sexual maturity. From birth until puberty, they appear as solid cords of epithelial cells, with only a suggestion of a lumen

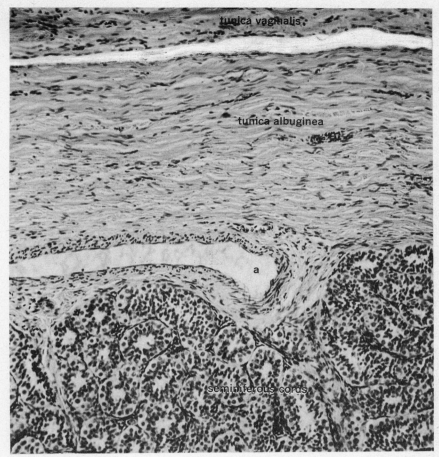

Figure 25-3 Testis of an immature monkey. The outer wall of the tunica vaginalis is above the cleft at the upper edge of the figure; below the cleft is the heavy tunica albuginea with an artery, *a*, in the lower part of it. Seminiferous cords (tubules), with lumens forming, are seen at the lower part of the figure.Photomicrograph, × 150.

here and there (Fig. 25.3). The cords develop true lumens during their metamorphosis at puberty, and this development converts them into tubules, lined with an unusual variety of stratified epithelium. A prominent basal lamina lies beneath the epithelium.

The convoluted seminiferous cords of the prepubertal testis consist of undifferentiated cells capable of forming the supportive and sex cells of the mature tubules. A few large, clear cells among them can be recognized as **spermatogonia,** or primary sex cells. None of these proceeds to a more advanced stage until puberty.

Puberty is signaled by the appearance of pubic hairs, but more than that is involved. All the reproductive organs rapidly mature, and there is a general spurt in the body growth rate. The stimulus for puberty originates in the brain where a change appears in responsiveness of the hypothalamic centers to prepubertal levels of testicular hormone. This leads to production of the releasing factor for gonadotropins of the adenohypophysis. An increase in gonadotropins precedes further testicular development and interstitial-cell secretion of testosterone.

Interstitial Cells   Endocrine function of the testis is vested in the **interstitial cells.**[1] These are clearly recognizable in the fetus and newborn infant, but they regress after birth and thence until puberty are represented by inconspicuous spindle-shaped cells. This change reflects the great reduction in hormone secretion prior to puberty.

Pubertal and postpubertal interstitial cells occur individually or in small clusters in the connective-tissue stroma between seminiferous tubules (Fig. 25.4). They are irregularly polyhedral epithelioid cells with indistinct boundaries, measuring about 15 to 20 μm in diameter. Thus they are distinctly contrasted with the smaller, connective-tissue cells.

The nucleus of a mature interstitial cell is surrounded by abundant acidophilic cytoplasm containing many cisternae of agranular endoplasmic reticulum. There are a well-formed golgi complex, centrioles, and mitochondria of variable shape, as well as some lipid and lipochrome pigment inclusions. Secretion granules are not seen, as a rule, but there are prominent crystalloid bodies in human interstitial cells.

The principal hormone secreted by interstitial cells is **testosterone,** a potent androgen. Small amounts of an estrogen also are formed. Testosterone is responsible for the various manifestations of maleness that start at puberty: growth and function of genital organs; increase in hair growth; central nervous expression of aggressiveness and libido; increase in muscle mass; and laryngeal growth (voice change).

Stimulation of testosterone secretion is effected by the central nervous system through hypothalamic hormones acting on the adenohypophysis. Negative feedback from the testis tends to inhibit the output of releasing factors and gonadotropic hormones.

The hypophyseal gonadotropins that stimulate male reproductive organs have the same chemical structure as those of the female. Therefore, they share the same names, which are indeed misnomers. **Follicle-stimulating hormone** (FSH) stimulates testicular tubule growth and meiosis of cells destined to become spermatozoa. **Luteinizing hormone** (LH) stimulates interstitial-cell function.[2] Both of these gonadotropins are required for complete spermatogenesis and emission of sperm. Both are influenced by their releasing factors from the hypothalamus.

---

[1]These are often called "cells of Leydig."
[2]Consequently, this is sometimes called **interstitial-cell-stimulating hormone** (ICSH).

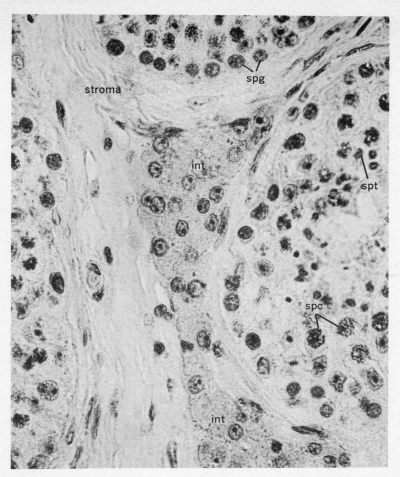

Figure 25-4 Interstitial cells, *int*, in testis of a 65-year-old man: *spc*, spermatocytes; *spg*, spermatogonia; *spt*, spermatids. Photomicrograph, × 600.

Adult Seminiferous Tubules The structure of the adult seminiferous tubule is complex because its cells are constantly changing. Like the bone marrow, the seminiferous epithelium is engaged in mass production of free cells. Its products are the sperm.

Not all cells of the tubular epithelium form sperm. Some are **supportive cells,**[3] of irregular shape. As they tower above the basal almina, they are recognizable in sections by a large vesicular nucleus with a prominent nucleolus, in contrast with the dark nuclei of developing sex cells. Supportive cells are indented from the side by the pressure of adjoining spermatogenic cells. Their

[3]Sometimes called "cells of Sertoli."

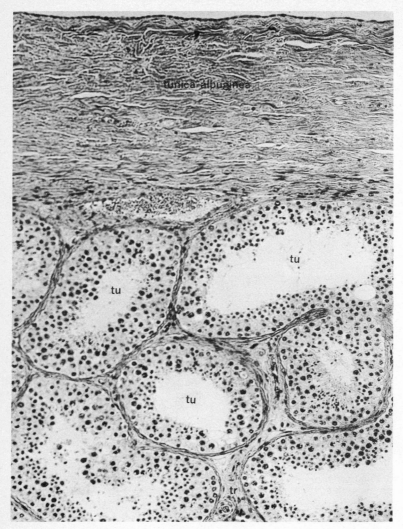

Figure 25-5 Testis of a young man. Note the thick tunica albuginea, trabeculae of connective tissue, *tr,* and seminiferous tubules, *tu.* Photomicrograph, × 150.

nuclei appear near the middle of the tubular epithelium. Tiny rod-shaped crystalloids are seen in the cytoplasm of these cells.

The appearance of seminiferous tubules is shown in Figs. 25.5 and 25.6. A variable number of layers of cells is concerned with sperm formation. Nearest the basal lamina are the **spermatogonia.** From their mitotic division other spermatogonia arise. Several irregular rows of them are distinguishable in the adult. After many divisions of this type, **primary spermatocytes** are formed. They are larger cells lying about midway between the basal lamina and the lumen. By their divisions, **secondary spermatocytes** arise, but few are seen in most tubules

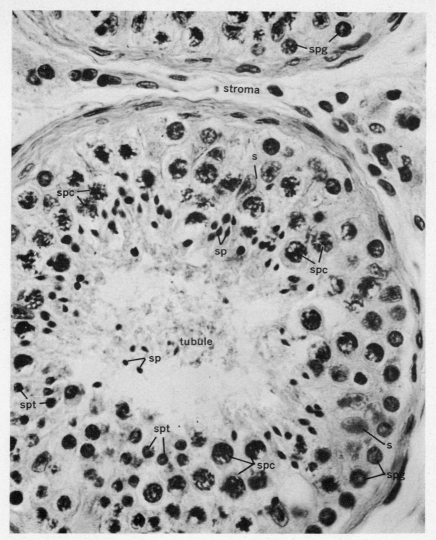

Figure 25-6 Testis of a young man; connective-tissue stroma surrounds seminiferous tubules. Abbreviations are s, supportive-cell nuclei; spg, nuclei of spermatogonia; spc, spermatocytes; spt, spermatids; sp, sperm cells; from the same specimen as Fig. 25-5. Photomicrograph, × 600.

because they quickly divide into **spermatids,** which are small cells with dark nuclei, found in several layers near the lumen.

Various stages in the transformation of spermatids into **sperm** are seen in different tubules. Groups of immature sperm with their heads indenting the cytoplasm of supporting cells can be found. Not every region in a tubule, nor even every cross section through a tubule, will show such groups of nearly ready sperm. Their development and maturation occurs periodically. When sperm at one site have matured, they detach and leave the testis to be stored in the epididymis. Sperm are nonmotile at this time. How they leave the seminiferous tubules and pass through the rete testis is unknown, but they appear to be flushed along in a fluid secreted by the tubules.

Spermatogenesis The final mitotic division of spermatogonia is incomplete cytoplasmically and produces two conjoined cells; these grow into primary spermatocytes during their intermitotic interval. Each has the full number of chromosomes, i.e., the number characterizing all body cells of the species. The normal number in human beings is 46. The chromosomes occur in pairs, and although the 23 pairs vary in shape and size, the two individuals of each pair are alike in 22 of the pairs. The twenty-third pair consists of two dissimilar chromosomes, called X and Y.

The intermitotic period, between the last spermatogonial and first spermatocytic divisions, is one of growth and preparation for an event that occurs nowhere else in the body. The pairs of chromosomes separate in a special **meiotic division** of the large primary spermatocytes, one member of each pair going to each of the two secondary spermatocytes. This applies also to the X and Y chromosomes. Thus there are two kinds of spermatocytes: those with an X chromosome plus 22 ordinary chromosomes and those with a Y chromosome plus 22 ordinary chromosomes. Complete division of the cytoplasm fails, leaving true intercellular bridges connecting four spermatocytes.

The secondary spermatocytes undergo another cell division in which each of the 23 chromosomes splits lengthwise in the manner of body-cell chromosomes during mitosis. Again, cytoplasmic division is incomplete. Thus, groups of eight interconnected spermatids are formed; each has the haploid number of chromosomes. No further cell divisions take place. The spermatids become transformed into separate mature sperm by a process called spermiogenesis.

Some stages in the maturation of spermatids are illustrated in Fig. 25.7. The electron microscope has revealed details of this remarkable process involving the cytoplasmic organelles.

The prominent golgi complex of the spermatid gives rise to a large vesicle containing granular electron-dense material. The granules coalesce to form a single round mass, or **acrosome**, within this acrosomal vesicle (Fig. 25.8). The membranes of the vesicle later fold over the nucleus of the spermatid, and the acrosome comes to lie on the nucleus; membranes and acrosome become the head cap of the sperm. The centrioles shift to the pole of the nucleus opposite the acrosome. One of them sends out a flagellum, the beginning of the sperm tail (Fig. 25.7). The other forms a ring-shaped structure just behind the nucleus.

The spermatid cytoplasm shifts tailward, gradually becoming attenuated by budding off unnecessary portions, until only a thin coat of it remains over the middle piece and tail of the sperm (Fig. 25.9). The nucleus changes shape, becoming flat. The middle piece, or neck, of the sperm is formed by the centrioles and mitochondria. The latter accumulate in a sheath around the tail filaments and take on a helical appearance (Fig. 25.7E and F). Mature sperm are shown in Fig. 25.10.

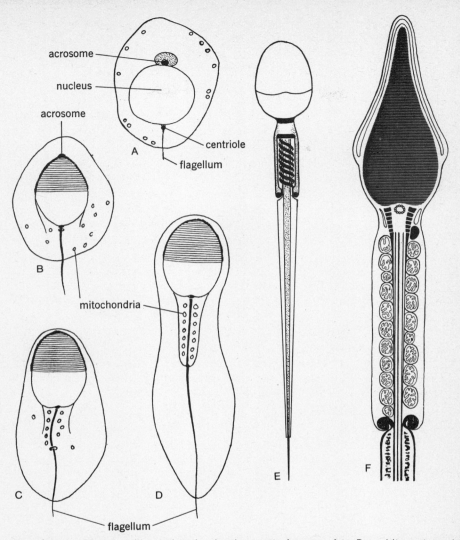

Figure 25-7 Diagrams illustrating the development of sperm, *A* to *D*, and its mature structure, as interpreted from observations under the light microscope, *E*, and as interpreted from electron micrographs, *F*. Diagrams *A* to *D* redrawn from Y. Clermont and C. P. Leblond; *E*, redrawn from Meves; *F*, redrawn from D. W. Fawcett. *(WEL)*

The two kinds of sperm in man cannot be told apart by inspection. One bears the X chromosome; the other, the Y chromosome. Ova have only X chromosomes. Fertilization of an ovum by an X-bearing sperm gives rise to a female offspring; fertilization by a Y-bearing sperm, to a male. Union of sperm and ovum restores the 46 somatic chromosomes.

The Y chromosome determines sexual differentiation up to the time of formation of the testes and beginning of androgen secretion. The X chromosome has on it a receptor protein at a specific locus. The hormone binds to this recep-

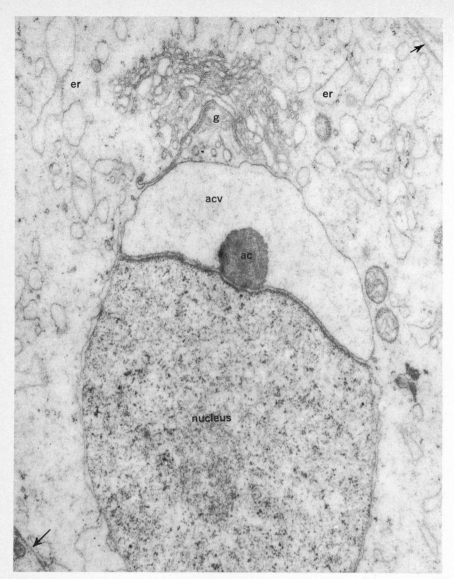

Figure 25-8 Part of a spermatid (cat) showing the nucleus, golgi complex, *g,* and elements of the endoplasmic reticulum, *er.* A prominent acrosomal vesicle, *acv,* containing the dark acrosomal granule, *ac,* has formed. Plasmolemma is marked by arrows. Electron micrograph, about × 40,000. *(Contributed by D. W. Fawcett.)*

tor protein, and, thereafter, male characteristics are produced. Should the binding be blocked, sexual differentiation stops and a genetic male with external appearance of a female results.

Under normal conditions, there is never a time when spermatogenesis ceases in man, once it has been initiated at puberty. Sperm formation becomes slower with age, but a definite climacteric comparable to the female menopause does not occur in normal males.

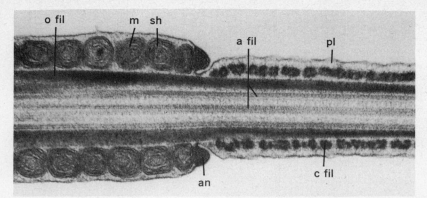

Figure 25-9 Sperm flagellum (guinea pig) at the junction of middle (left) and principal (right) pieces. Thin axial filaments, *a fil*, surrounded by larger and thicker outer ones (so-called "outer fibers"), *o fil*, traverse both components of the tail. The mitochondrial sheath, *m sh*, the middle piece, ends at a denser terminal ring or annulus, *an*. The principal piece has a sheath of circumferential filaments, *c fil*. The plasma membrane, *pl*, is continuous overall. Electron micrograph, ×70,000. (See also Fig. 2-21C.) *(Contributed by D. W. Fawcett.)*

Scrotum Spermatogenesis requires special conditions not present in the abdominal cavity, where the body temperature is too high. During development, the testes with their ducts and blood vessels descend into the scrotum, where the temperature is a degree or two lower than that of the abdominal viscera. Failure to descend is accompanied by inhibition of development of spermatogenesis.

The scrotum is made of connective tissue containing smooth muscle and covered by thin skin. The epidermis is similar to that of other parts of the body but contains somewhat more pigment in the stratum germinativum. The dermis is not sharply delineated from the subcutaneous tissue, both layers lacking adipose tissue. Many bundles of smooth muscle (dartos) are found (Fig. 25.11). Hair follicles are large and tend to be placed more obliquely in respect to the epidermis than those of other regions. The scrotum contains the **tunica vaginalis testis,** a sac of peritoneum separated from the abdominal cavity during development.

Cold and certain other stimuli cause the smooth muscle of the scrotum to contract, wrinkling the scrotal skin. Heat has the opposite effect. This is a protective temperature-regulating mechanism, important for maintaining healthy testicular function.

Straight Tubules and Rete Testis The convoluted seminiferous tubules end abruptly at the mediastinum testis by joining short straight tubules, lined with simple columnar epithelium. There is no smooth muscle around the tubules but only connective tissue.

The straight tubules enter anastomosing channels of similar structure, known as the rete testis (Fig. 25.12). The lining is low columnar epithelium, in which an occasional cell may show a single flagellum extending from its microvilli-studded surface.

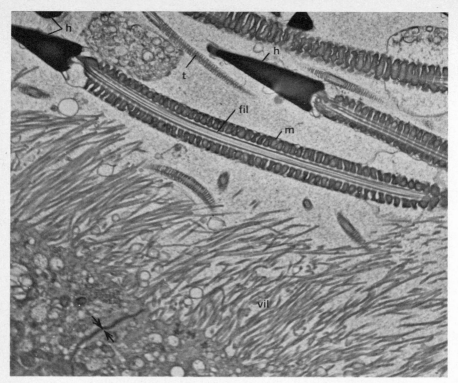

Figure 25-10 Mature sperm cells stored in the epididymis (bat). The dark pyramidal struc-tures are the nuclear head pieces, *h*. Body piece is ringed by densely packed mitochondria, *m*, and shows a core of filaments, *fil*. Tail pieces, *t*. The epithelial surface of two cells of the epididymis, at the lower left (*arrows*), show long microvilli, *vil*. Electron micrograph, about × 6,000. *(Contributed by D. W. Fawcett.)*

EPIDIDYMIS

The **efferent ductules,** a dozen or more in number, enter the head of the epididymis and join it with the **rete testis** (Fig. 25.12). They are convoluted tubes about 6 cm long. Some storage of sperm may take place in them. Along the path from the seminiferous tubules, they are the first components of the spermatic duct system to exhibit secretory characteristics.

The epithelium of the efferent ductules (Fig. 25.13) is composed of alter-nating longitudinal strips of low and high columnar cells, with some pseudostra-tified regions in which a few basal cells occur. The cells of the human ductules are ciliated. The cilia are active and beat toward the epididymis. Beneath the basal lamina are a few smooth-muscle cells forming a thin circular layer in the lamina propria, which is more prominent toward the epididymis. Sperm acquire the capacity for motility in the efferent ductules and epididymis.

The **epididymis** proper is the principal storage depot for sperm. Figure 25.14 shows sections of three convolutions filled with sperm. The mucous

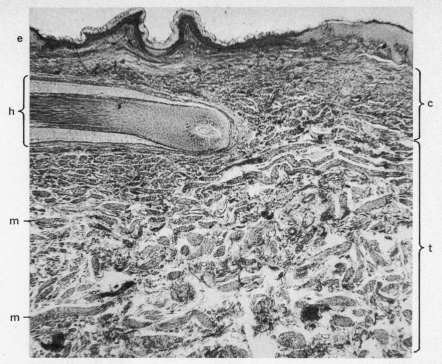

Figure 25-11 Human scrotum. The section shows the epidermis, *e*, and a prominent hair follicle, *h*, between the dermis, *c*, and subcutaneous layer, *t*, with dartos-muscle fibers, *m*. Photomicrograph, × 50.

membrane adds an essential secretion to the fluid medium in which the sperm are activated and stored.

The epididymis is a long (4 to 6m), narrow (0.4mm), convoluted tube, receiving the efferent ductules at the upper pole and joining the ductus deferens at the lower pole of the testis. The tube is lined with tall pseudostratified columnar epithelium displaying two rows of nuclei. The epithelium rests on a distinct basal lamina. On the free surface of the epithelium are unusually long and thin microvilli resembling cilia (Fig. 25.15).

The lamina propria of the epididymis consists of fibrous connective tissue containing a thin layer of smooth muscle (Fig. 25.14). Contraction of the muscle during ejaculation expresses the contents of the epididymis into the ductus deferens. Only at this time do sperm normally proceed through the excretory seminal ducts. In the intervals between emissions, sperm finding their way beyond the epididymis die in the ductus deferens.

SEMINAL DUCTS

The sperm-transporting passages are the ductus deferens, ejaculatory ducts, and urethra. They are not primarily concerned with secretion, although that function is not excluded.

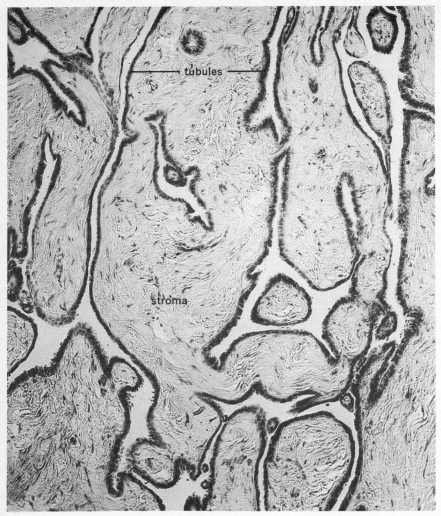

Figure 25-12 Rete testis of a 65-year-old man. The stroma lacks smooth muscle. Photomicrograph, × 150.

Ductus Deferens   The epididymis gradually changes in structure at the lower pole of the testis where it turns upward to become the **ductus deferens.**[4] Convolutions diminish, and the muscle increases in thickness. The epithelium changes from pseudostratified to tall simple columnar. Toward the ejaculatory duct, it may become stratified columnar. The lumen is wider than that of the epididymis and widens even more at the lower end to form the **ampulla** of the ductus deferens. The epithelium is thrown into longitudinal folds and has a little

[4]Formerly called "vas deferens," hence the term "vasectomy."

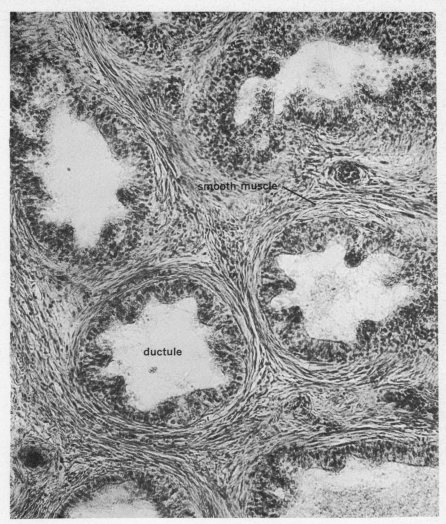

Figure 25-13   Efferent ductules of a young man.Photomicrograph, × 150.

connective tissue beneath it, forming a lamina propria. The rest of the wall is principally smooth muscle arranged in inner and outer longitudinal layers with a circular layer in between. The ductus deferens is illustrated in Fig. 25.16.

Surrounding the ductus deferens there is areolar connective tissue containing lymphatic vessels, an extensive venous plexus, and spermatic artery, nerves, and bundles of skeletal muscle (cremaster). The pampiniform veins have unusually thick walls with longitudinal and circular smooth muscle. These structures compose the **spermatic cord** that traverses the abdominal wall via the inguinal canal.

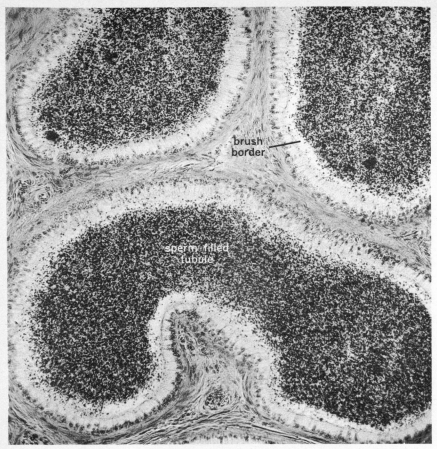

Figure 25-14 Epididymis of a young man. The tubules are full of sperm which stain darkly. The epithelium, of secretory columnar cells with wide brush border, stains lightly with a connective-tissue stain. Photomicrograph, × 150

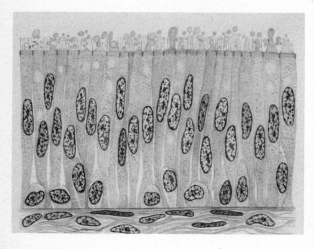

Figure 25-15 Pseudostratified epithelium of the epididymis (ram), actively secretory and showing surface projections with clumps of long microvilli covered with secretion. × 900. *(JFN)*

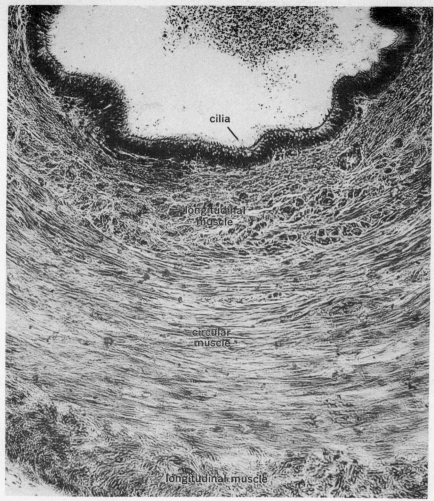

Figure 25-16 Human ductus deferens. Note surface epithelium, inner longitudinal muscle bundles, thick circular muscle layer, outer longitudinal muscle. Photomicrograph, × 150.

The ampulla of the ductus deferens is a dilatation, in which the longitudinal folds of mucosa are exaggerated and intervening depressions form deep valleys as well as diverticula. Some of the lining epithelium appears to be secretory. The surrounding muscular layers are irregularly arranged.

Ejaculatory Duct   The ampulla of the ductus deferens and the short duct of the seminal vesicle unite to form the **ejaculatory duct.** Its mucous membrane resembles that of the ampulla. It is thin, folded, and recessed, and is lined with simple columnar or pseudostratified epithelium, becoming transitional at the urethral end. Muscular layers are absent, and the wall is made up of dense fibrous connective tissue in the stroma of the prostate. The two ejaculatory ducts run for about 1.5 to 2 cm, converging toward the urethra where they open as shown in Fig. 25.17.

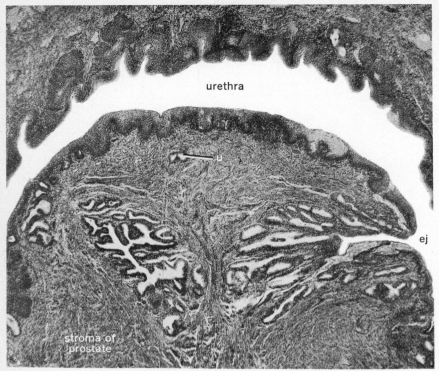

Figure 25-17 Colliculus seminalis in the human prostatic urethra. The crescentic cleft is the lumen of the urethra; the two fenestrated regions in the colliculus are the lower ends of the ampullae leading into the ejaculatory ducts, one of which is seen opening into the urethra on the right, *ej*. The blind end of the utriculus prostaticus may be seen at *u*. Photomicrograph, × 35.

Urethra The only part of the **male urethra** corresponding to that of the female lies between the bladder and the openings of the ejaculatory ducts. The structure of this part is the same in both sexes. The rest of the male urethra is a duct transporting semen as well as urine.

There are three parts of the male urethra: prostatic, membranous, and cavernous. Near the bladder the epithelium is transitional. Near the external orifice, where there is a dilatation called the **fossa navicularis urethrae,** it is stratified squamous. Elsewhere, throughout most of the length of the urethra, the mucous membrane has pseudostratified epithelium. Patches of stratified columnar and stratified squamous epithelium are commonly present. Mucous cells in the epithelium tend to form small glandular pouches, or lacunae, in some places (Fig. 25.18). Into these lacunae open the mucous **urethral glands.**

Muscle is present in the prostatic and membranous parts of the urethra as inner longitudinal and outer circular layers. Longitudinal muscle fibers continue into the proximal part of the cavernous urethra. Fibrous connective tissue, rich in elastic fibers, forms a lamina propria containing capillaries and venules.

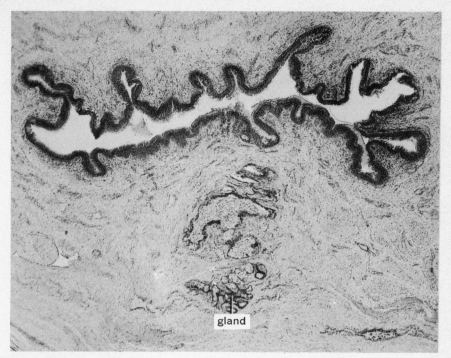

Figure 25-18 Human male urethra, cavernous portion. The lumen with branching lacunae is surrounded by erectile tissue in which is embedded a urethral gland. Photomicrograph, × 40.

A prominent dorsal longitudinal fold of mucosa in the prostatic urethra mounts an elevation known as the **colliculus seminalis** on which the openings of the ejaculatory ducts appear. At the middle of the colliculus there is a little blind pocket, the **utriculus prostaticus,** homologous with the vagina in the female (Fig. 25.17).

SEMINAL GLANDS

Three groups of glands contributing ingredients to the semen are the seminal vesicles, prostate, and bulbourethral glands. The first two provide an alkaline buffer solution, neutralizing the acid vaginal secretions and enhancing sperm activity.

Seminal Vesicles   The structure of the **seminal vesicle** is similar to that of the ampulla of the ductus deferens (Fig. 25.19). It is an irregularly coiled saccular appendage of the ductus deferens. The mucous membrane is extensively folded, and numerous crypts are formed. The epithelium of the seminal vesicles is mainly pseudostratified, and its cells usually contain lipofuscin pigment after puberty.

In and beneath the folds of epithelium, loose fibrous connective tissue forms a lamina propria. Muscular coats are mainly circular. An outer layer of

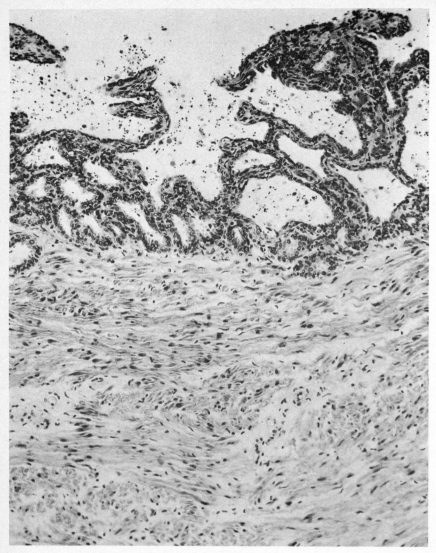

Figure 25-19   Human seminal vesicle. Photomicrograph, × 150.

connective tissue, blending with that of the bladder, may contain small autonomic ganglia.

   The seminal vesicles secrete a yellow viscous fluid. The presence of sperm
in the lumen of the seminal vesicles is no proof that they are stored in this
gland. Their appearance there after death is an artifact.

   Prostate   A mass of tissue surrounding the urethra at the neck of the bladder constitutes the **prostate gland.** It is a firm organ, lightly encapsulated with

fibrous connective tissue containing smooth-muscle fibers. Essentially, it consists of 30 to 50 small compound tubuloacinous serous glands. Lobulation is rather indistinct, but trabeculae of connective tissue containing many smooth-muscle fibers make up the major framework of the prostatic stroma, as can be observed in Fig. 25.20. The lamina propria of the glandular epithelium is formed by extensions of the stroma, providing a route for capillaries to supply the glandular tissue.

Alveoli of the glands vary in size and shape, their lumens being large and irregular. They are lined by simple columnar epithelium of varying height. Most of the cells are tall and have clear cytoplasm. They produce a thin, milky, alkaline secretion which imparts a distinctive odor to the semen. Eosinophilic

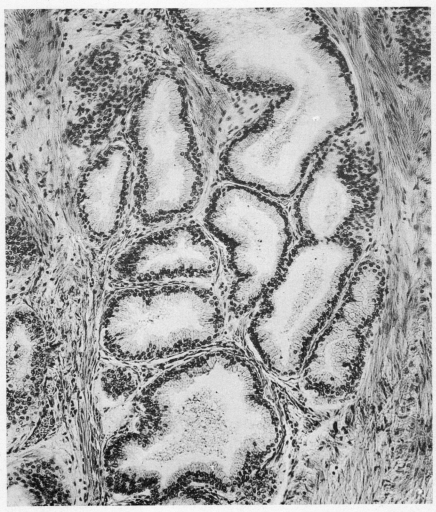

Figure 25-20   Lobule of the prostate of a young man. Photomicrograph, ×150.

prostatic concretions, frequently lamellated, are encountered in the glandular alveoli of old individuals. They may appear during middle age, but are rarely found in early life.

Before puberty the prostate and seminal vesicles are incompletely developed, but the production of testicular hormone brings about their full growth. Castration after puberty causes them to undergo atrophy. The prostate exhibits a tendency toward hypertrophy in later life.

Bulbourethral Glands   Two small compound tubuloacinous, mucous, **bulbourethral glands** empty into the beginning of the cavernous urethra by short ducts. They lie on either side of the membranous urethra.

Semen   Sperm and the secretions of the seminal ducts and glands, forming the mixture called **semen**, are expressed by joint action of the smooth muscles of the various passageways and by the striated bulbocavernous muscle of the penis. Semen is not a uniform mixture of ingredients. Secretion of the bulbourethral glands precedes that of the prostate, seminal vesicle, and the contents of the epididymis. Each ejaculate contains 200 to 300 million sperm and various other formed elements, such as desquamated epithelial cells and lymphocytes, as well as lipid droplets and products of the seminal glands.

Fertility depends upon a number of factors, including the excessive number of sperm in each ejaculate. A considerable number of sperm exhibit abnormal forms, and it is thought that the presence of more than 20 or 25 percent of these in the semen is indicative of impaired fertility. Sperm are rich in the enzyme hyaluronidase. It has been suggested that one function of the great excess of sperm in the ejaculate may be to provide an adequate amount of this enzyme to denude the unfertilized ovum of its surrounding cells and permit one sperm to penetrate it.

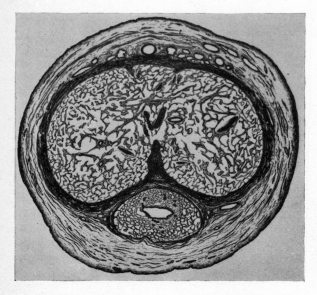

Figure 25-21 Cross section of the penis of a young man. Communication between corpora cavernosa through the septum is shown. About ×2. *(Reproduced from R. O. Greep, after Stieve.)*

PENIS

The essential parts of the copulatory organ are three cavernous bodies and the urethra (Fig. 25.21). The rest of the penis is composed of fibrous connective tissue and skin. A bone is present in some animals to supplement an inadequate vascular erectile mechanism. The penis is well supplied with afferent nerve end organs.

The **corpora cavernosa penis** are the two principal erectile bodies. Surrounded by a double layer of dense fibrous connective tissue, the **lamina albuginea,** they are incompletely separated by a septum of this same connective tissue.

The **corpus spongiosum penis** is a similar erectile mass surrounding the urethra (Fig. 25.18). It begins as a bulbous enlargement at the membranous urethra, has a narrow shaft, and spreads out at the end of the penis to form a cap, the **glans penis,** which is covered with thin skin.

The corpora cavernosa are supplied by unusual **tortuous arteries** that have bands of longitudinal smooth muscle bulging into the lumen (Fig. 25.22). Most

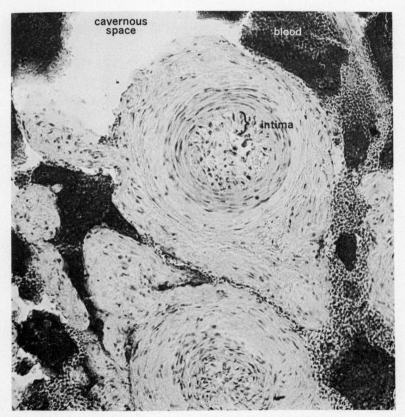

Figure 25-22 Arteries of the adult human penis surrounded by cavernous spaces containing darkly stained blood (clotted). Note the heavy intima with the lumen almost occluuded. Photomicrograph, × 150.

of the time, the circular smooth muscle is contracted, and the pads formed by the longitudinal muscle block the arterial lumen. Vasodilation of the arteries, initiated by the nervous system, brings about erection. The veins draining the cavernous bodies have valves that tend to retard blood flow. The intervening channels are mere endothelium-lined clefts in the flaccid penis. During erection, however, these fill with blood under arterial pressure and stiffen the cavernous bodies against the surrounding lamina albuginea. After ejaculation, vasodilatation is inhibited, the arterial muscle resumes its tonus, the cavernous spaces are no longer engorged by blood, and flaccidity is resumed.

SUGGESTED READING

Burgos, M. H., and D. W. Fawcett: Studies on the Fine Structure of the Mammalian Testis. *Journal of Biophysical and Biochemical Cytology,* vol. 1, pp. 287–300, 1955.

Clermont, Y.: The Cycle of the Seminiferous Epithelium in Man. *American Journal of Anatomy,* vol. 112, pp. 35–51, 1963.

Fawcett, D. W.: The Anatomy of the Mammalian Spermatozoan, with Particular Reference to the Guinea Pig. *Zeitschrift für Zellforschung,* vol. 67, pp. 279–296, 1965.

Kornano, M., and Snoranta: Microvascular Organization of the Adult Human Testis. *Anatomical Record,* vol. 170, pp. 31–40, 1971.

Riva, A.: Fine Structure of Human Seminal Vesicle Epithelium. *Journal of Anatomy,* vol. 102, pp. 71–86, 1967.

Rosenberg, E., and C. A. Paulsen (eds.): *The Human Testis* (Advances in Experimental Medicine and Biology, vol. 10. Plenum Press, Plenum Publishing Corporation, New York, 1970.

Van Wagenen, G., and M. E. Simpson: *Embryology of the Ovary and Testis; Homo Sapiens and Macaca Mulatta.* Yale University Press, New Haven, 1965.

Zamboni, I., R. Zemjanis, and M. Stefanini: The Fine Structure of Monkey and Human Spermatozoa. *Anatomical Record,* vol. 169, pp. 129–154, 1971.

Chapter 26

Female Reproductive Organs

The female reproductive organs are the ovaries, in which egg cells are formed and sex hormones secreted, and the uterine tubes, uterus, and vagina, for reception and transportation of ova and sperm (Fig. 26.1). Histologic study of the reproductive organs requires consideration of them at different ages. Furthermore, structural appearance of the ovaries and uterus varies with cyclicly functional states after puberty. There are notable species differences in structure and function. The human uterus displays changes correlated with endocrine activity of the ovary. Each month, during the childbearing period, it is prepared for implantation of a fertilized ovum. It exhibits remarkable adaptability in accommodating the growing fetus during pregnancy.

Determination of the female reproductive system occurs when a sperm bearing an X chromosome fertilizes an ovum (also X-bearing). Primodia of the female organs appear in the embryonal period when a primitive gonadal mass begins to form an ovary; but characteristic ovarian structure does not become recognizable until about 21 weeks of gestation.

The female embryo lacks Y chromosomes, which determine maleness, and no testis-inducing hormone is produced. Consequently, the primordial müllerian ducts do not undergo atrophy but proceed to develop into uterine tubes, uterus, and upper part of the vagina. One of the X chromosomes of the female embryo is partially inactivated between 12 and 18 days after fertilization and becomes the chromatin body of the nucleus.

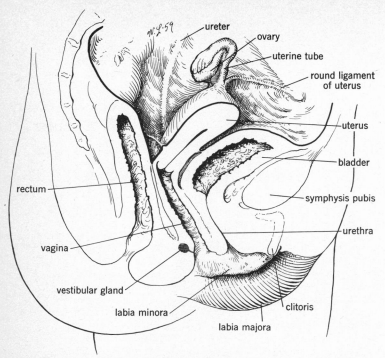

Figure 26-1   Diagram of the female reproductive system to illustrate relations of the organs to each other. *(WEL)*

OVARY

Cellular proliferation and growth lead to a gradual enlargement of the fetal ovary. At 7 months of gestation, each ovary contains 3 to 4 million potential oocytes, or **oogonia**. Some of these, with surrounding stromal cells, become primary follicles. About 300,000 to 400,000 are present at birth, and no more are formed thereafter. The nucleus of each oocyte in the fetus starts to divide, but stays in the late prophase of the first meiotic division until the follicle develops and ovulation occurs, which may be 12 to 47 years later.

The human ovary has little endocrine function before birth. It and the other reproductive organs remain relatively quiescent for the first decade. Hormonal stimulation of the ovaries begins in girls 10 or 11 years old, and **puberty** occurs about 2 years later. The prepubertal ovaries secrete a small amount of estrogen noncyclically, and the secretion increases and becomes cyclic after puberty. This stimulates further growth and maturation of the other reproductive organs and mammary glands and is marked by the appearance of pubic hair. Gonadotropins from the adenohypophysis, under influence of their hypothalamic releasing factors, induce the sequence of events leading to manifestations of puberty and menarche. Ovulation preceding menstruation begins erratically at first.

Basic Structure   The mature ovary is smaller and flatter than the male gonad. It lies in the peritoneal cavity, attached by a fold of peritoneum, the **mesovarium**, to the broad ligament of the uterus. It has no intrinsic duct or tubules and lacks a glandular appearance. Figure 26.2 illustrates the ovary in cross section.

The epithelium on the surface of the ovary is continuous with the mesothelium of the peritoneal cavity, but it is low simple columnar instead of simple squamous and lacks a basal lamina. A layer of dense fibrous connective tissue forms a collagenous capsule, the tunica albuginea, just beneath the ovarian epithelium. The mesovarium, or mesentery of the ovary, attaches to

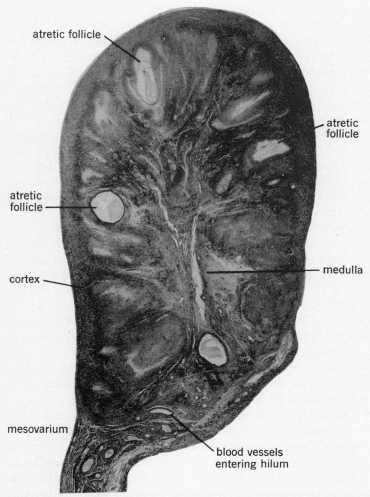

Figure 26-2   Human ovary during puberty. The cortex is full of primary follicles which are invisible at this low magnification. Several stages in atresia of prematurely developed follicles can be seen. Photomicrograph, × 5.

the hilum, and its looser connective tissue carries blood vessels, lymphatic vessels, and nerves through the hilum into a central portion, the medulla of the ovary.

The junction of medulla and cortex usually is indistinct (Fig. 26.2). The medulla contains a few small ductlike structures related embryologically to the rete testis. These are vestigeal, but may become cystic in later life.

Peripherally, the stroma of the ovarian cortex exhibits an unusual cellularity; this is so characteristic that, even when oocytes and follicles are not seen, one can recognize ovarian cortical tissue. It is filled with spindle-shaped connective-tissue cells, and although elastic fibers are scarce, collagenous fibers, reticular fibers, and ground substance are present in the cortical stroma. The spindle-shaped cells resemble smooth-muscle fibers, but they lack fibrils in their cytoplasm and are not contractile (Fig. 26.7).

Prepubertal Ovary   The size and appearance of the ovaries vary with age and functional state. Those of the infant and child are characterized by large numbers of primary oocytes, forming a cortical layer beneath the tunica albuginea (Fig. 26.3). Each oocyte as a rule has a single layer of flattened stromal cells around it. These become the follicular cells; together with the oocyte, they form a **primary follicle**.

The number of primary follicles decreases in the course of time. Only about 400 out of the original 300,000 to 400,000 will reach maturity and ovulate; few ova, indeed, will be fertilized. Most of the primary follicles degenerate at various stages in their development. Comparison of the cortex of an infantile ovary in Fig. 26.4 with that of a 10-year-old girl in Fig. 26.5 shows a marked difference in the number of primary follicles.

The prepubertal ovarian cortex has the characteristic stroma composed of spindle-shaped cells arranged often in whorls. Scattered throughout the stroma are primary follicles, few of which have undergone significant growth in size. Each measures about 40 μm in diameter, i.e., about twice that of the oocyte within it.

Postpubertal Ovary   During the years after puberty, throughout the childbearing period, and until the menopause, the ovary undergoes cyclic changes in structure. These are manifested by follicular enlargement, follicular atresia, ovulation, corpus-luteum formation and regression, and the scarring that follows (Figs. 26.5 and 26.6). The ovary, originally a smooth pink organ, is transformed into a wrinkled grayish body by the end of this period.

The stage of follicle enlargement coincides in general with prepubertal increase in hypothalamic and hypophyseal endocrine activities. After 10 to 12 years of intermitotic rest, some of the primary follicles begin to enlarge by proliferation of follicular cells, producing a stratified layer, the **stratum granulosum,** around the oocyte (Fig. 26.7). This layer is separated from surrounding ovarian stroma, the **theca,** by a basal lamina. The oocyte grows in size, and a clear, refractile membrane, the **zona pellucida**, appears between it and the follicular cells. As the follicle enlarges, this clear zone becomes wider, and microvilli

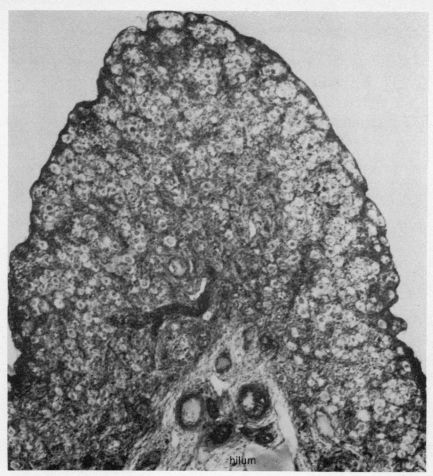

Figure 26-3 Part of an ovary of a 7-day-old human infant. The cortex is filled with oocytes. Photomicrograph, about × 75. *(Contributed by G. Van Wagenen.)*

project into it from the plasma membranes of the oocyte as well as from the follicular cells.

Small accumulations of tissue fluid appear among the follicular cells when the stratum granulosum attains a thickness of eight or ten layers. These coalesce, as the follicle grows, to form the **follicular antrum**, the enlargement of which converts the primary follicle into a **vesicular follicle**.

The fully developed vesicular follicle, commonly designated a "graafian follicle," contains an oocyte measuring nearly 0.15 mm in diameter. The whole follicle attains a diameter of 10 mm or more just before ovulation. A fortuitous section through a mature vesicular follicle (Fig. 26.8) shows the oocyte in a clump of follicular cells, called the **cumulus oophorus**, on one side of the relatively large cavity filled with **follicular fluid** and lined with stratified cells of the

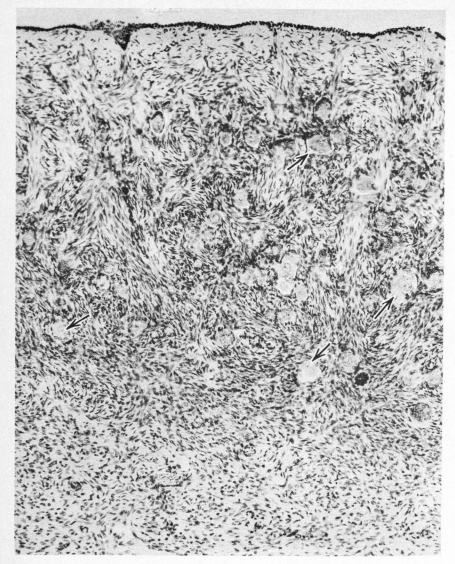

Figure 26-4 Cortex of the ovary of a newborn human infant. Note the ovarian epithelium and many primary follicles (*arrows*) embedded in the highly cellular stroma. Photomicrograph, × 125.

membrana granulosa. A thick basal lamina separates the stratified epithelium from the theca, which consists of internal vascular and external fibrous layers. The appearance of an antrum in the stratum granulosum marks the stage at which the follicle cells begin to secrete estrogens under control of gonadotropins from the adenohypophysis.

Many stages in development of follicles can be found in serial sections of

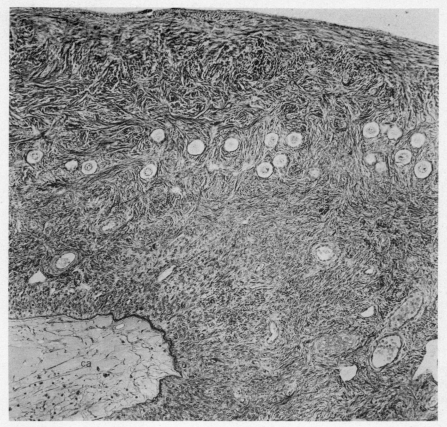

Figure 26-5 Cortex of an ovary of a 10-year-old child, showing a narrow band of primary follicles at the stage of early pubertal development. Part of a corpus albicans, *ca,* is visible. Photomicrograph, × 125. *(Contributed by G. Van Wagenen.)*

an ovary of a young woman. However, a single section, especially toward the end of the childbearing period, may display few if any follicles. Study confined to sections of ovaries of laboratory animals is apt to give a false impression of the number of follicles present in the human species (e.g., many oocytes appear in each section of a cat's ovary).

The vesicular follicle is no longer buried deeply in the ovarian stroma at the time of its maximum development, but is found near the surface of the ovary. The tunica albuginea becomes thin at one point, called the **stigma**, where rupture will occur. Additional tissue spaces form among the follicular cells of the cumulus oophorus, and the oocyte, with an encapsulating layer of follicular cells, is loosened from the membrana granulosa. The cells surrounding the mature oocyte are said to constitute its **corona radiata**. The luteinizing hormone (LH) is believed to function in the process of loosening the oocyte and its corona. The process of development of a follicle to maximum size requires about 2 weeks.

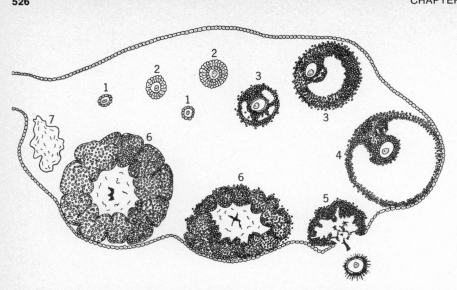

Figure 26-6   Schematic representation of the sequence of formation of ovum and corpus lu-teum. Primary follicles, *1;* growth of follicular cells, *2;* maturing follicles, *3; graafian follicle, 4;* ovulating follicle, *5;* corpus luteum, *6;* corpus albicans, *7. (CHP)*

Atresia is the fate of most ovarian follicles with their oocytes. The primary follicles, undergoing degeneration, simply disappear, but after a follicle has begun to grow, atresia is followed by formation of an appreciable scar in the ovarian stroma. The more advanced the follicle is when atresia occurs, the greater the size and the longer the persistence of the scar.

A number of follicles grow in each cycle, but only one wins the ovulatory race. The other nearly mature follicles become atretic. The zona pellucida becomes folded and may remain visible for some time. The degenerating membrana glomerulosa is replaced by fibrous connective tissue even before the zona pellucida has disappeared. Cells of the internal theca at first become swollen and are filled with lipid droplets; they become organized into cords or radial strands resembling the theca lutein cells of the corpus luteum, and consti-tute a **corpus atretica**. The thick basal lamina of the membrana granulosa per-sists. Corpora atretica in various stages of development and decline may be found in most sections of the ovary (Figs. 26.2 and 26.11*A*).

Only one mature follicle ordinarily reaches the stage of **ovulation** in each cycle, the two ovaries alternating, as a rule. This event takes place when the stigma becomes thin enough for the rupture point to be reached—about 2 weeks before onset of menstruation regardless of the length of the menstrual cycle. Follicular fluid oozes from the opening and causes the dislodged ovum, surrounded by its corona radiata, to be washed into the abdominal cavity (Fig. 26.9). The rupture is accompanied by a little hemorrhage, and, in some women, this is signaled by referred pain. The basal body temperature rises after ovula-tion and remains slightly elevated for 12 to 14 days, because of progesterone secretion.

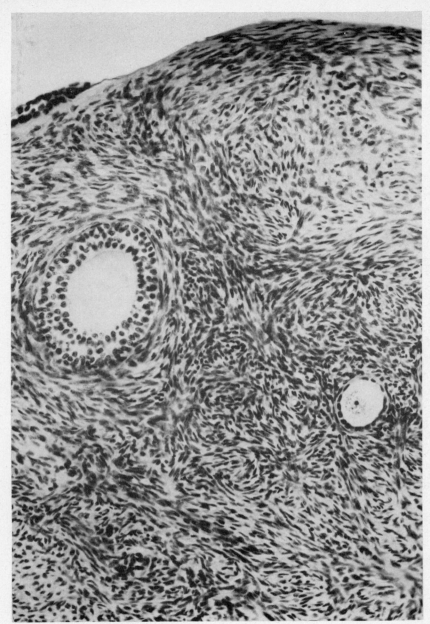

Figure 26-7 Cortex of an ovary of a 44-year-old woman on day 24 of the menstrual cycle. A primary follicle (lower right) and one undergoing enlargement with formation of a stratum granulosum (left) are seen. Part of the ovarian epithelium appears detached and folded over the intact portion. Photomicrograph, about ×300. *(Contributed by G. Van Wagenen.)*

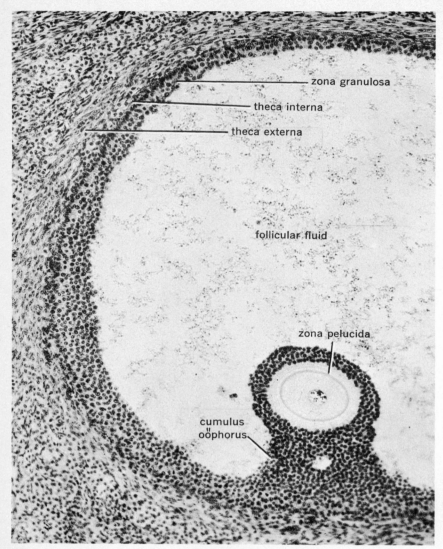

zona granulosa

theca interna

theca externa

follicular fluid

zona pelucida

cumulus oöphorus

Figure 26-8 Graafian follicle in a cat's ovary. Photomicrograph, × 150.

The ovum finds itself in close proximity to the fimbria of the uterine tube, which it enters immediately (Fig. 26.10). Fertilization takes place in the uterine tube by a sperm that has ascended it. The ovum at this stage has undergone reduction of chromosomes to the haploid number, which is 23 in the human species. The reduction began before the oocyte left its follicle, by formation of a **polar body** containing half of the chromosomes. A second polar body is produced by the next meiotic division, which occurs only after the ovum has been discharged, has entered the uterine tube, and has been penetrated by a

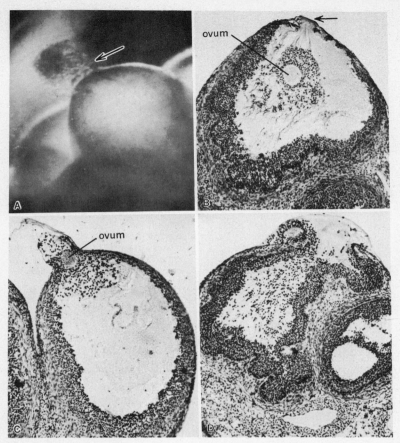

Figure 26-9 Ovuiation in the rat ovary: *A*, enlargement of a frame from a motion picture showing ripe follicles on the surface of the ovary, one of which has ruptured and exhibits a "cloud" of escaping follicular fluid containing the ovum; *B, C,* and *D*, sections illustrating three stages in ovulation: *B*, the cumulus separating; *C*, the ovum emerging; and *D*, the follicle collapsing. *(Photographs contributed by R. J. Blandau.)*

sperm. Both polar bodies degenerate. The 23 chromosomes from the sperm restore the diploid number (46), and development of a new human being begins.

A **corpus luteum** develops by transformation of the wall of the ruptured mature follicle (Fig. 26.11*B*). The wall of the follicle collapses and becomes folded. Its cells are rearranged by ingrowth of capillaries, separating them into cords. The cells enlarge and quickly assume the characteristics of endocrine cells. Their cytoplasm contains agranular endoplasmic reticulum and many lipid particles. The latter impart the yellow color to the corpus luteum in the fresh state.

Vascularity is provided by the internal theca. Cells of this layer enlarge and form masses in the recesses between folds of the transformed follicular cells. They constitute **thecal lutein cells**; those derived from follicular cells are called **granular lutein cells** (Fig. 26.13).

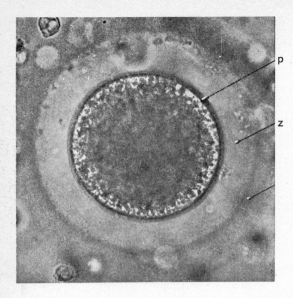

Figure 26-10 An unfertilized human ovum obtained from the uterine tube. The zona pellucida, z, and plasma membrane, p, are indicated. *(Reproduced with permission of A. J. Hertig.)*

The corpus luteum is a transient endocrine gland. When the ovum fails to be fertilized, the corpus luteum begins involution in about 2 weeks and is gradually replaced by connective tissue. Several weeks later, the site of a corpus luteum of menstruation is marked by a small dense scar called a **corpus albicans** (Fig. 26.12).

The corpus luteum of pregnancy differs from the more common type in size and duration of functional state. It may be 2 to 3 cm in diameter, producing a marked bulging on the ovarian surface. This gland remains functional through most of pregnancy, activity declining toward term. After delivery it undergoes involution with formation of a large corpus albicans.

The interfollicular stroma of the human ovary contains groups of epithelioid cells with structural characteristics of those in other endocrine glands. They tend to be arranged in cords closely related to capillaries. Collectively the cells are designated the **interstitial gland**. Although the cells secrete a progestin in rabbits, this function in the human female is unknown.

The normal human ovary produces hormones cyclically. The two principal varieties are **estrogens** and **progestins**. The former are secreted mainly during the follicular stage of the ovarian cycle, while the latter are produced in the luteal stage. The follicular cells and surrounding tissue produce mainly estrogens, while the corpus luteum secrets principally progestins. Furthermore, a minute amount of testosterone appears to be secreted by ovarian interstitial tissue, possibly from hilum cells. The principal active estrogen of the human ovary is 17B-estradiol. Its production is stimulated mainly by the hypophyseal gonadotropic hormone, LH, with FSH playing a supportive role. Estrogen increases sensitivity of the granulosa cells of follicles to the follicule-stimulating hor-

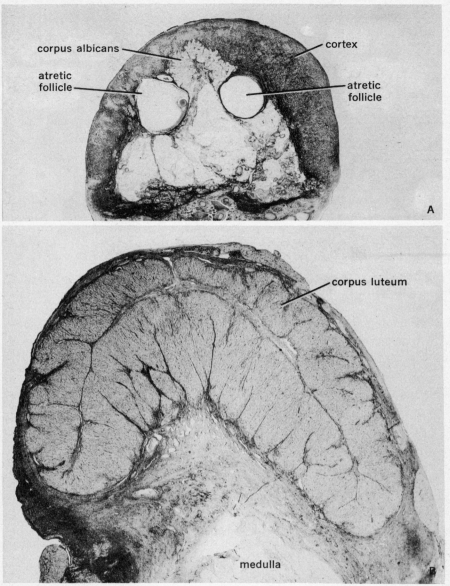

Figure 26-11 Human ovary showing, *A,* vesicular follicles undergoing atresia; *B,* corpus luteum of menstruation. Photomicrograph, × 6.

mone, FSH. The roles of these hormones in regulating the endometrial changes of the menstrual cycle are discussed later in this chapter. Estrogens induce female secondary sex characteristics and affect thresholds of neural activity in regions of the brain that influence hypothalamic functions.

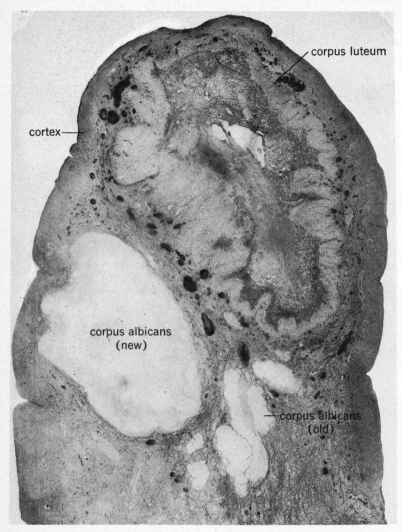

Figure 26-12 Adult human ovary showing degeneration of a corpus luteum of menstruation with many darkly stained blood vessels around it; a large corpus albicans and several older smaller ones are shown. Photomicrograph, × 6.

Postmenopausal Ovary   Cyclic production of ova continues for 30 to 40 years before it subsides and is followed by the **menopause**. Ovarian hormones are no longer secreted in significant quantities after cessation of ovulation. Gonadotropins continue to be produced by the adenohypophysis, the amounts increasing in absence of a negative feedback from the ovary. The postmenopausal ovary contains many scars but no follicles. The typical ovarian stroma is abundant even in the aged organ.

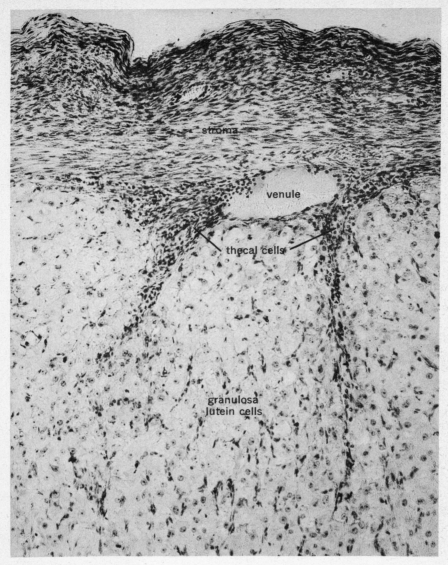

Figure 26-13 Corpus luteum; a detail from the specimen shown in Fig. 26-11*B*. Photomicrograph, × 150.

UTERINE TUBES

Each uterine tube[1] is about 15 cm long and 10 mm in diameter, has a free end near the ovary, and, at the other, buries itself in the upper end of the uterus. Structural appearance varies according to distance away from the uterus. Three regions are recognized in the uterine tube. A narrow **isthmus** forms the

[1]The names "oviduct" and "Fallopian tube" are widely used.

uterine one-third; a widening, the **ampulla**, makes up the outer two-thirds; and a dilated funnel opening, from which fingerlike processes (fimbria ovarica) project, composes the **infundibulum.** Like other tubular organs, the uterine tube has a mucous membrane, muscular layer, and a serosa, but lacks a submucosa, a muscularis mucosae being absent.

The mucous membrane of the uterine tube has a lamina propria composed of rather cellular and vascular fibrous connective tissue beneath a simple columnar epithelium. It is irregularly folded. In the ampulla, the folding is much exaggerated and becomes complex (Fig. 26.14*A*), but in the isthmus the folding is less marked (Fig. 26.14*B*).

Cells of the epithelium are of two types, many being ciliated. The nonciliated cells are secretory, providing the ovum with a fluid vehicle for its passage down the tube to the uterus. The height of the epithelium of the tubular mucosa changes cyclically, along with the mucous membrane of the uterus, in response to the ovarian hormones. Although the complicated mucosal foldings suggest a glandular structure, there are no true glands in the uterine tube.

Ciliated epithelial cells are more numerous on fimbria than farther down the tube. Their presence is related to ovarian endocrine activity. Fewer are present after the menopause. The fimbrial cilia beat toward the ampulla and tend to sweep the ovum into the uterine tube where peristaltic action provides the main force to carry it to the uterus. It takes only about 10 minutes from ovulation for the ovum to reach the ampulla, which is the usual site of fertilization. Thereafter, its passage is slower; it takes almost a week for it to appear in the uterus.

The tunica muscularis of the uterine tube consists of two layers: a thin outer longitudinal layer and a thicker inner circular or spiral layer. The two layers are not sharply delineated from each other. They are thickest at the uterine end of the isthmus.

UTERUS

The uterus is a thick tubular organ representing the fused lower part of two embryonic müllerian ducts from which the uterine tubes arise. Its basic structure—mucosa, muscularis, and serosa—resembles that of the uterine tubes. The epithelium of the uterus is similar to that lining the uterine tubes but is invaginated to form tubular glands. Beneath the epithelium there is a thick layer of highly cellular loose connective tissue somewhat resembling mesenchyme.

Two portions of the uterus differ markedly. The **cervix,** or lower end, including the part projecting into the vagina, maintains a fairly constant structure. The rest of the organ, made up of **isthmus** and **corpus** (including fundus), exhibits maximal variations during menstrual as well as pregnancy cycles.

Prepubertal Uterus   At birth, the uterus is larger in relation to the entire body than it is in the adult. It immediately undergoes a size reduction

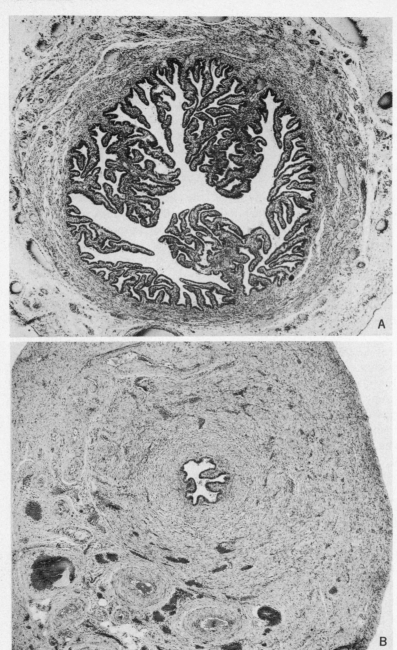

Figure 26-14 Human uterine tube sectioned, *A,* through the ampulla and, *B,* through the isthmus. Photomicrograph, × 35.

correlated with withdrawal of the influence of the mother's estrogen. Thenceforth until puberty, the uterus changes only slightly. Cervix and corpus are approximately of equal length.

Figure 26.15*B* illustrates the structure of the uterus in childhood. The prepubertal uterus has a thick muscular coat covered with peritoneum where it lies in the pelvic cavity. It is lined with a cellular lamina propria and simple columnar epithelium. Simple tubular glands project from the epithelium into the connective tissue of the lamina propria. The uterine lumen is small. The two principal layers of the uterine body and isthmus are known as **endometrium** and **myometrium**.

Postpubertal Uterus Enlargement of the uterus coincides with the increase in hormonal activity associated with puberty. This involves the myometrium as well as the endometrium, but the more characteristic structural and functional changes are in the latter. They are associated with menstrual cycles, which continue until the menopause.[2] The appearance of the uterine wall is illustrated in Fig. 26.15*A*.

The endometrium is lined with simple columnar epithelium containing groups of ciliated cells here and there. Most of the nonciliated cells are secretory. Simple tubular **uterine glands** are invaginations of the surface epithelium. They extend down into the deepest part of the endometrium where they end blindly adjacent to the myometrium. The glands are surrounded by a thick vascular and highly cellular lamina propria constituting the endometrial stroma. This is composed of two layers, a **superficial layer** that breaks down and is shed at menstruation and a **deep layer** that remains intact.

Branches of the uterine arteries traverse the myometrium, forming arcuate arteries from which many radial branches pass into the deep layer of the endometrium. The radial arteries send out **straight branches** that supply tissues of the deep layer, and coiled branches, the **spiral arteries**, that run on into the superficial layer to form extensive plexuses of thin-walled capillaries. The portions of spiral arteries that lie in the superficial layer degenerate at the time of menstruation and regenerate afterward, their activities being regulated hormonally by the ovaries. Bands of longitudinal smooth muscle lie beneath the tunica intima along one side of the lumen of spiral arteries. Contraction of this muscle bends the vessels and tends to retard the blood flow through them at the time of menstruation.

Changes in the endometrium during each menstrual cycle may be divided arbitrarily into three principal phases: proliferative, secretory, and menstrual. The secretory phase can be converted into a gravid phase. A brief postmenstrual phase is sometimes described.

---

[2]The length of normal menstrual cycles may vary widely from the traditionally accepted period of 28 days. This is especially the case during the early years after puberty and near the menopause. Although the median is about 28 days, only 15 percent of cycles are of this length, and the rest are longer or shorter.

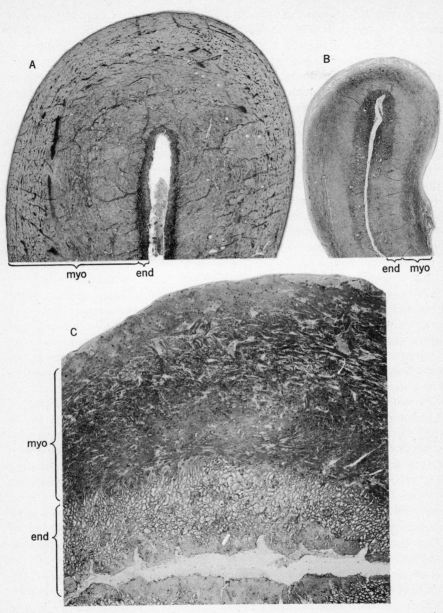

Figure 26-15 Human uterus: *A,* longitudinal section from a 38-year-old woman, showing heavy myometrium, *myo,* and thin endometrium, *end,* in proliferative phase of cycle; *B,* longitudinal section, 12-year-old girl, showing thinner myometrium; *C,* transverse section through body of uterus early in pregnancy. Photomicrographs, × 4.

The **proliferative phase** occupies the first part of the menstrual cycle and corresponds to the period of follicular-growth stimulation in the ovary. It is shorter in cycles of less than 28 days and longer in those of greater duration. It is brought about by an increasing secretion of estrogen. The proliferative phase consists of a reconstruction and slow growth in thickness of the endometrium, i.e., the portion that was not sloughed at the preceding menstrual phase. It continues until approximately the day of ovulation.

During the proliferative phase, the simple columnar epithelium of the uterus contains a few ciliated cells and many nonciliated cells, mostly secretory. The ends of the uterine glands in the deep layer of the endometrium are slightly convoluted. Secretion of a thin fluid is sparse. The endometrial stroma contains no spiral arteries in its outer portion during this phase. Only capillaries are present there. Figure 26.16 shows the endometrium at approximately the end of the proliferative phase.

The **secretory phase**, from approximately the day after ovulation until the beginning of menstrual flow—13 days—corresponds to the period of corpus luteum development and progesterone secretion in the ovary. The endometrium more than doubles in thickness, reaching 4 or even 5 mm by the end of this phase. Not only is it thick; it becomes edematous and full of long dilated and tortuous uterine glands, the abundant secretion of which contains glycogen. Spiral arteries make their appearance in the outer layer of the endometrium during the secretory phase. The amount of stroma between glands in the deep spongy portion is relatively reduced. Near the surface of the endometrium, the stroma becomes more compact. Figure 26.17 shows this phase of the endometrium at about its termination.

The endometrium is ready to receive a fertilized ovum in the secretory phase. Should fertilization and implantation take place, the secretory phase becomes a **gravid phase**, and the endometrium continues its development. Endometrial development is extended by pregnancy because the fetal trophoblast takes over maintenance of the corpus luteum. In the absence of an implanting ovum, the corpus luteum begins to undergo involution. This is the signal to break down the receptive endometrium and start again.

A significant change in vascularity of the endometrium occurs a day or so before the beginning of the menstrual flow. Intermittently, contraction of muscle in the spiral arteries deprives the outer compact zone of the endometrium of blood. This renders the superficial part ischemic for periods of time that gradually lengthen. These ischemic intervals initiate destruction of the outer part of the endometrium, and lymphocytes invade the stroma in numbers.

The **menstrual phase** occupies the first 3 or 4 days of bleeding. Figure 26.18 illustrates the second- or third-day endometrium. As the progesterone stimulus declines with the beginning of corpus luteum involution, walls of capillaries and some of the spiral arteries give way. Bleeding then takes place into the stroma of the superficial layer of the endometrium. Pieces of the superficial layer are split off by lakes of this blood. They tear away and open other vascular channels.

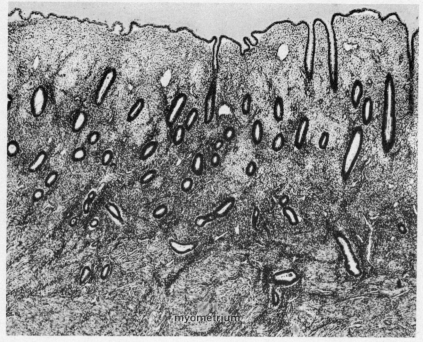

Figure 26-16 Endometrium of the human uterus in the proliferative phase. Photomicrograph, ×40.

Contraction of the musculature of the spiral arteries that produces the ischemia likewise prevents excessive hemorrhage. No more than 35 ml of blood is lost, as a rule. The blood oozes; it does not spurt. It clots, and the clot is liquefied by a proteolytic enzyme. The **menstruum** consists of the altered blood, glandular secretion, and sloughed superficial endometrial tissue. The deep layer of the endometrium, with stubs of the uterine glands, remains intact because it has a conventional blood supply separate from that of the superficial layer.

A brief **posmenstrual phase** precedes the next proliferative phase. It is illustrated in Fig. 26.19 at about the fifth day of the cycle. Even before menstrual discharge ceases, the epithelial cells of the uterine gland stubs in the deep layer proliferate and move out to reestablish a surface epithelium. The endometrium is only about one-sixth as thick as it was at the secretory phase.

The normal menstrual cycle requires an intact hypothalmus-adenohypophysis-ovary complex. Environmental and emotional stimuli activate the hypothalamus which responds to them by secreting releasing factors that stimulate the adenohypophysis. Thus the hypothalamus provides the key to regulation of endometrial activities. There are no structural differences between female and male hypophyses, but there are marked functional differences resulting from exposure to different hypothalamic stimuli.

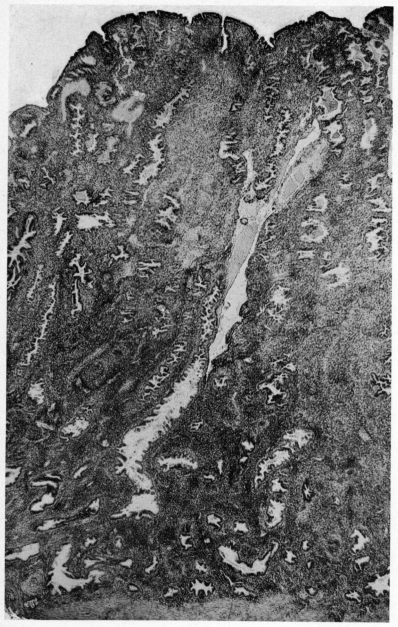

Figure 26-17 Endometrium of the human uterus in the secretory phase. Photo-micrograph, ×40.

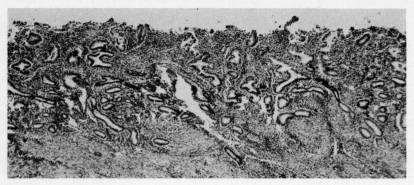

Figure 26-18 Endometrium of the human uterus in the menstrual phase. Photomicrograph, ×40.

The mechanisms by which the gonadotropic hormones regulate ovarian secretion of steroid hormones are not completely understood. However, the cyclic manner of their formation is known to be controlled in part by feedback from the ovary to the hypothalamus and hypophysis.

The quantity of circulating ovarian hormones is lowest during menstruation, at which time the hypothalamic releasing factors for the gonadotropic hormones, FSH and LH, begin to stimulate the adenohypophysis again. Sudden release of the luteinizing hormone (LH) from the hypophysis occurs at midcycle, and the ovarian follicle, which had been primed by FSH, releases its ovum. The rising level of ovarian hormones secreted in the first half of the menstrual cycle acts as a positive-feedback stimulus to release gonadotropic hormones. The activity of the center in the hypothalamus, once initiated, continues inevitably to ovulation, provided the ovary is normal.

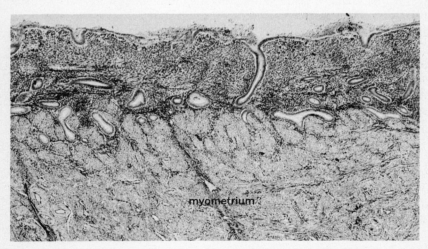

Figure 26-19 Endometrium of the human uterus in the postmenstrual phase of repair. Photomicrograph, × 40.

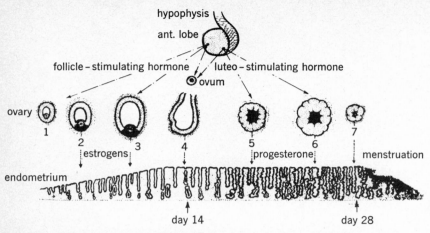

Figure 26-20 Schematic representation of the relationship between ovarian and "average" menstrual cycles. *(Modified from B. A. Houssay.) (MWS)*

Ovarian androgens and estrogens are released during the first half of the menstrual cycle. After ovulation, the corpus luteum secretes large amounts of progesterone and some estrogen. These maintain the endometrium until the corpus luteum ceases to function and hormone levels in the blood decline. Then the superficial layer of the endometrium degenerates, and menstruation occurs. Figure 26.20 illustrates these points schematically.

The **cervix uteri** differs from the rest of the uterus in respect to its mucous membrane. The surface is lined with simple columnar epithelium, made up of tall pale-staining mucous cells. Glands are large branched tubular structures, formed by tall cells like those of the surface epithelium. They are shown in Fig. 26.21. No cyclical changes occur in the mucous membrane of the cervix. The lumen opens onto the vaginal portion of the uterus; it is lined with stratified squamous epithelium continuous with that lining the vagina.

The **myometrium** is a thick tunic consisting of a number of layers of large smooth-muscle fibers interspersed with connective tissue carrying blood vessels, lymphatic vessels, and nerves. It is illustrated in the low-power photomicrograph shown in Fig. 26.15*A*. The myometrial connective tissue contains elastic fibers except in the region of the cervix. Muscle cells undergo some hypertrophy during the secretory phase of the endometrium and diminish again in size after menstruation. They attain phenomenal length during pregnancy.

Postmenopausal Uterus When estrogenic stimuli are no longer provided by ripening ovarian follicles, the uterus ceases to exhibit cyclic structural variations. After the menopause, the endometrium undergoes atrophic change. Uterine glands become short, fewer in number, and often appear cystic, as in Fig. 26.22, and fibrous connective tissue increases in amount in the myometrium.[3] The cervix loses prominence in old age and recedes, as it were, from its protrusion into the vagina.

[3]Fibrous tumors develop at this time in some women.

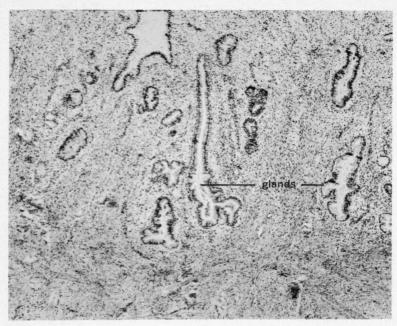

Figure 26-21 Mucous membrane of the human cervix showing large branched tubular glands that secrete mucus. Photomicrograph, × 40.

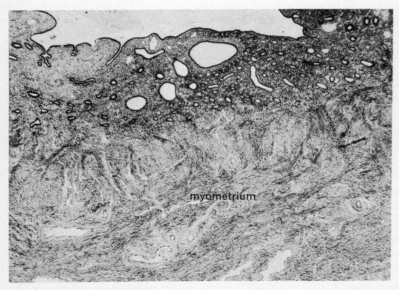

Figure 26-22 Endometrium and part of the myometrium of the human postmenopausal uterus. Photomicrograph, × 40.

PLACENTA

Achievement of pregnancy is the goal of the female reproductive organs. Figure 26.23 illustrates the marked glandular proliferation in the endometrium of its early gravid phase, sustained under influence of continued activity of the corpus luteum.

Fertilization of an ovulated egg cell takes place at the upper end of the uterine tube; cleavage begins at once, and by the time the uterus is reached, a **blastocyst** has been formed. The blastocyst contains a central cell mass, the embryo proper, separated from a surrounding layer of **trophoblast** cells by a small fluid-filled cavity. The blastocyst arrives at the site of implantation at the height of endometrial development and attaches to the epithelium of the uterine mucosa. There, erosion of the surface takes place, and the blastocyst quickly becomes buried in the stroma of the endometrium. The epithelium regenerates and closes over the embedded blastocyst.

The embryonic inner cell mass develops into the fetus. Description of this process is found in textbooks of embryology. However, the trophoblast cells participate in forming the placenta, a transient component of the uterus, providing for fetal respiratory, nutritional, and excretory processes. The histology of the placenta does require brief consideration.

The trophoblast rapidly increases in thickness. Its inner cells have distinct boundaries and form a layer called the "cytotrophoblast." Its outer, more basophilic, cells proliferate and come together in a syncytium called a "syncytial trophoblast."

The two layers of trophoblast compose an outer fetal membrane, known as the **chorion**. As development proceeds, the trophoblast sends processes out into endometrial stroma. Later on, blood vessels from the embryo grow into these to form the chorionic villi.

Growth of the trophoblast layer is uneven. The deep portion grows more rapidly than the part immediately beneath the surface of the endometrium; villi there are longer and are supported by more connective tissue, which forms a chorionic plate. The chorion in this region is known as the chorion frondosum, while the thinner part facing the uterine cavity becomes the chorion laeve. The chorionic plate and chorion frondosum constitute the fetal portion of the placenta.

The endometrium of the gravid uterus varies structurally in three regions. All but its deepest layer adjacent to the myometrium will be shed at parturition. The parts to be shed are referred to as **decidua**: that beneath the chorion frondosum is the decidua basalis; the thin part next to the uterine cavity is the decidua capsularis; and the lining of the rest of the uterus is called decidua parietalis. The **decidua basalis** forms the maternal part of the placenta. Figure 26.24 shows these relationships.

Structure of the placenta is illustrated semidiagrammatically in Fig. 26.25. The endometrium of the decidua basalis becomes modified, and its stromal cells are known as **decidual cells**. The endometrial glands are flattened horizontally against the subjacent myometrium. The spiral arteries open into wide

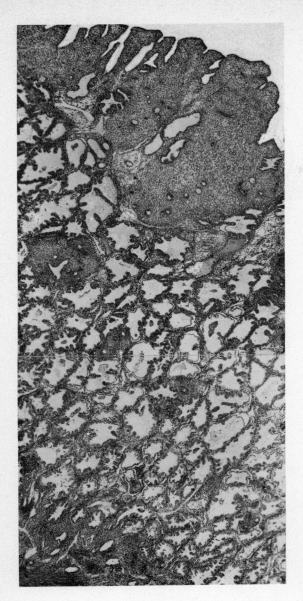

Figure 26-23 Endometrium of the uterus early in pregnancy. This is a detail from Fig. 26-15C. In comparing with other sections, note that the thickness of the endometrium has made it necessary to reduce the size of the photograph by about one-third. Photomicrograph, × 25.

blood sinusoids, the **intervillous spaces**. There is normally no direct communication between fetal and maternal blood streams. Capillaries in the chorionic villi are separated from the maternal blood of the intervillous spaces by (1) endothelium, (2) villous connective tissue (mesenchyme), and (3) the trophoblast layers. Oxygen, carbon dioxide, and other substances must be transported across these three tissues, collectively forming the "placental barrier."

The endocrine functions of the placenta differ widely among various species, but in general, mammals with short gestation periods depend less upon

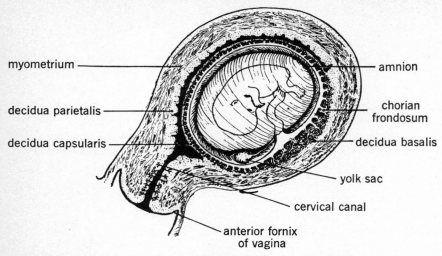

Figure 26-24 Diagram illustrating relationship of fetus to uterine endometrium at 2 months of gestation. *(Reproduced from B. M. Patten, Human Embryology, 2d ed., McGraw-Hill Book Company, New York, 1953.)*

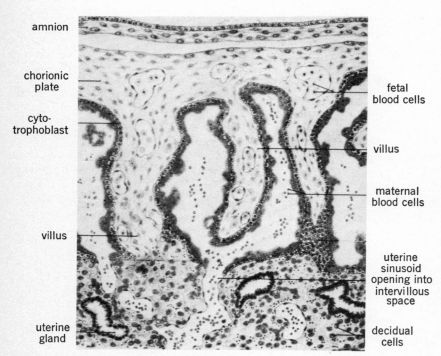

Figure 26-25 Semidiagrammatic representation of the relation of fetal membranes and chorionic villi to the maternal portion of the placenta. *(Reproduced from B. M. Patten, Human Embryology, 2d ed., McGraw-Hill Book Company, New York, 1953.)*

its secretions for maintenance of pregnancy than do those with long gestation periods. Maintenance of pregnancy requires that definite amounts of progesterone and estrogens be present in critical balance. Both of these are produced in the ovary, which is their only source in such animals as mice, rats, and rabbits. In primates, however, their production is taken over early in gestation by the placenta—at 5 weeks in the human placenta. Removal of the ovaries after that time does not cause the pregnancy to terminate.

Placental hormones are secreted by the syncytial trophoblast and are therefore products of fetal cells. The secretions pass into the intervillous spaces, thereby reaching the maternal circulation. The human placenta is the source of two principal hormones, **chorionic gonadotropin** and **placental lactogen**. Progesterone is synthesized from maternal precursor substances. The fetus, on the other hand, appears to provide the placenta, perhaps from its suprarenal cortex, with the substances needed for synthesis of estrogens.

The specific functional activity of placental hormones is still somewhat speculative. Chorionic gonadotropin has an incomplete lutenizing effect. It prevents the involution of the corpus luteum (which normally occurs in about 12 days in the nonpregnant woman). Thus, secretion of progesterone continues and pregnancy is maintained. Placental lactogen, otherwise known as "chorionic growth hormone prolactin," has actions similar to those of hypophyseal growth hormone.

So much chorionic gonadotropin is secreted by the trophoblast that it appears in the urine of the woman in early pregnancy. Advantage is taken of this fact to devise tests for pregnancy. One test uses small samples of the woman's urine or serum; injection of them into virgin estrus rabbits, for example, causes the animals to ovulate.

VAGINA

The vagina is a tubular organ connecting the uterus with the exterior and providing a receptacle for the semen at coitus. It is a flat channel lined with stratified squamous epithelium and surrounded by fibrous connective tissue and smooth muscle.

The epithelium of the vagina rests on a well-marked papillary zone of lamina propria, rich in blood vessels and containing lymphocytes. There are no glands, as a rule; the mucosa is moistened by secretions from the uterus. Figures 23.19 and 26.26 illustrate the structure of the vagina.

The thickness of the vaginal epithelium varies with age, and it is influenced by hormones. At birth it is thick because the mother's estrogen has acted through the placenta. Within 2 weeks after birth, the vaginal epithelium of the infant becomes a thin layer and remains so until estrogens are secreted by its own ovary after puberty. Again, after menstrual cycles cease at the menopause, the vaginal epithelium becomes thin.

The secretion of the uterus, moistening the vaginal mucosa, contains glycogen from the uterine glands. Bacterial fermentation of glycogen produces acid in the vagina, most marked during the progravid phase. If it were not for

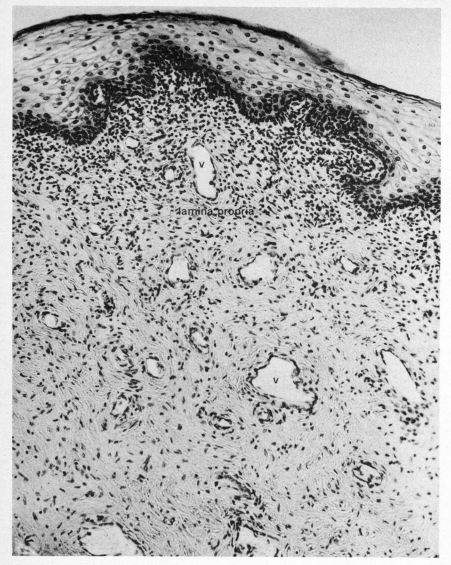

Figure 26-26 Human vaginal mucosa. Note the cellular lamina propria and many small venous channels, *v.* Photomicrograph, × 150.

seminal alkalinity and buffering action, sperm would die in the vagina before accomplishing their mission.

The tunica muscularis of the vagina lies external to the mucosa, there being no distinct submucous layer. The division into inner circular and outer longitudinal layers is indistinct. Much fibrous connective tissue is interspersed among the smooth-muscle bundles. A circular vaginal sphincter of skeletal-muscle fibers guards the external orifice.

EXTERNAL GENITALIA

The external genitalia of the female are shown diagramatically in Fig. 26.1. The **labia minora** are folds of thin skin, merging with the mucous membrane of vestibule and vaginal orifice. Hair follicles and adipose tissue are absent; sebaceous glands, sweat glands, and nerves are present. The **vestibule** lies between the labia minora. Several small glands empty onto its mucous membrane, as do the ducts of the large **vestibular glands,**[4] which are homologs of the male bulbourethral glands. The vestibular glands are tubuloacinous, each with a main duct lined with simple columnar epithelium. All secrete mucus. Anterior to the labia minora and vestibule lies the **clitoris** which is formed of two miniature erectile bodies corresponding to the corpora cavernosa penis. It contains rudimentary homologs of the glans and corpus spongiosum of the male, and is covered by a mucous membrane continuous with that of the vestibule.

The **labia majora** are large folds of skin with hair follicles, sweat glands and sebaceous glands. The hair follicles are especially well developed on the outer surface. Subcutaneous adipose tissue, a few smooth-muscle fibers, a venous plexus, and loose connective tissue are to be found in the labia majora. These bodies are homologs of the two halves of the scrotum.

SUGGESTED READING

Corner, G. W.: Development, Organization and Breakdown of the Corpus Luteum in the Rhesus Monkey. *Contributions to Embryology,* vol. 31, pp. 117–146, 1945.

Crisp, T. M., D. A. Dessonky, and F. R. Denys: The Finestructure of the Human Corpus Luteum of Early Pregnancy and During the Postgestational Phase of the Menstrual Cycle. *American Journal of Anatomy,* vol. 127, pp. 37–70, 1970.

Diamond, M. (ed.): *Perspective in Reproduction and Sexual Behavior.* Indiana University Press, Bloomington, 1968.

Greep, R. (ed.): *Female Reproductive System,* sec. 7, *Endocrinology,* vol. 2. American Physiological Society, The Williams & Wilkins Company, Baltimore, 1973.

Mossman, H. W., and K. L. Duke: *Comparative Morphology of the Mammalian Ovary.* University of Wisconsin Press, Madison, 1973.

Ramsey, E. M.: The Placenta Comes of Age. *American Journal of Anatomy,* vol. 133, pp. 389–390, 1972. (Editorial with key references.)

Sawyer, C. H., and R. A. Gorski (eds.): *Steroid Hormones and Brain Function.* University of California Press, Berkeley, 1971.

Van Wagenen, G., and M. E. Simpson: *Postnatal Development of the Ovary in Homo Sapiens and Macaca Mulatta and Induction of Ovulation in the Macaque.* Yale University Press, New Haven, 1973.

---

[4]At one time designated "Bartholin's glands."

Index

Index